STRENGTH TRAINING FOR SOCCER

Strength and power are key elements of soccer performance. A stronger player can sprint faster, jump higher, change direction more quickly, and kick the ball harder. *Strength Training for Soccer* introduces the science of strength training for soccer. Working from a sound evidence-base, it explains how to develop a training routine that integrates the different components of soccer performance, including strength, speed, coordination, and flexibility, and outlines modern periodization strategies that keep players closer to their peak over an extended period.

Dealing with themes of injury prevention, rehabilitation, and interventions, as well as performance, the book offers a uniquely focused guide to the principles of strength and conditioning in a footballing context. Fully referenced, and full of practical drills, detailed exercise descriptions, training schedules, and year plans, *Strength Training for Soccer* is essential reading for all strength and conditioning students and any coach or trainer working in football.

Bram Swinnen is a high-performance specialist at the *Move to Cure* rehabilitation center, Antwerp, Belgium, where he is responsible for the rehabilitation programs of several elite soccer players from across European football's top teams. He has more than 15 years' experience as a physical trainer and physical therapist in professional sport.

"I've experienced Bram's work in the field of strength and conditioning first hand whilst working with him at Anzhi Makhachkala. His methods are innovative, football-related, and based on expertise and experience. Anyone who reads this book will gain a lot of new insights into this important aspect of football training."

Rene Meulensteen, former Manchester United First Team Coach

STRENGTH TRAINING FOR SOCCER

Bram Swinnen

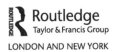
Routledge
Taylor & Francis Group

LONDON AND NEW YORK

First published 2016
by Routledge
2 Park Square, Milton Park, Abingdon, Oxon OX14 4RN

and by Routledge
711 Third Avenue, New York, NY 10017

Routledge is an imprint of the Taylor & Francis Group, an informa business

© 2016 B. Swinnen

British Library Cataloguing in Publication Data
A catalogue record for this book is available from the British Library

Library of Congress Cataloguing in Publication Data
A catalog record for this book has been requested

ISBN: 978-1-138-95714-5 (hbk)
ISBN: 978-1-138-95715-2 (pbk)
ISBN: 978-1-315-66527-6 (ebk)

Typeset in Bembo
by Out of House Publishing

CONTENTS

FIGURES

TABLES

FOREWORD

I have known Bram for almost a decade. I got to know him through a number of top athletes, who reaped success with the training methods described in this book. I saw those guys coming back really fit from injury or after a pre-season program with Bram. The results of his work spoke for themselves. As a consultant for the football team of Anzhi Makhachkala I also witnessed the fantastic job Bram did there. At the *Move to Cure* rehabilitation and performance center we work together closely. Bram mainly focuses on top players who are in the last phase of their rehabilitation.

Bram approaches the bodies of his athletes in their entirety to restore the ideal balance within the kinetic chain. He does not just strive for the ideal, but focuses on what works best for each player individually. Bram therefore starts from an in-depth functional analysis of the player to uncover the movement deficiencies and weaknesses in the kinetic chain. The player receives a training program, taking into account all possible perspectives: the kinetic chain, the different muscle chains, stability, mobility, strength, and other performance parameters. Bram excels in combining different training methodologies and puts his own accent on preparing his athletes in the most optimal way for competition. He works with the same attitude and mentality of a professional athlete. Perfection is not enough; he wants to do more and he wants to do it better. Bram has the ability to get the most out of the body. Through good planning and evidence-based training he optimizes the body's ability to recuperate, which prevents injuries and boosts performance. The book you are about to read represents Bram's cutting-edge method and deciphers the science, the different training methodologies, and practice on which it is based.

The great value of this book is that it is not only about strength training, but about optimizing the body's function and taxability. This text also addresses the injury mechanisms of the most common soccer injuries from a broad perspective, including local factors, activation patterns, muscle chains, and the entire kinetic chain. Strength training for soccer is a key resource that will set you on the path toward more effective rehabilitation, injury prevention, and performance training for soccer.

Lieven Maesschalck, founder/owner of the *Move to Cure*
rehabilitation and performance center.

ACKNOWLEDGMENTS

I dedicate this book to my gorgeous wife Adriana and daughter Yasmin, who fill my life with love and happiness and are a tremendous source of inspiration. You are wonderful and I love you.

I also want to acknowledge the people that have been of great help in the realization of this book. I want to express my gratitude to my dear brother Ruud who took and edited the photos. Thank you to Divock Origi and William Benka Davies for their help and flawless execution of the exercises. I want to thank my friend Free Van Heddegem for the making of the figures. I also want to express my thanks to the sports and leisure publisher Simon Whitmore, editor William Bailey, and the editing and production team of Routledge for their excellent job and advice.

My success as a strength and conditioning coach is a reflection of the hard work of the athletes I train. I thank all the athletes and colleagues I have worked with and learned from, in particular Lieven Maesschalck, who inspires me and always challenges me to think outside the box.

And last but not least a great thanks to my parents whom I love and who always supported me to keep going and finish strong.

INTRODUCTION

Soccer has increasingly evolved into a very athletic sport and soccer players are progressively becoming better athletes. Within a game, players repeatedly perform high-intensity actions in which muscle power is crucial (Stølen *et al.* 2005). These bursts of explosive actions, such as accelerating, sprinting, kicking, tackling, turning, changing direction, and jumping may be completed over 500 times during the game (Stølen *et al.* 2005). In particular, the decisive phases during the game require the player to perform at high intensity (Bangsbo *et al.* 2006; Rampinini *et al.* 2009). Speed, explosiveness, and the ability to intermittently repeat these high-intensity actions are fundamental to success in soccer (Cometti *et al.* 2001; Rampinini *et al.* 2009). Sprinting performance determines the outcome in match-winning actions (Cometti *et al.* 2001). A greater acceleration and sprinting ability increase the possibility to get to the ball first, to dribble past an opponent, to create or stop a goal-scoring opportunity. Straight sprinting is the most frequent action in goal situations in soccer, for both the assisting and the scoring player (Faude *et al.* 2012; Haugen *et al.* 2014).

Soccer is a fast-paced game and speed and explosiveness have become increasingly crucial in game situations (Barnes *et al.* 2014; Haugen *et al.* 2014). In the last decade the number of sprints and sprint distance per game increased in the English Premier league by 85 percent and 35 percent respectively (Barnes *et al.* 2014). Top-class players perform more high-intensity sprint actions during a game and cover a greater distance at very high speeds (Mohr *et al.* 2003). Professional soccer players have also become progressively faster over the last 15 years (Haugen *et al.* 2012, 2014). Sprinting speed, agility performance, and repeated-sprint ability can distinguish the elite from the sub-elite players (Cometti *et al.* 2001; Kaplan *et al.* 2009; Rampinini *et al.* 2009; Rebelo *et al.* 2013).

It is well established that strength and power are essential co-determinants of soccer performance (Haff 2012; Silva *et al.* 2013). Higher strength and power levels enable a player to sprint faster, jump higher, stop and change direction more quickly, and kick the ball harder (López-Segovia *et al.* 2011; Wisløff *et al.* 2004). Stronger players are able to better withstand the high forces associated with high-intensity actions. They are therefore better able to repeat the high-intensity actions with less decrement in performance (Ingebrigtsen and Jeffreys 2012; López-Segovia *et al.* 2014; Silva *et al.* 2013). This enhanced ability to resist fatigue enables stronger players to maintain a higher work rate during the game (Silva *et al.* 2013). They perform more high-intensity actions during the match and cover a greater distance while sprinting, especially during the second half (Silva *et al.* 2013). Players with greater strength levels also show less post-match fatigue despite the higher game load (Johnston *et al.* 2014).

Because stronger players are better able to maintain a high level of performance during the game, display less neuromuscular fatigue, and recover faster after a game it should come as no surprise that strength training has been shown to significantly reduce acute and overuse injuries (Askling *et al.* 2003; Hägglund *et al.* 2009, 2013; Lauersen *et al.* 2014; Petersen *et al.* 2011).

Strength training as a means to enhance soccer fitness and performance is still undervalued, however. In contrast to other team sports, many soccer teams still do not perform strength training year round and/or do not adhere to a periodized approach to address and develop the different strength qualities.

During the competitive season most of the training time is devoted to tactical and soccer-specific skill development. The time and volume that can be devoted to soccer conditioning is therefore limited. A time-consuming conditioning program will probably be rejected by the coach. Strength is only one aspect of performance. Dedicating time to develop the different motor abilities separately is time consuming and inefficient. Strength training needs therefore to be optimized and should ideally integrate multiple essential elements of soccer performance. The integrated strength training needs to improve the overall athletic performance and assure transference to soccer-specific technical skills.

This book provides guidelines how to develop a strength training routine that serves as a foundation for the integrated development of the different fitness components of soccer performance. The ultimate goal of strength training is not to increase absolute strength levels but to improve movement efficiency and soccer performance. Maximal strength forms the basis for the development of power, speed, athletic ability, and repeated-sprint ability. Incorporating exercises that mimic soccer-specific movement patterns will facilitate the transfer to soccer performance. A nonlinear periodization approach allows the various qualities of soccer to be addressed concurrently, provides greater flexibility to tailor training to the competition schedule, and will keep the players closer to their peak over an extended time period.

How this book is organized

This book is divided into six different parts. The first part describes how strength training can help create more efficient movement. The different motor abilities (strength, coordination, endurance, flexibility, and speed) are all integrated into athletic soccer performance. There is so much crossover and interaction between these abilities. Developing these different abilities separately will compromise the transfer to soccer performance. A proper strength training routine can serve as the foundation for the integrated development of all these different bio-motor abilities.

Chapter 1 defines the underlying mechanisms by which strength training improves performance, reduces post-match fatigue, and prevents injuries. This chapter will clarify why strength training is a key factor to optimize movement efficiency and to develop the dominant bio-motor abilities needed for soccer. Chapter 2 emphasizes how strength training can improve flexibility and stability. During soccer, movements are executed through a wide range of motion with great acceleration and production of power. Good athletic performance also requires the player to stabilize and control the movement. Strength training performed over the full range of motion improves flexibility and will help transfer the gained flexibility to athletic performance. In line with the focus on flexibility in Chapter 2, Chapter 3 summarizes the research on the effects of static and dynamic stretching on strength and athletic performance. This chapter also addresses the warm-up and how the specific warm-up can be tailored in function of the strength training workout. Chapter 4 is devoted to the interaction between strength and skill training. Motor control theories and principles that are relevant to strength training are outlined. Designing a strength program conforming to the laws of motor control will benefit movement mechanics and body control during soccer.

Part II is devoted to core training for the purpose of injury prevention and performance enhancement. The demands on the core during soccer occur in multiple positions and directions. To develop total core stability a range of different exercises should be incorporated. Traditional core exercises can enhance the low-threshold recruitment and endurance capacity of the stabilizing muscles, while free-weight, multiple-joint exercises can improve stability under high load or during high-speed movements, specific to the demands imposed on the core during soccer.

Part III presents a broad selection of strength exercises, which are categorized in terms of movement patterns. Classifying exercises according to the movement pattern can facilitate the exercise selection when designing a strength program. A total body workout should contain exercises from every movement pattern. A balanced strength training equally emphasises opposing movement patterns. Selecting a hip dominant exercise for each knee dominant exercise will help facilitate a more balanced quadriceps-to-hamstring strength ratio. Programming an upper body pull exercise for each push exercise can encourage proper shoulder function. While the focus in Part III is mainly on movement patterns, the anatomy and function of the gluteal muscles, hamstrings, hip adductors, and vastus medialis obliquus are also explained in high detail. These muscles play a crucial role in providing neuromuscular control of the lower extremity, and altered activation patterns of these muscles are a contributing factor for various lower extremity injuries (Hewett and Myer 2011; Mendiguchia *et al*. 2011).

Speed and explosiveness are considered the most important physical prerequisites for success in modern soccer (Reilly *et al*. 2000; Tomáš *et al*. 2014). Especially sprinting speed over short distances, agility, and vertical jump performance distinguish the elite players from the rest (Reilly *et al*. 2000). A major goal of strength training for soccer is therefore to enhance power performance and speed of movement. To increase the speed at which force is produced, speed-strength needs to be developed. Part IV is dedicated to speed-strength training and presents the available training methods and exercises to enhance speed and explosiveness of the soccer player. Olympic lifts, plyometrics, and ballistic exercises are high-velocity movements. Because of the potential to accelerate throughout the entire range of motion and produce high power outputs, these exercises are considered as some of the best exercises to maximize speed and explosiveness.

Part V is used to discuss blood flow restriction training and how it can be integrated into the strength training and rehabilitation of soccer players. Low-intensity strength training in combination with blood flow restriction can induce strength and hypertrophy gains similar to those observed with high-intensity strength training, without increasing indices of muscle damage or resulting in prolonged strength decrements. Blood flow restriction training can provide an effective training stimulus to maintain strength levels during competition periods that require unloading.

Training efficiency is impossible to achieve without a good organization. To make this book even more practical, Part VI encompasses all elements of program design: periodization methodology, training variables. Chapter 19 comprises sample training programs for soccer players of different levels. It also describes and gives a practical example of how to manipulate the training parameters to develop the different strength qualities and sequence the different strength training sessions to maintain a high level of performance throughout the entire competitive season.

References

Askling C, Karlsson J, Thorstensson A. Hamstring injury occurrence in elite soccer players after preseason strength training with eccentric overload. *Scand J Med Sci Sports*. 2003 Aug;13(4):244–50.

Bangsbo J, Mohr M, Krustrup P. Physical and metabolic demands of training and match-play in the elite football player. *J Sports Sci*. 2006 Jul;24(7):665–74.

Barnes C, Archer DT, Hogg B, Bush M, Bradley PS. The evolution of physical and technical performance parameters in the English premier league. *Int J Sports Med*. 2014 Dec;35(13):1095–100.

Cometti G, Maffiuletti NA, Pousson M, Chatard JC, Maffulli N. Isokinetic strength and anaerobic power of elite, subelite and amateur French soccer players. *Int J Sports Med*. 2001 Jan;22(1):45–51.

Faude O, Koch T, Meyer T. Straight sprinting is the most frequent action in goal situations in professional football. *J Sports Sci*. 2012;30(7):625–31.

Haff GG. Current research: training for strength, power, and speed. *Strength Cond J*. 2012 Apr;34(2):76–8.

Hägglund M, Waldén M, Atroshi I. Preventing knee injuries in adolescent female football players – design of a cluster randomized controlled trial. *BMC Musculoskelet Disord*. 2009 Jun;10:75.

Hägglund M, Atroshi I, Wagner P, Waldén M. Superior compliance with a neuromuscular training programme is associated with fewer ACL injuries and fewer acute knee injuries in female adolescent football players: secondary analysis of an RCT. *Br J Sports Med*. 2013 Oct;47(15):974–9.

Haugen TA, Tønnessen E, Seiler S. Speed and countermovement-jump characteristics of elite female soccer players, 1995–2010. *Int J Sports Physiol Perform*. 2012 Dec;7(4):340–9.

Haugen T, Tønnessen E, Hisdal J, Seiler S. The role and development of sprinting speed in soccer. *Int J Sports Physiol Perform*. 2014 May;9(3):432–41.

Hewett TE, Myer GD. The mechanistic connection between the trunk, hip, knee, and anterior cruciate ligament injury. *Exerc Sport Sci Rev*. 2011 Oct;39(4):161–6.

Ingebrigtsen J, Jeffreys I. The relationship between speed, strength and jumping abilities in elite junior handball players. *Serbian J of Sports Sci*. 2012;6(3):83–8.

Johnston RD, Gabbett TJ, Jenkins DG, Hulin BT. Influence of physical qualities on post-match fatigue in rugby league players. *J Sci Med Sport*. 2014 Feb 6. [Epub ahead of print]

Kaplan T, Erkmen N, Taskin H. The evaluation of the running speed and agility performance in professional and amateur soccer players. *J Strength Cond Res*. 2009 May;23(3):774–8.

Lauersen JB, Bertelsen DM, Andersen LB. The effectiveness of exercise interventions to prevent sports injuries: a systematic review and meta-analysis of randomised controlled trials. *Br J Sports Med*. 2014 Jun;48(11):871–7.

López-Segovia M, Marques MC, van den Tillaar R, González-Badillo JJ. Relationships between vertical jump and full squat power outputs with sprint times in u21 soccer players. *J Hum Kinet*. 2011 Dec;30:135–44.

López-Segovia M, Dellal A, Chamari K, González-Badillo JJ. Importance of muscle power variables in repeated and single sprint performance in soccer players. *J Hum Kinet*. 2014;40:201–11.

Mendiguchia J, Ford KR, Quatman CE, Alentorn-Geli E, Hewett TE. Sex differences in proximal control of the knee joint. *Sports Med*. 2011 Jul;41(7):541–57.

Mohr M, Krustrup P, Bangsbo J. Match performance of high-standard soccer players with special reference to development of fatigue. *J Sports Sci*. 2003 Jul;21(7):519–28.

Petersen J, Thorborg K, Nielsen MB, Budtz-Jørgensen E, Hölmich P. Preventive effect of eccentric training on acute hamstring injuries in men's soccer: a cluster-randomized controlled trial. *Am J Sports
Med*. 2011 Nov;39(11):2296–303.

Rampinini E, Sassi A, Morelli A, Mazzoni S, Fanchini M, Coutts AJ. Repeated-sprint ability in professional and amateur soccer players. *Appl Physiol Nutr Metab*. 2009 Dec;34(6):1048–54.

Rebelo A, Brito J, Maia J, Coelho-e-Silva MJ, Figueiredo AJ, Bangsbo J, Malina RM, Seabra A.
Anthropometric characteristics, physical fitness and technical performance of under-19 soccer players by competitive level and field position. *Int J Sports Med*. 2013 Apr;34(4):312–17.

Reilly T, Williams AM, Nevill A, Franks A. A multidisciplinary approach to talent identification in soccer.
J Sports Sci. 2000 Sep;18(9):695–702.

Silva JR, Magalhães J, Ascensão A, Seabra AF, Rebelo AN. Training status and match activity of professional soccer players throughout a season. *J Strength Cond Res*. 2013 Jan;27(1):20–30.

Stølen T, Chamari K, Castagna C, Wisløff U. Physiology of soccer: an update. *Sports Med*. 2005;35(6):
501–36.

Tomáš M, František Z, Lucia M, Jaroslav T. Profile, correlation and structure of speed in youth elite soccer
players. *J Hum Kinet*. 2014 Apr;40:149–59.

Wisløff U, Castagna C, Helgerud J, Jones R, Hoff J. Strong correlation of maximal squat strength
with sprint performance and vertical jump height in elite soccer players. *Br J Sports Med*. 2004
Jun;38(3):285–8.

PART I
Components of athletic training

1

MECHANISMS OF ENHANCED PERFORMANCE, INJURY PREVENTION, AND REDUCED POST-MATCH FATIGUE

The mechanisms by which strength training improves performance, reduces post-match fatigue, and prevents injury are basically the same. A powerful and highly coordinated player is better able to handle the forces on the pitch. More efficient movement results in enhanced performance and reduced fatigue and is the major injury prevention factor.

1.1 Enhanced performance

Speed, power, quickness, and strength are highly interrelated abilities (Delecluse 1997; Wisløff et al. 2004). Several studies show that there is a strong association between sprint ability and levels of strength and power in soccer players (López-Segovia et al. 2011; Wisløff et al. 2004). The correlations between strength and the ability to accelerate are greater than those between strength and maximal sprinting speed (Wisløff et al. 2004).

In soccer the vast majority of sprints are performed over shorter distances (<20 m) (Haugen et al. 2014). Contact times during the acceleration phase of sprinting, changing direction, and jumping are relatively higher, which means force can be exerted over a relatively longer time period (Dintiman and Ward 2003; Mero and Komi 1986). The longer the ground contact time, the stronger the association between strength and performance and the greater the impact of strength and power training will be on performance. Enhanced lower body strength has therefore excellent transference to agility performance, vertical jump height, and the ability to accelerate (Spiteri et al. 2014). Strength training in addition to soccer training is an effective training strategy to improve the player's sprint, agility, vertical jump, and kicking performance (Brito et al. 2014; Buchheit et al. 2010; Chelly et al. 2009; Garcia-Pinillos et al. 2014; Keiner et al. 2014; Maio Alves et al. 2010; Manolopoulos et al. 2013; Mujika et al. 2009). Although several authors state that strength training plays a key role to improve sprint performance, not all training routines are able to augment the player's maximal sprinting speed (Jullien et al. 2008; Shalfawi et al. 2013). The low level of exercise and velocity specificity might explain however the ineffectiveness of some of the programs used to enhance sprinting speed. Improving the maximal sprinting speed of players with a higher training status requires velocity-specific strength training. Explosive-type strength training is needed to optimally develop athletic performance.

It is also recommended to include explosive strength training to improve the ability to recover between high-intensity actions (Bishop *et al.* 2011). Repeated-sprint ability is positively correlated with lower body strength and power, agility performance, acceleration ability, and the initial sprint performance (Brocherie *et al.* 2014; Girard *et al.* 2011; Ingebrigtsen and Jeffreys 2012; López-Segovia *et al.* 2014; Mendez-Villanueva *et al.* 2008; Spencer *et al.* 2011). Stronger and more powerful soccer players are able to sprint faster and sprint more times without a decrement in speed (Brocherie *et al.* 2014; López-Segovia *et al.* 2014).

The consensus is that the ability to maintain performance and attenuate fatigue for a prolonged period of time is usually related to the individual's endurance capability. Fatigue is affected however by multiple factors and repeated-sprint ability has been related to neuromuscular and metabolic factors (López-Segovia *et al.* 2014; Rampinini *et al.* 2009; Silva *et al.* 2013). Training that enhances neuromuscular and/or metabolic function can therefore improve repeated-sprint ability. Fatigue and the performance decline during subsequent sprints are manifested by a decreased sprint speed or power output (Bishop and Girard 2011; Girard *et al.* 2011). The decline in power output during repeated sprints has also been attributed to a reduced neural drive and motor unit recruitment (Bishop and Girard 2011; Girard *et al.* 2011). The potential to activate more motor units as a result of strength training can therefore attenuate fatigue and reduce the loss of power output when repeating high-intensity actions (Silva *et al.* 2013).

Stronger players have also a greater ability to maintain a high level of force production and power output toward the final stages of the game due to the positive relation between strength and muscular endurance (Silva *et al.* 2013; Zatsiorsky 1995).

Repeated-sprint ability and long-term endurance performance have also been related to musculotendinous stiffness (Bishop and Girard 2011; Girard *et al.* 2011). Strength and plyometric training significantly increase the stiffness of the muscle–tendon unit, which enables the muscles and tendons to store and release more elastic energy and reduce the amount of wasted energy (Saunders *et al.* 2004). The reduced energy demand results in less oxygen consumption, which explains the strong association between running economy and endurance performance (Saunders *et al.* 2004). An improved running economy and running performance following strength or plyometric training have been reported frequently (Jung 2003; Saunders *et al.* 2006; Spurrs *et al.* 2003; Turner *et al.* 2003).

The improvements in motor unit activation and synchronization, musculotendinous stiffness, and stretch-shortening efficiency as a result of strength training can have a beneficial impact on both sprint performance and repeated-sprint ability (Aagaard and Andersen 2010; Bishop and Girard 2011; Buchheit *et al.* 2010; Girard *et al.* 2011; Nummela *et al.* 2006; Silva *et al.* 2013).

1.2 Injury prevention

A large meta-analysis including over 26000 participants revealed that strength training reduces acute injuries by more than two-thirds and almost halves the number of overuse injuries (Lauersen *et al.* 2014). Several other studies that examined the effectiveness of strength training on reducing injury incidence and recurrence in soccer had similar results (Askling *et al.* 2003; Hägglund *et al.* 2009, 2013; Petersen *et al.* 2011). Various reasons can help explain the effectiveness of strength training to prevent injuries.

Most acute sports injuries occur in the early phase of ground contact (Krosshaug *et al.* 2007). Fast movement reaction times and the potential to quickly produce force will benefit stability and balance during this initial phase of ground contact (Krosshaug *et al.* 2007). Resistance and plyometric training enhance the ability to rapidly produce force, through a reduced mechanical delay and an increased rate of force development (Aagaard *et al.* 2002; Wu *et al.* 2010). The higher musculotendinous stiffness and neuromuscular drive following strength training will shorten the time between muscle activation and contraction (mechanical delay) and increase the speed at which force is produced after the onset of contraction (rate of force development) (Waugh *et al.* 2014). The ability to faster produce force will not only benefit movement reaction times, but can also reduce the injury incidence through an enhanced co-activation potential during the initial phase of ground contact (Waugh *et al.* 2014).

Strength training can also increase the size and strength of the ligaments and tendons. As increases in muscular strength occur with strength training, ligaments and tendons also need to adapt in order to support and efficiently transmit these greater forces to the bones (Fleck and Kraemer 1987; Waugh *et al.* 2014).

Strength and plyometric training also improve the neuromuscular control of the lower extremities. The altered muscle activation patterns that have been reported following plyometric training include a higher pre-activation and a more symmetric co-activation between the quadriceps and hamstrings and also between the hip abductor and adductor muscles (Chimera *et al.* 2004; Hewett *et al.* 1996). These altered motor control patterns result in a better lower limb alignment and more stable knee position upon landing (Chimera *et al.* 2004; Cuoco and Tyler 2012). The enhanced pre-activation and stiffness of the muscle-tendon complex will increase the load absorbed by the muscles and tendons and diminish the load transmitted through the joints and ligaments (Chimera *et al.* 2004; Fouré *et al.* 2010, 2011).

A stronger musculoskeletal system and enhanced pre-activation will also improve the reactive stability and restraint against sudden movement perturbations, such as being pushed, contact with the opponent, or unforeseen game situations (Blazevich *et al.* 2007; Blickhan *et al.* 2007; Bosch 2012).

Players with higher strength levels are also less prone to injury due to a higher muscular endurance and resistance to fatigue. Muscular and central fatigue negatively affect neuromuscular control and alter landing mechanics (Cortes *et al.* 2013). As the level of fatigue increases, hip extension, knee valgus, and ankle supination angles progressively increase during deceleration, landing, and cutting actions (Borotikar *et al.* 2008; Chappell *et al.* 2005; McLean and Samorezov 2009; McLean *et al.* 2007). These altered kinematics as a result of fatigue decrease movement efficiency and augment the risk of injury (Blackburn and Padua 2008; Koga *et al.* 2010; Krosshaug *et al.* 2007; Olsen *et al.* 2004). This is in accordance with the increased injury incidence during the final 15 minutes of the first half and final 30 minutes of the second half of a soccer match (Hawkins *et al.* 2001; Woods *et al.* 2004).

Muscle imbalances, expressed as the agonist/antagonist ratio, and core weakness increase the risk of injury (Herman *et al.* 2012; Maffey and Emery 2007). An effective strength routine will correct these agonist/antagonist muscle imbalances and enhance the strength and neuromuscular control of the core.

1.3 Enhanced recovery

Repeatedly performing high-intensity actions over the course of a match induces neuromuscular fatigue and muscle damage (Nédélec *et al.* 2012; Silva *et al.* 2013). The magnitude of the post-match fatigue response also depends to a great extent on the player's training status

(Johnston *et al.* 2014). Developing a sound strength base can moderate the neuromuscular fatigue and muscle damage following match-play. That post-match fatigue is reduced in players with greater lower body strength can be attributed to neural, connective tissue, and cellular adaptations (Johnston *et al.* 2014).

Strength training results in an enhanced neural drive, which will transfer to similar movements in soccer (Zatsiorsky 1995). Because more motor units can be activated simultaneously, the contractile stress during these high-intensity actions is distributed over a larger number of contracting muscle fibers, which will limit the amount of muscle damage incurred (McHugh *et al.* 1999).

The high-intensity actions during soccer involve repeated bouts of stretch-shortening cycles in which a rapid lengthening of a muscle is followed by an immediate shortening. Stronger players possess greater eccentric strength and ability to utilize the stretch-shortening cycle (Miyaguchi and Demura 2006, 2008). Strength and plyometric training induce changes in connective tissue and elastic properties of the muscle that increase the ability of the muscle–tendon complex to store and release more elastic energy (Fouré *et al.* 2010, 2011; Kubo *et al.* 2007; Markovic and Mikulic 2010; Vissing *et al.* 2008). More efficient movement mechanics and an increased dependence on passive elastic force production can decrease the stress imposed on the contractile elements and reduce the neuromuscular fatigue and muscle damage (Byrne *et al.* 2004; Johnston *et al.* 2014).

Ballistic, full range of motion, and eccentric strength training result in greater muscle lengths through an increase of the number of sarcomeres connected in series (Alegre *et al.* 2006; O'Sullivan *et al.* 2012; Seynnes *et al.* 2007; Wyon *et al.* 2013). An increased number of sarcomeres in series will diminish the possibility that sarcomeres are lengthened to the point of disruption, which is the initial stage of muscle damage (Proske and Morgan 2001). An increased number of sarcomeres in series will therefore reduce the sarcomere strain during repeated bouts of active muscle lengthening and limit the subsequent muscle damage (McHugh *et al.* 1999).

Post-match fatigue is reduced in players with greater lower body strength because they can better handle the forces associated with the high-intensity actions during soccer (Johnston *et al.* 2014; López-Segovia *et al.* 2014). These lower levels of neuromuscular fatigue can positively influence the recovery time following match-play (Nédélec *et al.* 2012).

References

Aagaard P, Andersen JL. Effects of strength training on endurance capacity in top-level endurance athletes. *Scand J Med Sci Sports.* 2010 Oct;20 Suppl 2:39–47.

Aagaard P, Simonsen EB, Andersen JL, Magnusson P, Dyhre-Poulsen P. Increased rate of force development and neural drive of human skeletal muscle following resistance training. *J Appl Physiol (1985).* 2002 Oct;93(4):1318–26.

Alegre LM, Jiménez F, Gonzalo-Orden JM, Martín-Acero R, Aguado X. Effects of dynamic resistance training on fascicle length and isometric strength. *J Sports Sci.* 2006 May;24(5):501–8.

Askling C, Karlsson J, Thorstensson A. Hamstring injury occurrence in elite soccer players after preseason strength training with eccentric overload. *Scand J Med Sci Sports.* 2003 Aug;13(4):244–50.

Bishop D, Girard O. Repeated-sprint ability (RSA). In: Cardinale M, Newton R, Nosaka K, editors. *Strength and conditioning: biological principles and practical applications.* Oxford: Wiley-Blackwell; 2011. pp. 223–41.

Bishop D, Girard O, Mendez-Villanueva A. Repeated-sprint ability – part II: recommendations for training. *Sports Med.* 2011 Sep;41(9):741–56.

Blackburn JT, Padua DA. Influence of trunk flexion on hip and knee joint kinematics during a controlled drop landing. *Clin Biomech (Bristol, Avon)*. 2008 Mar;23(3):313–19.

Blazevich AJ, Cannavan D, Coleman DR, Horne S. Influence of concentric and eccentric resistance training on architectural adaptation in human quadriceps muscles. *J Appl Physiol (1985)*. 2007 Nov;103(5):1565–75.

Blickhan R, Seyfarth A, Geyer H, Grimmer S, Wagner H, Günther M. Intelligence by mechanics. *Philos Trans A Math Phys Eng Sci*. 2007 Jan;365(1850):199–220.

Borotikar BS, Newcomer R, Koppes R, McLean SG. Combined effects of fatigue and decision making on female lower limb landing postures: central and peripheral contributions to ACL injury risk. *Clin Biomech (Bristol, Avon)*. 2008;23(1):81–92.

Bosch F. *Krachttraining en coördinatie, een integratieve benadering*. Rotterdam: 2010 Uitgevers; 2012. 352 pp.

Brito J, Vasconcellos F, Oliveira J, Krustrup P, Rebelo A. Short-term performance effects of three different low-volume strength-training programmes in college male soccer players. *J Hum Kinet*. 2014 Apr;40:121–8.

Brocherie F, Girard O, Forchino F, Al Haddad H, Dos Santos GA, Millet GP. Relationships between anthropometric measures and athletic performance, with special reference to repeated-sprint ability, in the Qatar national soccer team. *J Sports Sci*. 2014;32(13):1243–54.

Buchheit M, Mendez-Villanueva A, Delhomel G, Brughelli M, Ahmaidi S. Improving repeated sprint ability in young elite soccer players: repeated shuttle sprints vs. explosive strength training. *J Strength Cond Res*. 2010 Oct;24(10):2715–22.

Byrne C, Twist C, Eston R. Neuromuscular function after exercise-induced muscle damage: theoretical and applied implications. *Sports Med*. 2004;34(1):49–69.

Chappell JD, Herman DC, Knight BS, Kirkendall DT, Garrett WE, Yu B. Effect of fatigue on knee kinetics and kinematics in stop-jump tasks. *Am J Sports Med*. 2005;33(7):1022–9.

Chelly MS, Fathloun M, Cherif N, Ben Amar M, Tabka Z, Van Praagh E. Effects of a back squat training program on leg power, jump, and sprint performances in junior soccer players. *J Strength Cond Res*. 2009 Nov;23(8):2241–9.

Chimera NJ, Swanik KA, Swanik CB, Straub SJ. Effects of plyometric training on muscle-activation strategies and performance in female athletes. *J Athl Train*. 2004 Mar;39(1):24–31.

Cortes N, Greska E, Kollock R, Ambegaonkar J, Onate JA. Changes in lower extremity biomechanics due to a short-term fatigue protocol. *J Athl Train*. 2013 May–Jun;48(3):306–13.

Cuoco A, Tyler TF. Plyometric training and drills. In: Andrews J, Harrelson G, Wilk K, editors. *Physical rehabilitation of the injured athlete*. 4th ed. Philadelphia: Elsevier Saunders; 2012. pp. 571–95.

Delecluse C. Influence of strength training on sprint running performance. Current findings and implications for training. *Sports Med*. 1997 Sep;24(3):147–56.

Dintiman G, Ward B. *Sports speed*. 3rd ed. Champaign, IL: Human Kinetics. 2003. 280 p.

Fleck SJ, Kraemer WJ. *Designing resistance training programs*. 2nd ed. Champaign, IL: Human Kinetics; 1987. 275 p.

Fouré A, Nordez A, Cornu C. Plyometric training effects on Achilles tendon stiffness and dissipative properties. *J Appl Physiol (1985)*. 2010 Sep;109(3):849–54.

Fouré A, Nordez A, McNair P, Cornu C. Effects of plyometric training on both active and passive parts of the plantarflexors series elastic component stiffness of muscle-tendon complex. *Eur J Appl Physiol*. 2011 Mar;111(3):539–48.

García-Pinillos F, Martínez-Amat A, Hita-Contreras F, Martínez-López EJ, Latorre-Román PA. Effects of a contrast training program without external load on vertical jump, kicking speed, sprint, and agility of young soccer players. *J Strength Cond Res*. 2014 Sep;28(9):2452–60.

Girard O, Mendez-Villanueva A, Bishop D. Repeated-sprint ability – part I: factors contributing to fatigue. *Sports Med*. 2011 Aug 1;41(8):673–94.

Hägglund M, Waldén M, Atroshi I. Preventing knee injuries in adolescent female football players – design of a cluster randomized controlled trial. *BMC Musculoskelet Disord*. 2009 Jun;10:75.

Hägglund M, Atroshi I, Wagner P, Waldén M. Superior compliance with a neuromuscular training programme is associated with fewer ACL injuries and fewer acute knee injuries in female adolescent football players: secondary analysis of an RCT. *Br J Sports Med*. 2013 Oct;47(15):974–9.

Haugen T, Tønnessen E, Hisdal J, Seiler S. The role and development of sprinting speed in soccer. *Int J Sports Physiol Perform*. 2014 May;9(3):432–41.

Hawkins RD, Hulse MA, Wilkinson C, Hodson A, Gibson M. The association football medical research programme: an audit of injuries in professional football. *Br J Sports Med*. 2001 Feb;35(1):43–7.

Herman K, Barton C, Malliaras P, Morrissey D. The effectiveness of neuromuscular warm-up strategies, that require no additional equipment, for preventing lower limb injuries during sports participation: a systematic review. *BMC Med*. 2012 Jul;10:75.

Hewett TE, Stroupe AL, Nance TA, Noyes FR. Plyometric training in female athletes. Decreased impact forces and increased hamstring torques. *Am J Sports Med*. 1996 Nov–Dec;24(6):765–73.

Ingebrigtsen J, Jeffreys I. The relationship between speed, strength and jumping abilities in elite junior handball players. *Serbian J of Sports Sci*. 2012;6(3):83–8.

Johnston RD, Gabbett TJ, Jenkins DG, Hulin BT. Influence of physical qualities on post-match fatigue in rugby league players. *J Sci Med Sport*. 2014 Feb 6. [Epub ahead of print]

Jullien H, Bisch C, Largouët N, Manouvrier C, Carling CJ, Amiard V. Does a short period of lower limb strength training improve performance in field-based tests of running and agility in young professional soccer players? *J Strength Cond Res*. 2008 Mar;22(2):404–11.

Jung AP. The impact of resistance training on distance running performance. *Sports Med*. 2003;33(7):539–52.

Keiner M, Sander A, Wirth K, Schmidtbleicher D. Long-term strength training effects on change-of-direction sprint performance. *J Strength Cond Res*. 2014 Jan;28(1):223–31.

Koga H, Nakamae A, Shima Y. et al. Mechanisms for noncontact anterior cruciate ligament injuries: knee joint kinematics in 10 injury situations from female team handball and basketball. *Am J Sports Med*. 2010;38(11):2218–25.

Krosshaug T, Nakamae A, Boden BP, Engebretsen L, Smith G, Slauterbeck JR, Hewett TE, Bahr R. Mechanisms of anterior cruciate ligament injury in basketball: video analysis of 39 cases. *Am J Sports Med*. 2007 Mar;35(3):359–67.

Kubo K, Morimoto M, Komuro T, Yata H, Tsunoda N, Kanehisa H, Fukunaga T. Effects of plyometric and weight training on muscle-tendon complex and jump performance. *Med Sci Sports Exerc*. 2007 Oct;39(10):1801–10.

Laursen JB, Bertelsen DM, Andersen LB. The effectiveness of exercise interventions to prevent sports injuries: a systematic review and meta-analysis of randomised controlled trials. *Br J Sports Med*. 2014 Jun;48(11):871–7.

López-Segovia M, Marques MC, van den Tillaar R, González-Badillo JJ. Relationships between vertical jump and full squat power outputs with sprint times in u21 soccer players. *J Hum Kinet*. 2011 Dec;30:135–44.

López-Segovia M, Dellal A, Chamari K, González-Badillo JJ. Importance of muscle power variables in repeated and single sprint performance in soccer players. *J Hum Kinet*. 2014 Apr;40:201–11.

Maffey L, Emery C. What are the risk factors for groin strain injury in sport? A systematic review of the literature. *Sports Med*. 2007;37(10):881–94.

Maio Alves JM, Rebelo AN, Abrantes C, Sampaio J. Short-term effects of complex and contrast training in soccer players' vertical jump, sprint, and agility abilities. *J Strength Cond Res*. 2010 Apr;24(4):936–41.

Manolopoulos E, Katis A, Manolopoulos K, Kalapotharakos V, Kellis E. Effects of a 10-week resistance exercise program on soccer kick biomechanics and muscle strength. *J Strength Cond Res*. 2013 Dec;27(12):3391–401.

Markovic G, Mikulic P. Neuro-musculoskeletal and performance adaptations to lower-extremity plyometric training. *Sports Med*. 2010 Oct 1;40(10):859–95.

McHugh MP, Connolly DA, Eston RG, Gleim GW. Exercise-induced muscle damage and potential mechanisms for the repeated bout effect. *Sports Med*. 1999 Mar;27(3):157–70.

McLean SG, Samorezov JE. Fatigue-induced ACL injury risk stems from a degradation in central control. *Med Sci Sports Exerc*. 2009 Aug;41(8):1661–72.

McLean SG, Felin RE, Suedekum N, Calabrese G, Passerallo A, Joy S. Impact of fatigue on gender-based high-risk landing strategies. *Med Sci Sports Exerc*. 2007 Mar;39(3):502–14.

Mendez-Villanueva A, Hamer P, Bishop D. Fatigue in repeated-sprint exercise is related to muscle power factors and reduced neuromuscular activity. *Eur J Appl Physiol*. 2008 Jul;103(4):411–19.

Mero A, Komi PV. Force-, EMG-, and elasticity-velocity relationships at submaximal, maximal and supramaximal running speeds in sprinters. *Eur J Appl Physiol Occup Physiol*. 1986;55(5):553–61.

Miyaguchi K, Demura S. Muscle power output properties using the stretch-shortening cycle of the upper limb and their relationships with a one-repetition maximum bench press. *J Physiol Anthropol*. 2006 May;25(3):239–45

Miyaguchi K, Demura S. Relationships between stretch-shortening cycle performance and maximum muscle strength. *J Strength Cond Res*. 2008 Jan;22(1):19–24.

Mujika I, Santisteban J, Castagna C. In-season effect of short-term sprint and power training programs on elite junior soccer players. *J Strength Cond Res*. 2009 Dec;23(9):2581–7.

Nédélec M, McCall A, Carling C, Legall F, Berthoin S, Dupont G. Recovery in soccer: part I – post-match fatigue and time course of recovery. *Sports Med*. 2012 Dec;42(12):997–1015.

Nummela AT, Paavolainen LM, Sharwood KA, Lambert MI, Noakes TD, Rusko HK. Neuromuscular factors determining 5 km running performance and running economy in well-trained athletes. *Eur J Appl Physiol*. 2006 May;97(1):1–8.

Olsen OE, Myklebust G, Engebretsen L, Bahr R. Injury mechanisms for anterior cruciate ligament injuries in team handball: a systematic video analysis. *Am J Sports Med*. 2004 Jun;32(4):1002–12.

O'Sullivan K, McAuliffe S, Deburca N. The effects of eccentric training on lower limb flexibility: a systematic review. *Br J Sports Med*. 2012 Sep;46(12):838–45.

Petersen J, Thorborg K, Nielsen MB, Budtz-Jørgensen E, Hölmich P. Preventive effect of eccentric training on acute hamstring injuries in men's soccer: a cluster-randomized controlled trial. *Am J Sports Med*. 2011 Nov;39(11):2296–303.

Proske U, Morgan DL. Muscle damage from eccentric exercise: mechanism, mechanical signs, adaptation and clinical applications. *J Physiol*. 2001 Dec 1;537(Pt 2):333–45.

Rampinini E, Sassi A, Morelli A, Mazzoni S, Fanchini M, Coutts AJ. Repeated-sprint ability in professional and amateur soccer players. *Appl Physiol Nutr Metab*. 2009 Dec;34(6):1048–54.

Saunders PU, Pyne DB, Telford RD, Hawley JA. Factors affecting running economy in trained distance runners. *Sports Med*. 2004;34(7):465–85.

Saunders PU, Telford RD, Pyne DB, Peltola EM, Cunningham RB, Gore CJ, Hawley JA. Short-term plyometric training improves running economy in highly trained middle and long distance runners. *J Strength Cond Res*. 2006 Nov;20(4):947–54.

Seynnes OR, de Boer M, Narici MV. Early skeletal muscle hypertrophy and architectural changes in response to high-intensity resistance training. *J Appl Physiol (1985)*. 2007 Jan;102(1):368–73.

Shalfawi SA, Haugen T, Jakobsen TA, Enoksen E, Tønnessen E. The effect of combined resisted agility and repeated sprint training vs. strength training on female elite soccer players. *J Strength Cond Res*. 2013 Nov;27(11):2966–72.

Silva JR, Magalhães J, Ascensão A, Seabra AF, Rebelo AN. Training status and match activity of professional soccer players throughout a season. *J Strength Cond Res*. 2013 Jan;27(1):20–30.

Spencer M, Pyne D, Santisteban J, Mujika I. Fitness determinants of repeated-sprint ability in highly trained youth football players. *Int J Sports Physiol Perform*. 2011 Dec;6(4):497–508.

Spiteri T, Nimphius S, Hart NH, Specos C, Sheppard JM, Newton RU. Contribution of strength characteristics to change of direction and agility performance in female basketball athletes. *J Strength Cond Res*. 2014 Sep;28(9):2415–23.

Spurrs RW, Murphy AJ, Watsford ML. The effect of plyometric training on distance running performance. *Eur J Appl Physiol*. 2003 Mar;89(1):1–7.

Turner AM, Owings M, Schwane JA. Improvement in running economy after 6 weeks of plyometric training. *J Strength Cond Res*. 2003 Feb;17(1):60–7.

Vissing K, Brink M, Lønbro S, Sørensen H, Overgaard K, Danborg K, Mortensen J, Elstrøm O, Rosenhøj N, Ringgaard S, Andersen JL, Aagaard P. Muscle adaptations to plyometric vs. resistance training in untrained young men. *J Strength Cond Res*. 2008 Nov;22(6):1799–810.

Waugh CM, Korff T, Fath F, Blazevich AJ. Effects of resistance training on tendon mechanical properties and rapid force production in prepubertal children. *J Appl Physiol (1985)*. 2014 Aug;117(3):257–66.

Wisløff U, Castagna C, Helgerud J, Jones R, Hoff J. Strong correlation of maximal squat strength with sprint performance and vertical jump height in elite soccer players. *Br J Sports Med*. 2004 Jun;38(3):285–8.

Woods C, Hawkins RD, Maltby S, Hulse M, Thomas A, Hodson A, Football Association Medical Research Programme. The Football Association Medical Research Programme: an audit of injuries in professional football – analysis of hamstring injuries. *Br J Sports Med*. 2004 Feb;38(1):36–41.

Wu YK, Lien YH, Lin KH, Shih TT, Wang TG, Wang HK. Relationships between three potentiation effects of plyometric training and performance. *Scand J Med Sci Sports*. 2010 Feb;20(1):e80–6.

Wyon MA, Smith A, Koutedakis Y. A comparison of strength and stretch interventions on active and passive ranges of movement in dancers: a randomized controlled trial. *J Strength Cond Res*. 2013 Nov;27(11):3053–9.

Zatsiorsky VM. *Science and practice of strength training*. Champaign, IL: Human Kinetics; 1995. 243 pp.

2

THE ROLE OF STRENGTH TRAINING IN THE ENHANCEMENT OF STABILITY AND MOBILITY

Introduction

Joint stability and mobility have long been regarded as opposites. Increased mobility would result in a decrease of stability and vice versa. The focus on extremes gave rise to this erroneous way of thinking. Joint laxity absolutely compromises stability, and in a rigid joint that can barely move past its neutral zone, ligament and membrane stretch as a result of extreme range of motion is less likely to occur. But joint laxity and rigidity are opposite from good, clean full range of motion joint movement and both augment the risk of injuries in sports (Taimela *et al.* 1990; Vaishya and Hasija 2013). Soccer, identical to most other sports, requires the expression of both stability and mobility. Imagine the ankle, knee, and hip angles of a soccer player changing direction at high speed and the forces that these joints simultaneously have to absorb and produce. Olympic weightlifters and gymnasts are known to be the most flexible athletes in the Olympics, while both groups of athletes require a great amount of stability, strength, and power to be successful in their sport.

More and more research also points in the direction that joint flexibility and stability are not opposites but complement each other. Strength training plays an important role in both the development and expression of stability and flexibility, or to quote Dr. Eric Cobb: "Strength training cements your posture and mobility." A well-designed strength training will enhance both stability and mobility. The body needs stability in order to move.

2.1 Local stabilizers, global stabilizers, and global movers

Based on muscle functional roles, muscles can be divided into three categories: local stabilizers, global stabilizers, and global movers (Comerford and Mottram 2001a; Comerford *et al.* 2004; Table 2.1).

Local stabilizers: Local stabilizers are responsible for segmental stabilization and control of the spinal curvature and posture (Danneels *et al.* 2001; McGill 2004). Contraction increases the intersegmental stiffness of the spine and decreases excessive intersegmental motion. These muscles do not significantly change length during contraction nor contribute to movement or limit the range of motion (Hodges and Richardson 1997). The local stabilizer muscles consist

TABLE 2.1 Function and dysfunction of the local and global muscles

	Local stabilizer	*Global stabilizer*	*Global mover*
Function/ characteristics	- Segmental stabilization - Deep location with insertion close to the joint → limited lever arm and torque - Control neutral joint position - Does not produce ROM - Activity is independent from the direction of movement - Anticipatory feedforward recruitment: contract prior to movement - Consist mainly of low-threshold motor units: low-load recruitment with low susceptibility to fatigue - Continuous activity	- Isometrically hold position, eccentrically control ROM, and provide gross stability - located more superficial → larger lever arm and torque - Stability function when the body is under load or during high-speed movements - Control of rotational forces - Activity depends on direction of movement - Noncontinuous activity	- Produce high force or power - Bi- or multi-articular - Contract concentrically to generate powerful movements and acceleration - Consist mainly of high-threshold motor units: high-load recruitment with high susceptibility to fatigue - Mainly generate movement in the sagittal plane of motion (flexion/ extension) - Shock absorption of high loads - Intermittent activity: contract– relax
Muscle	- Transversus abdominis - Multifidus - Vastus medialis obliquus	- External oblique abdominis - Internal oblique abdominis - Gluteus medius	- Rectus femoris - Hamstrings
Dysfunction	- Inhibition - Delayed timing of recruitment - Decreased stiffness and control of neutral zone	- Hypermobile - Poor low-threshold recruitment - Diminished control of excessive ROM - Poor rotational control - Poor hip/spine dissociation	- Overactive low-threshold recruitment - Decreased flexibility

mainly of low-threshold motor units that are recruited with low loads and remain active throughout the entire movement with low susceptibility to fatigue (Cholewicki *et al.* 1996). Their activity is independent from the direction of the movement (Hodges and Richardson 1997). The muscles of the local system are small muscles that are located deep and inserted close to the joint, which limits their torque-generating capacity (Carter *et al.* 2006; Liemohn *et al.* 2005). The anticipatory feedforward recruitment of the local stabilizer muscles is critical for proper stabilization (Bouisset and Zattara 1981; Zattara and Bouisset 1988). The ability of these muscles to contract prior to movement of the body or extremities, independent of the direction, range of motion, or load, is more important than their force of contraction (Barr *et al.* 2005). These muscles also have a high density of receptors and their muscle stiffness is mediated by the proprioceptive input of movement and joint position (McGill 2007).

The transversus abdominis, multifidus, and vastus medialis obliquus are examples of muscles that have a very specific global stabilizer role.

Global stabilizers: The global stabilizer muscles are located more superficially than the local stabilizers and their larger lever and moment arm allow them to produce a large torque (Bergmark 1989; Janda 1996; Sahrmann 2002). These muscles have an important stability function when the body is under load (lifting weights) or during high-speed movements (Barr *et al.* 2005; Bergmark 1989). The global stabilizers isometrically hold position, eccentrically control range of motion, and provide gross stability (Bergmark 1989; Danneels *et al.* 2001). These muscles play especially an important role in controlling rotational forces (McGill 2007). Their activity is noncontinuous throughout the movement and is direction-dependent (Aruin and Latash 1995; Cordo and Nashner 1982; Hodges and Richardson 1997). The external oblique abdominis is a muscle that acts as a global stabilizer.

Global movers: Global movers are biarticular or multi-articular muscles that show phasic patterns of muscle activity (Bergmark 1989; Janda 1996; Sahrmann 2002). These muscles contract concentrically to generate powerful movements and acceleration (Bergmark 1989). Because these muscles consist mainly of high-threshold motor units, they are recruited to generate great force or fast movement with high susceptibility to fatigue (Richardson and Bullock 1986). The global movers mainly generate movement in the sagittal plane of motion (flexion/extension) and also play an important role in the shock absorption of high loads (Comerford and Mottram 2001a). The rectus femoris and the hamstrings are examples of global mobilisers.

2.2 Proximal stability for distal mobility

The integration of the local and global system plays an important role in efficient movement and biomechanical function. The local muscles provide segmental stability to maintain a neutral spine posture, while the global stabilizers together with the thoracolumbar fascia form a corset surrounding the trunk (McGill 2007, 2010). The stability provided by the stabilizer muscles minimizes joint loads, transfers forces from the ground, and allows the global movers to efficiently produce great force and power in all types of activities ranging from running to throwing (Behm *et al.* 2005; Kibler *et al.* 2006).

2.3 Instability and dysfunction

Instability, injury, or pain can alter the coordination between the local and global systems, resulting in an exaggerated recruitment of the superficial multi-joint muscles over the deeper segmental muscles (Comerford and Mottram 2001a; Hodges and Moseley 2003). These altered recruitment strategies are associated with delayed activation and inhibition of the local and global stabilizers (Comerford and Mottram 2001a). The local stabilizers lose stiffness resulting in decreased control of the neutral zone (Comerford and Mottram 2001a). The global stabilizer muscles become hypermobile, which leads to diminished control of excessive range of motion and poor rotational control (Comerford and Mottram 2001a; Gossman *et al.* 1982). As compensation the global movers are recruited with low loads (Comerford and Mottram 2001a). As a result of this overactive low-threshold recruitment the global mover muscles will shorten and become less flexible (Comerford and Mottram 2001a).

As a metaphor we can say that when the stabilizer muscles are weak and unable to control the range of motion, they need a wingman to get the job done. The multi-articular prime movers need to shorten in order to effectively help the stabilizers control and prevent excessive range of motion (Comerford and Mottram 2001a). For every tight muscle there is a weak one.

The body will compensate for the loss of flexibility with increased movement elsewhere in the kinetic chain to maintain function (Comerford and Mottram 2001a, 2001b). When this compensatory movement, higher or lower in the kinetic chain, is controlled by the synergist of the global and local systems, the body can cope well. Poorly controlled compensation however will decrease movement efficiency and place higher stress on the body, increasing the risk of injury.

People that suffer from low back pain have been shown to have atrophied deep trunk musculature, tight hamstrings, and diminished hip rotation (Barbee-Ellison *et al.* 1990; Chesworth *et al.* 1994; Ellison *et al.* 1990; Hides *et al.* 1994; McClure *et al.* 1997; Vad *et al.* 2004; Van Dillen *et al.* 2008). Low back pain is also associated with inhibition of the gluteus maximus and a dominance of the hamstring muscles during hip extension (Janda 1985; Leinonen *et al.* 2000; Nelson-Wong *et al.* 2012; Sahrmann 2002). Stretching only, without proper training to address the weakness of the stabilizers, will not or only temporarily result in an enhanced hamstring length and range of motion at the hip.

2.4 Training stability and mobility as separate bio-motor abilities compromise transfer to athletic performance

The increased range of motion as a result of stretching has been attributed to an enhanced tolerance of the stretch sensation or decreased musculotendinous unit stiffness (Halbertsma and Göeken 1994; Halbertsma *et al.* 1996; Magnusson *et al.* 1996a, 1996b; Mahieu *et al.* 2009; Morse *et al.* 2008; Nakamura *et al.* 2011; Samukawa *et al.* 2011). The musculotendinous unit consists of the muscle fibers, tendon, and connective tissue. The altered stiffness of the musculotendinous unit can therefore be the result of changes in tendon, connective, or muscle fascicle properties. Several studies showed that a large percentage (54–73 percent) of the overall length change during passive stretching occurs at the tendon (Morse *et al.* 2008; Nakamura *et al.* 2011; Samukawa *et al.* 2011). No studies with humans found that the enhanced range of motion due to flexibility training was caused by changes in muscle fascicle length. Riley and Van Dyke (2012) conclude that an active stretch is necessary to regulate muscle fascicle length. This is in accordance with research showing that eccentric training and full range of motion strength training increase muscle length through the addition of the number of sarcomeres in series (Aquino *et al.* 2010; Blazevich *et al.* 2007; Leighton 1964; Mahieu *et al.* 2008; O'Sullivan *et al.* 2012; Seynnes *et al.* 2007; Wyon *et al.* 2013).

A study involving athletes with tight hamstring muscles showed that the optimal length of the hamstrings was shifted toward shorter muscle lengths (Alonso *et al.* 2009; Magnusson *et al.* 1997). Stretching does not affect the active length–tension curve and the majority of these athletes were already performing stretching exercises on a regular basis (Magnusson *et al.* 1997).

To recover proper fascicle length, restore normal movement, and minimize the give (increased compensatory motion) elsewhere in the kinetic chain, proper stability function has to be re-established. In addition to stability training, active techniques like eccentric training and strength exercises performed in full range of motion can help restore optimal fascicle length of the tightened global mobilizer muscles (Aquino *et al.* 2010; Blazevich *et al.* 2007; Leighton 1964; McMahon *et al.* 2014; Mahieu *et al.* 2008; O'Sullivan *et al.* 2012; Seynnes *et al.* 2007; Wyon *et al.* 2013). These active techniques also concurrently develop stability and mobility. When performing a lunge or a Bulgarian split squat, the hip flexors lengthen while the lumbopelvic stabilizers control the position of the pelvis in the three planes of motion and counteract the pull of the lengthening hip flexors. Hurdle mobility drills take the muscles of the lower body through the full range of motion and require good balance, core, and single-leg stability.

A study by Wyon *et al.* showed that full range of motion strength training was equally effective at improving passive range of motion compared to moderate-intensity or high-intensity stretching, but was superior to both static stretching interventions at increasing active range of motion (Wyon *et al.* 2013). The strengthening of agonists and stabilizer muscles and training of reciprocal inhibition of the antagonist muscles can explain the larger gains in active range of motion as a result of strength training (Wyon *et al.* 2013). Active range of motion is also a better predictor of performance and the propensity for injury (Angioi *et al.* 2009; Henderson *et al.* 2010; Twitchett *et al.* 2011). It is therefore no surprise that active techniques, which develop both stability and mobility, result in an enhanced transfer to athletic performance (Amiri-Khorasani and Sotoodeh 2013; Amiri-Khorasani *et al.* 2011, 2012; Wyon *et al.* 2013).

When stretching alters the stiffness of the musculotendinous unit, the passive length–tension curve shifts to the right (Morse *et al.* 2008; Nakamura *et al.* 2011; Samukawa *et al.* 2011).

Some studies observed only an increase in end-range joint angles without a shift of the passive length–tension curve to the right (Halbertsma and Göeken 1994; Halbertsma *et al.* 1996; Magnusson *et al.* 1996a, 1996b; Mahieu *et al.* 2009; Figs 2.1 and 2.2). This indicates that the increased muscle length following a stretching routine cannot be caused by an increase in the number of sarcomeres in series or permanent lengthening of the connective tissue, but is the result of an increased tolerance to the uncomfortable stretch sensation (Weppler and Magnusson 2010).

2.5 Stability positively affects mobility

Moreside and McGill (2012) compared the effect of three different interventions on the hip range of motion. A group of young men with limited hip range of motion were divided into four groups: 1) stretch only; 2) stretch and motor control exercises for the hip and trunk;

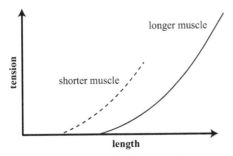

FIGURE 2.1 Increased end-range joint angles with a shift of the length–tension curve

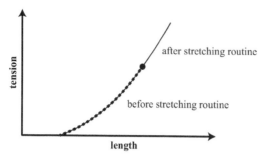

FIGURE 2.2 Increased end-range joint angles without a shift of the length–tension curve

3) core endurance and motor control exercises; 4) control group (no stretch or exercise). The group that performed core stability exercises without a concurrent stretching routine displayed an improvement in internal and total hip rotation. Stretching combined with core stability also resulted in greater improvements of hip mobility compared to stretching alone.

The outcome of this study can be explained by the proximal stability for distal mobility concept (Kibler *et al.* 2006). The pre-programmed integration of local, single-joint muscles and multi-joint muscles will provide stability and produce motion (Kibler *et al.* 2006). Improved core stability results in an enhanced ability to dissociate the hip from the spine. This means more hip movement can be produced without affecting the neutral lumbopelvic position.

2.6 Mobility positively affects stability

Also mobility can enhance strength through the arthrokinetic reflex (Warmerdam 1999; Wyke 1985). Articular mechanoreceptors can facilitate or inhibit muscle function (Warmerdam 1999; Wyke 1985). The increased mechanoreceptive information input due to mobilization can increase the activation and force output of the muscles attaching to that joint (Warmerdam 1999; Wyke 1985). Hip mobilizations have been shown to result in a 17 percent increase in hip abduction force output and an enhanced force output from the gluteus maximus (Makofsky *et al.* 2007; Yerys *et al.* 2002). Mobilizing a restricted joint can enhance muscular strength by down-regulating the reflexogenic inhibition from the joint mechanoreceptors (Warmerdam 1999; Wyke 1985). In case of restricted hip abduction and tight hip adductors, the hip abductor muscles become inhibited every time movement approaches the limits of hip abduction range of motion.

Dynamic stretching has also been shown to enhance strength and power output as well as improve vertical jump and sprinting performance (Fletcher and Anness 2007; Hough *et al.* 2009; McMillian *et al.* 2006; Manoel *et al.* 2008; Yamaguchi and Ishii 2005). The authors concluded that the improvements may be linked to enhanced nervous system stimulation and motor unit excitability, proprioceptive input, core and muscle temperature (Fletcher and Anness 2007; Hough *et al.* 2009; McMillian *et al.* 2006; Manoel *et al.* 2008; Yamaguchi and Ishii 2005).

2.7 Integrated training of stability and mobility

Frans Bosch questions the idea of training the different bio-motor abilities (strength, coordination, endurance, flexibility, speed) separately because there is so much crossover between

these properties and they are all integrated in athletic performance (Bosch 2012). By training them separately we compromise the transfer of training (Bosch 2012). This way of
thinking certainly applies to the development of mobility and stability. Both depend on
proprioceptive input, central nervous system facilitation or inhibition, and proper motor
control patterns. Only focusing on flexibility does not have an effect on the mechanical
muscle properties and results in a progressive reduction in the gained range of motion when
the stretching protocol is not maintained (Cipriani *et al.* 2012). Increased range of motion
following static stretching does also not transfer automatically to improved dynamic, functional, sport-specific flexibility (Amiri-Khorasani *et al.* 2011, 2012; Moreside and McGill
2013; Young *et al.* 2004).

Stability affects mobility and vice versa. The integrated training of mobility and stability
through dynamic flexibility drills, eccentric training, or full range of motion strength exercises
will elicit better results and transfer to athletic performance compared to developing either
skill independently (Amiri-Khorasani *et al.* 2011, 2012).

Active movement through the full range of motion will not only increase flexibility but
will also get the global and local stabilizer muscles firing and improve movement quality.
The obtained improvement in range of motion is also more likely to be grooved into a new
motor pattern and enhance functional sport-specific mobility compared to passive stretching
techniques (Amiri-Khorasani *et al.* 2011). Strength training performed over the full range
of motion improves mobility due to an increased number of sarcomeres in series. Athletes
that integrated dynamic stretching into the warm-up also showed superior long-term power,
strength, muscular endurance, and agility performance enhancements, compared to the athletes that performed static stretching (Herman and Smith 2008).

The literature is also conflictive whether stretching included in the warm-up or at another
time is effective for reducing the risk of injury (Leppänen *et al.* 2014; McHugh and Cosgrave
2010; Small *et al.* 2008; Thacker *et al.* 2004; Witvrouw *et al.* 2004). The research is more con-
sistent, however in that limited flexibility is a risk factor for various strain, overuse, and non-
contact injuries (Jones and Knapik 1999; Messier *et al.* 2008; Tabrizi *et al.* 2000; Tainaka *et al.*
2014; Witvrouw *et al.* 2003). This discrepancy may also indicate the necessity of an integrated
development of stability and mobility through strength training or other active techniques.

References

Alonso J, McHugh MP, Mullaney MJ, Tyler TF. Effect of hamstring flexibility on isometric knee flexion
   angle-torque relationship. *Scand J Med Sci Sports*. 2009 Apr;19(2):252–6.
Amiri-Khorasani M, Sotoodeh V. The acute effects of combined static and dynamic stretch protocols on
   fitness performances in soccer players. *J Sports Med Phys Fitness*. 2013 Oct;53(5):559–65.
Amiri-Khorasani M, Abu Osman NA, Yusof A. Acute effect of static and dynamic stretching on hip
   dynamic range of motion during instep kicking in professional soccer players. *J Strength Cond Res*.
   2011 Jun;25(6):1647–52.
Amiri-Khorasani M, Mohammadkazemi R, Sarafrazi S, Riyahi-Malayeri S, Sotoodeh V, Kinematics analyses related to stretch-shortening cycle during soccer instep kicking after different acute stretching.
   J Strength Cond Res. 2012 Nov;26(11):3010–17.
Angioi M, Metsios GS, Twitchett E, Koutedakis Y, Wyon M. Association between selected physical fitness
   parameters and esthetic competence in contemporary dancers. *J Dance Med Sci*. 2009;13(4):115–23.
Aquino CF, Fonseca ST, Goncalves GG, Silva PL, Ocarino JM, Mancini MC. Stretching versus strength
   training in lengthened position in subjects with tight hamstring muscles: a randomized controlled
   trial. *Man Ther*. Feb 2010;15(1):26–31.

Aruin AS, Latash ML. Directional specificity of postural muscles in feed-forward postural reactions during fast voluntary arm movements. *Exp Brain Res.* 1995;103(2):323–32.

Barbee-Ellison JB, Rose SJ, Sahrmann SA. Patterns of hip rotation range of motion: comparisons between healthy subjects and patients with low back pain. *Phys Ther.* 1990 Sep;70(9):537–41.

Barr KP, Griggs M, Cadby T. Lumbar stabilization: core concepts and current literature, Part 1. *Am J Phys Med Rehabil.* 2005 Jun;84(6):473–80.

Behm DG, Leonard AM, Young WB, Bonsey WA, MacKinnon SN. Trunk muscle electromyographic activity with unstable and unilateral exercises. *J Strength Cond Res.* 2005 Feb;19(1):193–201.

Bergmark A. Stability of the lumbar spine. A study in mechanical engineering. *Acta Orthop Scand Suppl.* 1989;230:1–54.

Blazevich AJ, Cannavan D, Coleman DR, Horne S. Influence of concentric and eccentric resistance training on architectural adaptation in human quadriceps muscles. *J Appl Physiol (1985).* 2007 Nov;103(5):1565–75.

Bosch F. *Krachttraining en coördinatie, een integratieve benadering.* Rotterdam: 2010 Uitgevers; 2012. 352 pp.

Bouisset S, Zattara M. A sequence of postural adjustments precedes voluntary movement. *Neurosci Lett.* 1981;22:263–70.

Carter JM, Beam WC, McMahan SG, Barr ML, Brown LE. The effects of stability ball training on spinal stability in sedentary individuals. *J Strength Cond Res.* 2006 May;20(2):429–35.

Chesworth BM, Padfield BJ, Helewa A, Stitt LW. A comparison of hip mobility in patients with non-specific low back pain. *Physiother Can.* 1994;46:267–74.

Cholewicki J, McGill SM. Mechanical stability of the in vivo lumbar spine: implications for injury and chronic low back pain. *Clin Biomech (Bristol, Avon).* 1996 Jan;11(1):1–15.

Cipriani DJ, Terry ME, Haines MA, Tabibnia AP, Lyssanova O. Effect of stretch frequency and sex on the rate of gain and rate of loss in muscle flexibility during a hamstring-stretching program: a randomized single-blind longitudinal study. *J Strength Cond Res.* 2012 Aug; 26(8):2119–29.

Comerford MJ, Mottram SL. Movement and stability dysfunction–contemporary developments. *Man Ther.* 2001a Feb;6(1):15–26.

Comerford MJ, Mottram SL. Functional stability re-training: principles and strategies for managing mechanical dysfunction. *Man Ther.* 2001b Feb;6(1):3–14.

Comerford MJ, Mottram SL, Gibbons SG. Understanding movement and function 'concepts'. *Kinetic control movement dysfunction course.* Southampton: Kinetic Control; 2004.

Cordo PJ, Nashner LM. Properties of postural adjustments associated with rapid arm movements. *J Neurophysiol.* 1982 Feb;47(2):287–302.

Danneels LA, Vanderstraeten GG, Cambier DC, Witvrouw EE, Stevens VK, De Cuyper HJ. A functional subdivision of hip, abdominal, and back muscles during asymmetric lifting. *Spine (Phila Pa 1976).* 2001 Mar;26(6):E114–21.

Ellison, JB, Rose SJ, Sahrmann SA. Patterns of hip rotation range of motion: a comparison between healthy subjects and patients with low back pain. *Phys Ther.* 1990 Sep;70(9):537–41.

Fletcher IM, Anness R. The acute effects of combined static and dynamic stretch protocols on fifty-meter sprint performance in track-and-field athletes. *J Strength Cond Res.* Aug 2007;21(3):784–7.

Gossman MR, Sahrmann SA, Rose SJ. Review of length-associated changes in muscle. Experimental evidence and clinical implications. *Phys Ther.* 1982 Dec;62(12):1799–808.

Halbertsma JP, Göeken LN. Stretching exercises: effect on passive extensibility and stiffness in short hamstrings of healthy subjects. *Arch Phys Med Rehabil.* 1994 Sep;75(9):976–81.

Halbertsma JP, van Bolhuis AI, Göeken LN. Sport stretching: effect on passive muscle stiffness of short hamstrings. *Arch Phys Med Rehabil.* 1996 Jul;77(7):688–92.

Henderson G, Barnes CA, Portas MD. Factors associated with increased propensity for hamstring injury in English Premier League soccer players. *J Sci Med Sport.* 2010 Jul;13(4):397–402.

Herman SL, Smith DT. Four-week dynamic stretching warm-up intervention elicits longer-term performance benefits. *J Strength Cond Res.* 2008 Jul;22(4):1286–97.

Hides JA, Stokes MJ, Saide M, Jull GA, Cooper DH. Evidence of lumbar multifidus muscle wasting ipsilateral to symptoms in patients with acute/subacute low back pain. *Spine (Phila Pa 1976).* 1994 Jan;19(2):165–72.

Hodges PW, Moseley GL. Pain and motor control of the lumbopelvic region: effect and possible mechanisms. *J Electromyogr Kinesiol.* 2003 Aug;13(4):361–70.

Hodges PW, Richardson CA. Feedforward contraction of transversus abdominis is not influenced by the direction of arm movement. *Exp Brain Res.* 1997 Apr;114(2):362–70.

Hough PA, Ross EZ, Howatson G. Effects of dynamic and static stretching on vertical jump performance and electromyographic activity. *J Strength Cond Res.* Mar 2009;23(2):507–12.

Janda V. Pain in the locomotor system – a broad approach. In: Glasgow EF, Twomey LT, Scull ER, Kleynhans AM, Idczak RM, editors. *Aspects of manipulative therapy.* Edinburgh: Churchill Livingstone; 1985. pp. 148–51.

Janda V. Evaluation of muscular imbalance, In: Liebenson C, editor. *Rehabilitation of the spine: a practitioner's manual.* Baltimore, MD: Lippincott Williams & Wilkins; 1996. pp. 97–112.

Jones BH, Knapik JJ. Physical training and exercise-related injuries. Surveillance, research and injury prevention in military populations. *Sports Med.* 1999 Feb;27(2):111–25.

Kibler WB, Press J, Sciascia A. The role of core stability in athletic function. *Sports Med.* 2006;36(3):189–98.

Leighton JR. A study of the effect of progressive weight training on flexibility. *J Assoc Phys Ment Rehabil.* 1964 Jul–Aug;18:101–4.

Leinonen V, Kankaanpää M, Airaksinen O, Hänninen O. Back and hip extensor activities during trunk flexion/extension: effects of low back pain and rehabilitation. *Arch Phys Med Rehabil.* 2000 Jan;81(1):32–7.

Leppänen M, Aaltonen S, Parkkari J, Heinonen A, Kujala UM. Interventions to prevent sports related injuries: a systematic review and meta-analysis of randomised controlled trials. *Sports Med.* 2014 Apr;44(4):473–86.

Liemohn WP, Baumgartner TA, Gagnon LH. Measuring core stability. *J Strength Cond Res.* 2005 Aug;19(3):583–6.

McClure PW, Esola M, Schreier R, Siegler S. Kinematic analysis of lumbar and hip motion while rising from a forward, flexed position in patients with and without a history of low back pain. *Spine (Phila Pa 1976).* 1997 Mar 1;22(5):552–8.

McGill SM. *Ultimate back fitness and performance.* 3rd ed. Ontario: Wabuno; 2004. Chapter 6, Fundamental principles of movement and causes of movement error; pp. 127–49.

McGill SM. *Low back disorders: evidence-based prevention and rehabilitation.* 2nd ed. Champaign, IL: Human Kinetics; 2007. 328 pp.

McGill SM. Core training: evidence translating to better performance and injury prevention. *Strength Cond J.* 2010 Jun;32(3):33–46.

McHugh MP, Cosgrave CH. To stretch or not to stretch: the role of stretching in injury prevention and performance. *Scand J Med Sci Spor.* 2010 Apr;20(2):169–81.

McMahon GE, Morse CI, Burden A, Winwood K, Onambélé GL. Impact of range of motion during ecologically valid resistance training protocols on muscle size, subcutaneous fat, and strength. *J Strength Cond Res.* 2014 Jan;28(1):245–55.

McMillian D, Moore J, Hatler B, Taylor D. Dynamic vs. static-stretching warm up: the effect on power and agility performance. *J Strength Cond Res.* 2006 Aug;20(3):492–9.

Magnusson SP, Simonsen EB, Aagaard P, Dyhre-Poulsen P, McHugh MP, Kjaer M. Mechanical and physical responses to stretching with and without preisometric contraction in human skeletal muscle. *Arch Phys Med Rehabil.* 1996a Apr;77(4):373–8.

Magnusson SP, Simonsen EB, Aagaard P, Sørensen H, Kjaer M. A mechanism for altered flexibility in human skeletal muscle. *J Physiol.* 1996b Nov 15;497 (Pt 1):291–8.

Magnusson SP, Simonsen EB, Aagaard P, Boesen J, Johannsen F, Kjaer M. Determinants of musculoskeletal flexibility: viscoelastic properties, cross-sectional area, EMG and stretch tolerance. *Scand J Med Sci Sports.* 1997 Aug;7(4):195–202.

Mahieu NN, McNair P, Cools A, D'Haen C, Vandermeulen K, Witvrouw E. Effect of eccentric training on the plantar flexor muscle-tendon tissue properties. *Med Sci Sports Exerc.* 2008 Jan;40(1):117–23.

Mahieu NN, Cools A, De Wilde B, Boon M, Witvrouw E. Effect of proprioceptive neuromuscular facilitation stretching on the plantar flexor muscle-tendon tissue properties. *Scand J Med Sci Sports.* 2009 Aug;19(4):553–60.

Makofsky H, Panicker S, Abbruzzese J, Aridas C, Camp M, Drakes J, Franco C, Sileo R, Immediate effect of grade IV inferior hip joint mobilization on hip abductor torque: a pilot study. *J Man Manip Ther.* 2007;15(2):103–10.

Manoel ME, Harris-Love MO, Danoff JV, Miller TA. Acute effects of static, dynamic, and proprioceptive neuromuscular facilitation stretching on muscle power in women. *J Strength Cond Res.* 2008 Sep;22(5):1528–34.

Messier SP, Legault C, Schoenlank CR, Newman JJ, Martin DF, DeVita P. Risk factors and mechanisms of knee injury in runners. *Med Sci Sports Exerc.* 2008 Nov;40(11):1873–9.

Moreside JM, McGill SM. Hip joint range of motion improvements using three different interventions. *J Strength Cond Res.* 2012 May;26(5):1265–73.

Moreside JM, McGill SM. Improvements in hip flexibility do not transfer to mobility in functional movement patterns. *J Strength Cond Res.* 2013 Oct;27(10):2635–43.

Morse CI, Degens H, Seynnes OR, Maganaris CN, Jones DA. The acute effect of stretching on the passive stiffness of the human gastrocnemius muscle tendon unit. *J Physiol.* 2008 Jan;586(1):97–106.

Nakamura M, Ikezoe T, Takeno Y, Ichihashi N. Acute and prolonged effect of static stretching on the passive stiffness of the human gastrocnemius muscle tendon unit in vivo. *J Orthop Res.* 2011 Nov;29(11):1759–63.

Nelson-Wong E, Alex B, Csepe D, Lancaster D, Callaghan JP. Altered muscle recruitment during extension from trunk flexion in low back pain developers. *Clin Biomech.* 2012 Dec;27(10):994–8.

O'Sullivan K, McAuliffe S, Deburca N. The effects of eccentric training on lower limb flexibility: a systematic review. *Br J Sports Med.* 2012 Sep;46(12):838–45.

Richardson C, Bullock MI. Changes in muscle activity during fast, alternating flexion-extension movements of the knee. *Scand J Rehabil Med.* 1986;18(2):51–8.

Riley DA, Van Dyke JM. The effects of active and passive stretching on muscle length. *Phys Med Rehabil Clin N Am.* 2012 Feb;23(1):51–7.

Sahrmann S. *Diagnosis and treatment of movement impairment syndromes.* St Louis, MO: Mosby; 2002. 384 pp.

Samukawa M, Hattori M, Sugama N, Takeda N. The effects of dynamic stretching on plantar flexor muscle-tendon tissue properties. *Man Ther.* 2011 Dec;16(6):618–22.

Seynnes OR, de Boer M, Narici MV. Early skeletal muscle hypertrophy and architectural changes in response to high-intensity resistance training. *J Appl Physiol (1985).* 2007 Jan;102(1):368–73.

Small K, McNaughton NL, Matthews M. A systematic review into the efficacy of static stretching as part of a warm-up for the prevention of exercise-related injury. *Res Sports Med.* 2008 Jul;16(3):213–31.

Tabrizi P, McIntyre WM, Quesnel MB, Howard AW. Limited dorsiflexion predisposes to injuries of the ankle in children. *J Bone Joint Surg Br.* 2000;82:1103–6.

Taimela S, Kujala UM, Osterman K. Intrinsic risk factors and athletic injuries. *Sports Med.* 1990 Apr;9(4):205–15.

Tainaka K, Takizawa T, Kobayashi H, Umimura M. Limited hip rotation and non-contact anterior cruciate ligament injury: a case-control study. *Knee.* 2014 Jan;21(1):86–90.

Thacker SB, Gilchrist J, Stroup DF, Kimsey CD Jr. The impact of stretching on sports injury risk: a systematic review of the literature. *Med Sci Sports Exerc.* 2004 Mar;36(3):371–8.

Twitchett EA, Angioi M, Koutedakis Y, Wyon M. Do increases in selected fitness parameters affect the aesthetic aspects of classical ballet performance? *Med Probl Perform Art.* 2011 Mar;26(1):35–8.

Vad VB, Bhat AL, Basrai D, Gebeh A, Aspergren DD, Andrews JR. Low back pain in professional golfers: the role of associated hip and low back range-of-motion deficits. *Am J Sports Med.* 2004 Mar;32(2):494–7.

Vaishya R, Hasija R. Joint hypermobility and anterior cruciate ligament injury. *J Orthop Surg (Hong Kong).* 2013 Aug;21(2):182–4.

Van Dillen LR, Bloom NJ, Gombatto SP, Susco TM. Hip rotation range of motion in people with and without low back pain who participate in rotation-related sports. *Phys Ther Sport.* 2008 May;9(2):72–81.

Warmerdam A. *Arthrokinematic therapy: improving muscle performance through joint manipulation.* Wantagh, NY: Pine Publications; 1999. pp. 32–44.

Weppler CH, Magnusson SP. Increasing muscle extensibility: a matter of increasing length or modifying sensation? *Phys Ther.* 2010 Mar;90(3):438–49.

Witvrouw E, Danneels L, Asselman P, D'Have T, Cambier D. Muscle flexibility as a risk factor for developing muscle injuries in male professional soccer players. A prospective study. *Am J Sports Med.* 2003 Jan-Feb;31(1):41–6.

Witvrouw E, Mahieu N, Danneels L, McNair P. Stretching and injury prevention: an obscure relationship. *Sports Med.* 2004;34(7):443–9.

Wyke BD. Articular neurology. In: Glasgow EF, Twoney LT, Scull ER, Kleynhams AM, editors. *Aspects of manipulative therapy.* New York: Churchill Livingstone, 1985:72–7.

Wyon MA, Smith A, Koutedakis Y. A comparison of strength and stretch interventions on active and passive ranges of movement in dancers: a randomized controlled trial. *J Strength Cond Res.* 2013 Nov;27(11):3053–9.

Yamaguchi T, Ishii K. Effects of static stretching for 30 seconds and dynamic stretching on leg extension power. *J Strength Cond Res.* 2005 Aug;19(3):677–83.

Yerys S, Makofsky H, Byrd C, Pennachio J, Cinkay J. Effect of mobilization of the anterior hip capsule on gluteus maximus strength. *J Manual Manipulative Ther.* 2002;10:218–24.

Young W, Clothier P, Otago L, Bruce L, Liddell D. Acute effects of static stretching on hip flexor and quadriceps flexibility, range of motion and foot speed in kicking a football. *J Sci Med Sport.* 2004 Mar;7(1):23–31.

Zattara M, Bouisset S. Posturo-kinetic organisation during the early phase of voluntary upper limb movement. 1. Normal subjects. *J Neurol Neurosurg Psychiatry.* 1988 Jul;51(7):956–65.

3

EFFECTIVE WARM-UP ROUTINE

The purpose of the warm-up is to gradually increase heart rate, core temperature, and blood flow. But a proper warm-up does not only prepare the body for the increased demands of exercise but also reduces the risk of injury and optimizes performance through neural activation and rehearsal of sport-specific movement patterns (Fletcher and Anness 2007; Hough et al. 2009; McMillian et al. 2006; Manoel et al. 2008; Yamaguchi and Ishii 2005). A well-designed warm-up will also elicit long-term performance benefits (Herman and Smith 2008). Ideally a warm-up is tailored to the subsequent workout and individual needs of the player.

Warm-ups are typically composed of a submaximal aerobic activity, stretching, and a sport-specific activity (Behm and Chaouachi 2011).

3.1 General warm-up

The purpose of the general warm-up is to elevate core, muscle temperature, and tissue suppleness while avoiding fatigue (Barroso et al. 2013). The general warm-up can consist of low- to moderate-intensity jogging, skipping exercises, running technique drills, or sport-specific technical drills performed at low intensity (e.g., dribbling the ball in soccer). A short duration of two to three minutes to raise a light sweat prior to stretching can already be sufficient (Sports Medicine Australia 2005).

3.2 Stretching

There is a vivid discussion going on in the literature about the acute effects of static and dynamic stretching on performance. This is an important discussion because the purpose of the warm-up is to enhance performance in the subsequent activities. But the discussion is narrowed down to short-term effects without much attention for the long-term development of these bio-motor abilities and the transfer to functional movement and athletic performance (Tables 3.1, 3.2).

ROM/transfer: Both dynamic and static stretching are equally effective at increasing range of motion prior to exercise or longer term. The range of motion in these studies was tested static however, and gained flexibility from static stretching does not automatically transfer

TABLE 3.1 Overview of studies that compare static and dynamic stretching routines

	Static — Better than dynamic and no stretching ↑	Static — Worse than no stretching →	No difference between static and dynamic	Dynamic — Better than static and no stretching ↑	Dynamic — Worse than no stretching →
ROM Acute	Covert et al. 2010 (ballistic) Morrin and Redding 2013 O'Sullivan et al. 2009 (ballistic) Samson et al. 2012		Beedle and Mann 2007 Behm et al. 2011 (↑) Curry et al. 2009 (↑) Chow and Ng 2010 (↑) (active) Perrier et al. 2011 (↑)	Aguilar et al. 2012 Amiri-Khorasani et al. 2011	
Training	Bandy et al. 1998 (active)		Chow and Ng 2010 (↑) (active) Herman and Smith 2008 (↑) Mahieu et al. 2007 (↑) Nelson and Bandy 2004 (↑) Webright et al. 1997 (↑) Winters et al. 2004 (↑) (active)	Meroni et al. 2010 (active)	
Strength Acute		**Isometric:** Herda et al. 2008 **Isokinetic:** Sekir et al. 2010	**Isometric:** Curry et al. 2009 (NC) Torres et al. 2008 (NC) **Eccentric isokinetic:** Ayala et al. 2013 (NC)	**Isokinetic:** Aguilar et al. 2012 Manoel et al. 2008 Sekir et al. 2010 Yamaguchi and Ishii 2005 **Power, strength, endurance:** Herman and Smith 2008	
Training					

TABLE 3.1 (cont.)

		Static		No difference between static and dynamic	Dynamic	
		Better than dynamic and no stretching ↑	Worse than no stretching ↓		Better than static and no stretching ↑	Worse than no stretching ↓
Performance	Acute		**Vertical jump:** Behm et al. 2011 Carvalho et al. 2012 Fletcher and Monte-Colombo 2010 Haddad et al. 2014 Holt and Lambourne 2008 Hough et al. 2009 Taylor et al. 2009 **Sprint 10–30m:** Fletcher and Jones 2004 Holt and Lambourne 2008 Haddad et al. 2014 Fletcher and Monte-Colombo 2010 **Agility:** Fletcher and Monte-Colombo 2010 Amiri-Khorasani et al. 2010	**Vertical jump:** Curry et al. 2009 (NC) Dalrymple et al. 2010 (NC) Little and Williams 2006 (NC) **Agility:** McMillian et al. 2006 (NC) **Medicine ball throw:** McMillian et al. 2006 (NC) Torres et al. 2008 (NC) **Reaction time:** Perrier et al. 2011 (NC)	**Vertical jump:** Aguilar et al. 2012 Cè et al. 2008 Haddad et al. 2014 Holt and Lambourne 2008 Hough et al. 2009 McMillian et al. 2006 Morrin and Redding 2013 Needham et al. 2009 Pagaduan et al. 2012 Pearce et al. 2009 Perrier et al. 2011 Kruse et al. 2013 Carvalho et al. 2012 Behm et al. 2011 **Sprint 10–50m:** Fletcher and Jones 2004 Fletcher and Anness 2007 Little and Williams 2006 Haddad et al. 2014 Needham et al. 2009 **Agility:** Little and Williams 2006 Van Gelder and Bartz 2011 Fletcher and Monte-Colombo 2010	

		Static		No difference between static and dynamic	Dynamic	
		↑ Better than dynamic and no stretching	↓ Worse than no stretching		↑ Better than static and no stretching	↓ Worse than no stretching
Performance	Acute				Amiri-Khorasani et al.2010 **Anaerobic power:** Franco et al. 2012 **Soccer kick velocity:** Amiri-Khorasani et al. 2011 **Golf perf. & ball speed:** Moran et al. 2009	
	Training				**Power, strength, muscular endurance, anaerobic capacity, agility:** Herman and Smith 2008 **Soccer kick ROM:** Amiri-Khorasani et al. 2011, 2012	
Sport-specific transfer	Acute					
	Training					
General warm-up – specific stretch – specific warm-up			**Vertical jump:** Pearce et al. 2009 **Repeated-sprint ability:** Taylor et al. 2013	**Vertical jump:** Taylor et al. 2009 **Sprint 20m:** Samson et al. 2012 Taylor et al. 2009	**Vertical jump:** Pearce et al. 2009 **Sprint 50–100m:** Fletcher and Anness 2007 Kistler et al. 2010 **Repeated-sprint ability:** Taylor et al. 2013	

NC: No change, ↑: Enhanced performance, ↓: Impaired performance.

TABLE 3.2 Overview of studies that verify the effect of a combination of static and dynamic stretching on performance

DS > CS > SS	DS = CS > SS	CS > DS
Vertical jump:	**Vertical jump:**	**Balance:**
Amiri-Khorasani and Sotoodeh 2013 (soccer players)	Morrin and Redding 2013 (dancers)	Morrin and Redding 2013 (dancers)
Pagaduan et al. 2012 (college football players)	Wallmann et al. 2008**	**ROM:**
Cè et al. 2008	**Sprint 50m:**	Morrin and Redding 2013 (dancers)
Sprint 10–100m:	Fletcher and Anness 2007 (track and field athletes)	
Amiri-Khorasani and Sotoodeh 2013 (soccer players)		
Kistler et al. 2010 (track and field athletes)*		
Agility:		
Amiri-Khorasani et al. 2010 (professional soccer players)		
Amiri-Khorasani and Sotoodeh 2013 (soccer players)		
Repeated-sprint ability:		
Taylor et al. 2013 (soccer players)		

DS: dynamic stretching – CS: combination of dynamic and static stretching – SS: static stretching.
* DS > CS (SS alone not tested).
** DS = CS (SS alone not tested).

to functional or sport-specific movement (Amiri-Khorasani *et al.* 2011, 2012; Moreside and McGill 2013). Moreside and McGill conclude that improvements in passive range of motion as a result of static stretching do not automatically transfer to functional movement, but require an additional focus on new motor pattern grooving (Moreside and McGill 2013). This is in accordance with Schache *et al.*, who found that static hip extension flexibility is not correlated with hip extension range of motion nor anterior pelvic tilt during running (Schache *et al.* 2000). Static stretching involves a slow, controlled lengthening of the muscle, stimulating the Golgi tendon organ, which results in further relaxation of the muscle being stretched (Miller 1995; Table 3.3). Functional and sport-specific movement in contrast, are ballistic in nature and activate the stretch reflex, which is regulated by the muscle spindles type Ia and II receptors (Guissard *et al.* 1988; Miller 1995; Witvrouw *et al.* 2007). Activation of the stretch reflex will result in contraction of the muscles being stretched and a relaxation of the antagonists (Prochazka 1996). Ballistic sport-specific and functional movements and static stretching stress different stretch receptors (Miller 1995). Facilitation of these different stretch receptors induces an opposite reaction of the muscles and antagonists being stretched (Miller 1995; Prochazka 1996). This explains the compromised transfer from static stretching to functional and sport-specific movement. The SAID principle (specific adaptations to imposed demands) states that to express fluidness of motion and sport-specific flexibility, dynamic stretches and movement that resemble the sports activities, need to form part of the warm-up.

Performance: From the overview of studies that compare static and dynamic stretching we can conclude that a warm-up to minimize impairments and enhance performance should consist of dynamic stretching (Behm and Chaouachi 2011).

TABLE 3.3 The roles of spindles and the Golgi tendon organ

	Muscle spindles	*Golgi tendon organ*
Location	In muscle belly, aligned parallel with muscle fibers	In the muscle tendon, oriented in series with the muscle fibers
Stimulus	Ballistic movement	Static stretching
	Changes in muscle length and velocity	Changes in muscle tension
Reflex	Stretch reflex:	Inverse stretch reflex:
	- Facilitation of contraction of stretched muscle	- Autogenic inhibition: Relaxation of stretched muscle
	- Reciprocal inhibition: Relaxation of antagonists	- Activation of antagonists
Purpose	Protecting the muscle from rapid lengthening	Protecting the muscle from excessive load

Static stretching has a detrimental or no effect on performance. Dynamic stretching has either no effect or improves subsequent vertical jump, sprint, agility, strength, power, and sport-specific performance. Integrating dynamic stretching into the warm-up will also result in superior long-term power, strength, muscular endurance, and agility performance enhancements, compared to a warm-up that consists of static stretching (Herman and Smith 2008).

Explanations for the impaired performance following a bout of static stretching include reduced muscle activation and decreased stiffness of the musculo-tendinous unit (Avela *et al.* 1999; Behm *et al.* 2001; Fowles *et al.* 2000; Guissard *et al.* 1988, 2001; Power *et al.* 2004; Taylor *et al.* 1990). A study by Avela *et al.* showed that the sensitivity of the muscle spindles to stretch is decreased due to the increased muscle compliance following a static stretching routine (Avela *et al.* 1999). The inhibition of the muscle spindles and stretch reflex activity compromises the ability of the muscles to store and release elastic energy (Fletcher and Anness 2007). This is in accordance with several studies that found increased contact times during running or jumping, following static stretching (Behm *et al.* 2006; Di Cagno *et al.* 2010; Lowery *et al.* 2014; Power *et al.* 2004; Young *et al.* 2006).

The performance impairments have been reported to occur as early as one minute after the static stretching routine and may last up to two hours (Behm *et al.* 2004; Power *et al.* 2004). Power *et al.* found the duration in enhanced range of motion following an acute bout of stretching to be parallel in duration with impaired isometric force output (Power *et al.* 2004). There is no relationship between the level of flexibility and the extent of force and power reductions that occur following a static stretching protocol (Behm *et al.* 2006).

It may not be concluded however that static stretching is detrimental to performance. Regular stretching may even benefit long-term strength, jump, and sprint performance (Hunter and Marshall 2002; Rees *et al.* 2007; Rubini *et al.* 2007; Shrier 2004; Wilson *et al.* 1992). Wilson *et al.* found that the increased muscle compliance and storage capacity of elastic energy as a result of flexibility training enhanced the bench press performance of experienced power lifters. Due to the detrimental effect on strength and power output, static stretching drills should not be incorporated into the warm-up of a strength workout however.

Combined stretching/sport-specific warm-up: A specific warm-up or dynamic stretching may attenuate the detrimental effect of static stretching on performance (Fletcher and

Anness 2007; Morrin and Redding 2013; Samson *et al.* 2012; Taylor *et al.* 2009; Wallmann *et al.* 2008). Static stretching of shorter duration and lower intensity performed before the dynamic stretches and specific warm-up minimizes the detrimental effect on performance (Behm *et al.* 2011; Kay and Blazevich 2012). A specific warm-up or dynamic stretching without static stretching however seem to have a more beneficial effect on performance compared to a combination with static stretching (Amiri-Khorasani *et al.* 2010, 2012; Cè *et al.* 2008; Kistler *et al.* 2010; Pagaduan *et al.* 2012; Pearce *et al.* 2009; Taylor *et al.* 2013).

3.3 Specific warm-up

The purpose of the specific warm-up is to enhance athletic performance in the subsequent workout using exercises that replicate sport-specific movement patterns, enhance coordination, and provide stimuli that result in improved force and power output through the post-activation potentiation effect.

Post-activation potentiation is the phenomenon by which the force and power a muscle produces is increased due to its previous contraction (Robbins 2005). High-intensity, low-volume muscle contractions that do not induce fatigue can enhance muscle performance through the stimulation of the central nervous system, which results in enhanced high-threshold motor unit recruitment (Docherty *et al.* 2004; Hilfiker *et al.* 2007; Stone *et al.* 2008). This enables the athlete to exert more force and power and move faster (Sale 2002). On the cellular level, post-activation potentiation enhances the sensitivity and the binding rate of the contractile proteins (actin and myosin), which means faster muscle contractions (increased myosin light-chain phosphorylation) (Hilfiker *et al.* 2007; Sahlin and Ren 1989; Yetter and Moir 2008).

Research demonstrates that incorporating some series of plyometric exercises, low-load exercises targeting the gluteal muscles, and sub-maximal strength exercises improve force and power performance through post-activation potentiation (Brandenburg and Czajka 2010; Crow *et al.* 2012; Gourgoulis *et al.* 2003; Tobin and Delahunt 2014).

The specific warm-up before strength training can benefit from the integration of a few plyometric series (Brandenburg and Czajka 2010). Plyometrics mainly affect the fast-twitch muscle fibers (Macaluso *et al.* 2012; Twist and Eston 2005). Performing some plyometric sets prior to strength training can facilitate the activation of more fast-twitch fibers and enhance force and power output (Brandenburg and Czajka 2010; Macaluso *et al.* 2012; Tobin and Delahunt 2014; Twist and Eston 2005).

The goal of strength training is not only increased force and power output, but also to improve movement pattern efficiency through enhanced coordination, stability, and balance. The effectiveness of unstable surface training to improve sport performance has been questioned. Several studies implementing a higher degree of instability showed decreased muscle activation and force output (Behm *et al.* 2002, 2012). Critics of unstable surface training also state that unstable surface training is not functional because the vast majority of sports are played on a stable surface. Other authors suggest that strength training on unstable surfaces cannot provide the necessary overload trained athletes require to improve strength and performance (Baechle *et al.* 2008; Behm *et al.* 2010; Kraemer *et al.* 2002).

Although sports are played on a stable surface, unstable situations occur. Imagine playing soccer on a wet pitch or sudden perturbations from contact or stepping on an opponent's foot. A distinction also has to be made between highly and mild to moderate unstable surface training. We do not need research to tell us that squatting on a stability ball can only help the circus acrobat and can be dangerous and counterproductive for a soccer player. Strength training on mild to moderate unstable surfaces on the other hand has been shown to enhance the activation of the core muscles, increase co-contraction and stability (Anderson and Behm 2004; Arjmand and Shirazi-Adi 2005; Holtzmann *et al.* 2004; Marshall and Murphy 2006; Vera-Garcia *et al.* 2007). The Canadian Society for Exercise Physiology state in their position stand that free weight ground-based exercises augment core and stabilizer activation while still providing maximal force and power outputs (Behm et al. 2010). The purpose of the warm-up is to gradually increase intensity, preparing the athlete to lift weights of 80 percent or more of their 1RM (repetition maximum). Next to strength and endurance of the core and stabilizer muscles, their anticipatory (feedforward) and reflexive (feedback) response to movement are vital (Akuthota and Nadler 2004; Hodges and Richardson 1996, 1998). Unstable surface training can decrease the latency time between perturbation and contraction of the stabilizing muscles (Kay and Blazevich 2012; Lowery *et al.* 2014; Robbins 2005). Unstable surface training has also been shown to reduce the incidence of ankle, knee, and back injuries (Caraffa *et al.* 1996; Carter *et al.* 2006; Durall *et al.* 2009; Fredericson *et al.* 2000; Leetun *et al.* 2004; Verhagen *et al.* 2005).

Integrating some unstable surface work in the warm-up can help prevent injuries and may positively affect movement quality during the subsequent ground-based strength training through increased activation of the stabilizer muscles (Behm *et al.* 2010; Caraffa *et al.* 1996; Leetun *et al.* 2004; Verhagen *et al.* 2005).

References

Aguilar AJ, DiStefano LJ, Brown CN, Herman DC, Guskiewicz KM, Padua DA. A dynamic warm-up model increases quadriceps strength and hamstring flexibility. *J Strength Cond Res*. 2012 Apr;26(4):1130–41.

Akuthota V, Nadler SF. Core strengthening. *Arch Phys Med Rehabil*. 2004 Mar;85(3 Suppl 1):S86–92.

Amiri-Khorasani M, Sotoodeh V. The acute effects of combined static and dynamic stretch protocols on fitness performances in soccer players. *J Sports Med Phys Fitness*. 2013 Oct;53(5):559–65.

Amiri-Khorasani M, Sahebozamani M, Tabrizi KG, Yusof AB. Acute effect of different stretching methods on Illinois agility test in soccer players. *J Strength Cond Res*. 2010 Oct;24(10):2698–704.

Amiri-Khorasani M, Abu Osman NA, Yusof A. Acute effect of static and dynamic stretching on hip dynamic range of motion during instep kicking in professional soccer players. *J Strength Cond Res*. 2011 Jun;25(6):1647–52.

Amiri-Khorasani M, Mohammadkazemi R, Sarafrazi S, Riyahi-Malayeri S, Sotoodeh V. Kinematics analyses related to stretch-shortening cycle during soccer instep kicking after different acute stretching. *J Strength Cond Res*. 2012 Nov;26(11):3010–17.

Anderson K, Behm DG. Maintenance of EMG activity and loss of force output with instability. *J Strength Cond. Res*. 2004 Aug;18(3):637–40.

Arjmand N, Shirazi-Adl A. Biomechanics of changes in lumbar posture in static lifting. *Spine (Phila Pa 1976)*. 2005 Dec 1;30(23):2637–48.

Avela J, Kyröläinen H, Komi PV. Altered reflex sensitivity after repeated and prolonged passive muscle stretching. *J Appl Physiol (1985)*. 1999 Apr;86(4):1283–91.

Ayala F, De Ste Croix M, Sainz De Baranda P, Santonja F. Acute effects of static and dynamic stretching on hamstring eccentric isokinetic strength and unilateral hamstring to quadriceps strength ratios. *J Sports Sci*. 2013;31(8):831–9.

Baechle TR, Earle RW, Wathen D. Resistance training. In: Baechle TR, Earle RW, editors. *Essentials of strength training and conditioning*. Champaign, IL: Human Kinetics; 2008. pp. 381–411.

Bandy WD, Irion JM, Briggler M. The effect of static stretch and dynamic range of motion training on the flexibility of the hamstring muscles. *J Orthop Sports Phys Ther*. 1998 Apr;27(4):295–300.

Barroso R, Silva-Batista C, Tricoli V, Roschel H, Ugrinowitsch C. The effects of different intensities and durations of the general warm-up on leg press 1RM. *J Strength Cond Res*. 2013 Apr;27(4):1009–13.

Beedle BB, Mann CL. A comparison of two warm-ups on joint range of motion. *J Strength Cond Res*. 2007 Aug;21(3):776–9.

Behm DG, Chaouachi A. A review of the acute effects of static and dynamic stretching on performance. *Eur J Appl Physiol*. 2011 Nov;111(11):2633–51.

Behm D, Colado JC. The effectiveness of resistance training using unstable surfaces and devices for rehabilitation. *Int J Sports Phys Ther*. 2012 Apr;7(2):226–41.

Behm DG, Button DC, Butt JC. Factors affecting force loss with prolonged stretching. *Can J Appl Physiol*. 2001 Jun;26(3):261–72.

Behm DG, Anderson K, Curnew RS. Muscle force and activation under stable and unstable conditions. *J Strength Cond Res*. 2002 Aug;16(3):416–22.

Behm DG, Bambury A, Cahill F, Power K. Effect of acute static stretching on force, balance, reaction time, and movement time. *Med Sci Sports Exerc*. 2004 Aug;36(8):1397–402.

Behm DG, Bradbury EE, Haynes AT, Hodder JN, Leonard AM, Paddock NR. Flexibility is not related to stretch-induced deficits in force or power. *J Sports Sci Med*. 2006 Mar;5(1):33–42.

Behm DG, Drinkwater EJ, Willardson JM, Cowley PM. The use of instability to train the core musculature. *Appl Physiol Nutr Metab*. 2010 Feb;35(1):91–108.

Behm DG, Plewe S, Grage P, Rabbani A, Beigi HT, Byrne JM, Button DC. Relative static stretch-induced impairments and dynamic stretch-induced enhancements are similar in young and middle-aged men. *Appl Physiol Nutr Metab*. 2011 Dec;36(6):790–7.

Brandenburg J, Czajka A. The acute effects of performing drop jumps of different intensities on concentric squat strength. *J Sports Med Phys Fitness*. 2010 Sep;50(3):254–61.

Caraffa A, Cerulli G, Projetti M, Aisa G, Rizzo A. Prevention of anterior cruciate ligament injuries in soccer. A prospective controlled study of proprioceptive training. *Knee Surg Sports Traumatol Arthrosc*. 1996;4(1):19–21.

Carter JM, Beam WC, McMahan SG, Barr ML, Brown LE. The effects of stability ball training on spinal stability in sedentary individuals. *J Strength Cond Res*. 2006 May;20(2):429–35.

Carvalho FL, Carvalho MC, Simão R, Gomes TM, Costa PB, Neto LB, Carvalho RL, Dantas EH. Acute effects of a warm-up including active, passive, and dynamic stretching on vertical jump performance. *J Strength Cond Res*. 2012 Sep;26(9):2447–52.

Cè E, Margonato V, Casasco M, Veicsteinas A. Effects of stretching on maximal anaerobic power: the roles of active and passive warm-ups. *J Strength Cond Res*. May 2008;22(3):794–800.

Chow TP, Ng GY. Active, passive and proprioceptive neuromuscular facilitation stretching are comparable in improving the knee flexion range in people with total knee replacement: a randomized controlled trial. *Clin Rehabil*. 2010 Oct;24(10):911–18.

Covert CA, Alexander MP, Petronis JJ, Davis DS. Comparison of ballistic and static stretching on hamstring muscle length using an equal stretching dose. *J Strength Cond Res*. 2010 Nov;24(11):3008–14.

Crow JF, Buttifant D, Kearny SG, Hrysomallis C. Low load exercises targeting the gluteal muscle group acutely enhance explosive power output in elite athletes. *J Strength Cond Res*. 2012 Feb;26(2):438–42.

Curry BS, Chengkalath D, Crouch GJ, Romance M, Manns PJ. Acute effects of dynamic stretching, static stretching, and light aerobic activity on muscular performance in women. *J Strength Cond Res*. 2009 Sep;23(6):1811–19.

Dalrymple KJ, Davis SE, Dwyer GB, Moir GL. Effect of static and dynamic stretching on vertical jump performance in collegiate women volleyball players. *J Strength Cond Res*. 2010 Jan;24(1):149–55.

Di Cagno A, Baldari C, Battaglia C, Gallotta MC, Videira M, Piazza M, Guidetti L. Preexercise static stretching effect on leaping performance in elite rhythmic gymnasts. *J Strength Cond Res*. 2010 Aug;24(8):1995–2000.

Docherty D, Robbins D, Hodgson M. Complex training revisited: A review of its current status as a viable training approach. *Strength Cond J*. 2004 Dec;26(6):52–7.

Durall CJ, Udermann BE, Johansen DR, Gibson B, Reineke DM, Reuteman P. The effects of preseason trunk muscle training on low-back pain occurrence in women collegiate gymnasts. *J Strength Cond Res.* 2009 Jan;23(1):86–92.

Fletcher IM, Anness R. The acute effects of combined static and dynamic stretch protocols on fifty-meter sprint performance in track-and-field athletes. *J Strength Cond Res.* 2007 Aug;21(3):784–7.

Fletcher IM, Jones B. The effect of different warm-up stretch protocols on 20 meter sprint performance in trained rugby union players. *J Strength Cond Res.* 2004 Nov;18(4):885–8.

Fletcher IM, Monte-Colombo MM. An investigation into the effects of different warm-up modalities on specific motor skills related to soccer performance. *J Strength Cond Res.* 2010 Aug;24(8):2096–101.

Fowles JR, Sale DG, MacDougall JD. Reduced strength after passive stretch of the human plantarflexors. *J Appl Physiol (1985).* 2000 Sep;89(3):1179–88.

Franco BL, Signorelli GR, Trajano GS, Costa PB, de Oliveira CG. Acute effects of three different stretching protocols on the Wingate test performance. *J Sports Sci Med.* 2012 Mar 1;11(1):1–7.

Fredericson M, Cookingham CL, Chaudhari AM, Dowdell BC, Oestreicher N, Sahrmann SA. Hip abductor weakness in distance runners with iliotibial band syndrome. *Clin J Sport Med.* 2000 Jul;10(3):169–75.

Gourgoulis V, Aggeloussis N, Kasimatis P, Mavromatis G, Garas A. Effect of a submaximal half-squats warm-up program on vertical jumping ability. *J Strength Cond Res.* 2003 May;17(2):342–4.

Guissard N, Duchateau J, Hainaut K. Muscle stretching and motoneuron excitability. *Eur J Appl Physiol Occup Physiol.* 1988;58(1–2):47–52.

Guissard N, Duchateau J, Hainaut K. Mechanisms of decreased motoneurone excitation during passive muscle stretching. *Exp Brain Res.* 2001 Mar;137(2):163–9.

Haddad M, Dridi A, Chtara M, Chaouachi A, Wong del P, Behm D, Chamari K. Static stretching can impair explosive performance for at least 24 hours. *J Strength Cond Res.* 2014 Jan;28(1):140–6.

Herda TJ, Cramer JT, Ryan ED, McHugh MP, Stout JR. Acute effects of static versus dynamic stretching on isometric peak torque, electromyography, and mechanomyography of the biceps femoris muscle. *J Strength Cond Res.* 2008 May;22(3):809–17.

Herman SL, Smith DT. Four-week dynamic stretching warm-up intervention elicits longer-term performance benefits. *J Strength Cond Res.* 2008 Jul;22(4):1286–97.

Hilfiker R, Hübner K, Lorenz T, Marti B. Effects of drop jumps added to the warm-up of elite sport athletes with a high capacity for explosive force development. *J Strength Cond Res.* 2007 May;21(2):550–5.

Hodges PW, Richardson CA. Inefficient muscular stabilization of the lumbar spine associated with low back pain. A motor control evaluation of transversus abdominis. *Spine (Phila Pa 1976).* 1996 Nov 15;21(22):2640–50.

Hodges PW, Richardson CA. Delayed postural contraction of transversus abdominis in low back pain associated with movement of the lower limb. *J Spinal Disord.* 1998 Feb;11(1):46–56.

Holt BW, Lambourne K. The impact of different warm-up protocols on vertical jump performance in male collegiate athletes. *J Strength Cond Res.* 2008 Jan;22(1):226–9.

Holtzmann M, Gaetz M, Anderson G. EMG activity of trunk stabilizers during stable and unstable push-ups. *Can J Appl Physiol.* 2004 Oct;29(S1):S55.

Hough PA, Ross EZ, Howatson G. Effects of dynamic and static stretching on vertical jump performance and electromyographic activity. *J Strength Cond Res.* 2009 Mar;23(2):507–12.

Hunter JP, Marshall RN. Effects of power and flexibility training on vertical jump technique. *Med Sci Sports Exerc.* 2002 Mar;34(3):478–86.

Kay AD, Blazevich AJ. Effect of acute static stretch on maximal muscle performance: a systematic review. *Med Sci Sports Exerc.* 2012 Jan;44(1):154–64.

Kistler BM, Walsh MS, Horn TS, Cox RH. The acute effects of static stretching on the sprint performance of collegiate men in the 60- and 100-m dash after a dynamic warm-up. *J Strength Cond Res.* 2010 Sep;24(9):2280–4.

Kraemer WJ, Adams K, Cafarelli E, Dudley GA, Dooly C, Feigenbaum MS, Fleck SJ, Franklin B, Fry AC, Hoffman JR, Newton RU, Potteiger J, Stone MH, Ratamess NA, Triplett-McBride T, American

College of Sports Medicine. American College of Sports Medicine position stand. Progression models in resistance training for healthy adults. *Med Sci Sports Exerc.* 2002 Feb;34(2):364–80.

Kruse NT, Barr MW, Gilders RM, Kushnick MR, Rana SR. Using a practical approach for determining the most effective stretching strategy in female college division I volleyball players. *J Strength Cond Res.* 2013 Nov;27(11):3060–7.

Leetun DT, Ireland ML, Willson JD, Ballantyne BT, Davis IM. Core stability measures as risk factors for lower extremity injury in athletes. *Med Sci Sports Exerc.* 2004 Jun;36(6):926–34.

Little T, Williams AG. Effects of differential stretching protocols during warm-ups on high-speed motor capacities in professional soccer players. *J Strength Cond Res.* 2006 Feb;20(1):203–7.

Lowery RP, Joy JM, Brown LE, Oliveira de Souza E, Wistocki DR, Davis GS, Naimo MA, Zito GA, Wilson JM. Effects of static stretching on 1-mile uphill run performance. *J Strength Cond Res.* 2014 Jan;28(1):161–7.

McMillian DJ, Moore JH, Hatler BS, Taylor DC. Dynamic vs. static-stretching warm up: the effect on power and agility performance. *J Strength Cond Res.* 2006 Aug;20(3):492–9.

Macaluso F, Isaacs AW, Myburgh KH. Preferential type II muscle fiber damage from plyometric exercise. *J Athl Train.* 2012 Jul–Aug;47(4):414–20.

Mahieu NN, McNair P, De Muynck M, Stevens V, Blanckaert I, Smits N, Witvrouw E. Effect of static and ballistic stretching on the muscle-tendon tissue properties. *Med Sci Sports Exerc.* 2007 Mar;39(3):494–501.

Manoel ME, Harris-Love MO, Danoff JV, Miller TA. Acute effects of static, dynamic, and proprioceptive neuromuscular facilitation stretching on muscle power in women. *J Strength Cond Res.* 2008 Sep;22(5):1528–34.

Marshall P, Murphy B. Changes in muscle activity and perceived exertion during exercises performed on a Swiss ball. *Appl Physiol Nutr Metab.* 2006 Aug;31(4):376–83.

Meroni R, Cerri CG, Lanzarini C, Barindelli G, Morte GD, Gessaga V, Cesana GC, De Vito G. Comparison of active stretching technique and static stretching technique on hamstring flexibility. *Clin J Sport Med.* 2010 Jan;20(1):8–14.

Miller PD. *Fitness programming and physical disability.* Champaign, IL: Human Kinetics; 1995. Chapter 3, Skeletal muscle physiology and anaerobic exercise; 232 pp.

Moran KA, McGrath T, Marshall BM, Wallace ES. Dynamic stretching and golf swing performance. *Int J Sports Med.* 2009 Feb;30(2):113–18.

Moreside JM, McGill SM. Improvements in hip flexibility do not transfer to mobility in functional movement patterns. *J Strength Cond Res.* 2013 Oct;27(10):2635–43.

Morrin N, Redding E. Acute effects of warm-up stretch protocols on balance, vertical jump height, and range of motion in dancers. *J Dance Med Sci.* 2013;17(1):34–40.

Needham RA, Morse CI, Degens H. The acute effect of different warm-up protocols on anaerobic performance in elite youth soccer players. *J Strength Cond Res.* 2009 Dec;23(9):2614–20.

Nelson RT, Bandy WD. Eccentric training and static stretching improve hamstring flexibility of high school males. *J Athl Train.* 2004 Sep;39(3):254–8.

O'Sullivan K, Murray E, Sainsbury D. The effect of warm-up, static stretching and dynamic stretching on hamstring flexibility in previously injured subjects. *BMC Musculoskelet Disord.* 2009 Apr;10:37.

Pagaduan JC, Pojskić H, Užičanin E, Babajić F. Effect of various warm-up protocols on jump performance in college football players. *J Hum Kinet.* 2012 Dec;35:127–32.

Pearce AJ, Kidgell DJ, Zois J, Carlson JS. Effects of secondary warm up following stretching. *Eur J Appl Physiol.* 2009 Jan;105(2):175–83.

Perrier ET, Pavol MJ, Hoffman MA. The acute effects of a warm-up including static or dynamic stretching on countermovement jump height, reaction time, and flexibility. *J Strength Cond Res.* 2011 Jul;25(7):1925–31.

Power K, Behm D, Cahill F, Carroll M, Young W. An acute bout of static stretching: effects on force and jumping performance. *Med Sci Sports Exerc.* 2004 Aug;36(8):1389–96.

Prochazka A. Proprioceptive feedback and movement regulation. In: Rowell L, Sheperd JT, editors. *Handbook of physiology: section 12: exercise: regulation and integration of multiple systems.* New York: American Physiological Society; 1996. pp. 89–127.

Rees SS, Murphy AJ, Watsford ML, McLachlan KA, Coutts AJ. Effects of proprioceptive neuromuscular facilitation stretching on stiffness and force-producing characteristics of the ankle in active women. *J Strength Cond Res.* 2007 May;21(2):572–7.

Robbins DW. Postactivation potentiation and its practical applicability: a brief review. *J Strength Cond Res.* 2005 May;19(2):453–8.

Rubini EC, Costa AL, Gomes PS. The effects of stretching on strength performance. *Sports Med.* 2007;37(3):213–24.

Sahlin K, Ren JM. Relationship of contraction capacity to metabolic changes during recovery from a fatiguing contraction. *J Appl Physiol* (1985). 1989 Aug;67(2):648–54.

Sale DG. Postactivation potentiation: role in human performance. *Exerc Sport Sci Rev.* 2002 Jul;30(3):138–43.

Samson M, Button DC, Chaouachi A, Behm DG. Effects of dynamic and static stretching within general and activity specific warm-up protocols. *J Sports Sci Med.* 2012 Jun;11(2):279–85.

Schache AG, Blanch PD, Murphy AT. Relation of anterior pelvic tilt during running to clinical and kinematic measures of hip extension. *Br J Sports Med.* 2000 Aug;34(4):279–83.

Sekir U, Arabaci R, Akova B, Kadagan SM. Acute effects of static and dynamic stretching on leg flexor and extensor isokinetic strength in elite women athletes. *Scand J Med Sci Sports.* 2010 Apr;20(2):268–81.

Shrier I. Does stretching improve performance? A systematic and critical review of the literature. *Clin J Sport Med.* 2004 Sep;14(5):267–73.

Sports Medicine Australia (SMA). Recommendations for Warm-Up – Stretching. 2005.

Stone MH, Sands WA, Pierce KC, Ramsey MW, Haff GG. Power and power potentiation among strength-power athletes: preliminary study. *Int J Sports Physiol Perform.* 2008 Mar;3(1):55–67.

Taylor DC, Dalton JD Jr, Seaber AV, Garrett WE Jr. Viscoelastic properties of muscle-tendon units. The biomechanical effects of stretching. *Am J Sports Med.* 1990 May–Jun;18(3):300–9.

Taylor JM, Weston M, Portas MD. The effect of a short practical warm-up protocol on repeated sprint performance. *J Strength Cond Res.* 2013 Jul;27(7):2034–8.

Taylor KL, Sheppard JM, Lee H, Plummer N. Negative effect of static stretching restored when combined with a sport specific warm-up component. *J Sci Med Sport.* 2009 Nov;12(6):657–61.

Tobin DP, Delahunt E. The acute effect of a plyometric stimulus on jump performance in professional rugby players. *J Strength Cond Res.* 2014 Feb;28(2):367–72.

Torres EM, Kraemer WJ, Vingren JL, Volek JS, Hatfield DL, Spiering BA, Ho JY, Fragala MS, Thomas GA, Anderson JM, Häkkinen K, Maresh CM. Effects of stretching on upper-body muscular performance. *J Strength Cond Res.* 2008 Jul;22(4):1279–85.

Twist C, Eston R. The effects of exercise-induced muscle damage on maximal intensity intermittent exercise performance. *Eur J Appl Physiol.* 2005 Aug;94(5–6):652–8.

Van Gelder LH, Bartz SD. The effect of acute stretching on agility performance. *J Strength Cond Res.* 2011 Nov;25(11):3014–21.

Vera-Garcia FJ, Elvira JL, Brown SH, McGill SM. Effects of abdominal stabilization maneuvers on the control of spine motion and stability against sudden trunk perturbations. *J Electromyogr Kinesiol.* 2007 Oct;17(5):556–67.

Verhagen EA, van Tulder M, van der Beek AJ, Bouter LM, van Mechelen W. An economic evaluation of a proprioceptive balance board training programme for the prevention of ankle sprains in volleyball. *Br J Sports Med.* 2005 Feb;39(2):111–15.

Wallmann HW, Mercer JA, Landers MR. Surface electromyographic assessment of the effect of dynamic activity and dynamic activity with static stretching of the gastrocnemius on vertical jump performance. *J Strength Cond Res.* 2008 May;22(3):787–93.

Webright WG, Randolph BJ, Perrin DH. Comparison of nonballistic active knee extension in neural slump position and static stretch techniques on hamstring flexibility. *J Orthop Sports Phys Ther.* 1997 Jul;26(1):7–13.

Wilson GJ, Elliott BC, Wood GA. Stretch shorten cycle performance enhancement through flexibility training. *Med Sci Sports Exerc.* 1992 Jan;24(1):116–23.

Winters MV, Blake CG, Trost JS, Marcello-Brinker TB, Lowe LM, Garber MB, Wainner RS. Passive versus active stretching of hip flexor muscles in subjects with limited hip extension: a randomized clinical trial. *Phys Ther.* 2004 Sep;84(9):800–7.

Witvrouw E, Mahieu N, Roosen P, McNair P. The role of stretching in tendon injuries. *Br J Sports Med.* 2007 Apr;41(4):224–6.

Yamaguchi T, Ishii K. Effects of static stretching for 30 seconds and dynamic stretching on leg extension power. *J Strength Cond Res.* 2005 Aug;19(3):677–83.

Yetter M, Moir GL. The acute effects of heavy back and front squats on speed during forty-meter sprint trials. *J Strength Cond Res.* 2008 Jan;22(1):159–65.

Young W, Elias G, Power J. Effects of static stretching volume and intensity on plantar flexor explosive force production and range of motion. *J Sports Med Phys Fitness.* 2006 Sep;46(3):403–11.

4

STRENGTH TRAINING CONSIDERED AS SKILL TRAINING WITH RESISTANCE

There is a fundamental difference between sports in which the athlete has to quickly react to the actions of the opponent and changes in the environment and sports in which the movement outcome is predetermined. The game of soccer is fundamentally different from sprinting in athletics or swimming. Sprinting and swimming are cyclic sports. This means the same movement is constantly repeated. Soccer and team sports are acyclic sports, in which many different motor patterns are executed over the course of the game. Split-second decisions and reactions determine success in soccer. The higher the level of competition the quicker the game and the more time pressure there is on the player to make an adequate action. The best players make quicker and better tactical decisions, remain technically sound under pressure, and are more agile and move better. Just like the aspects of soccer technique, fluid and explosive movement is also a matter of coordination. It is considered that an athlete needs 10000 hours of practice to excel in a skill (Coyle 2009). Coaches are creative in providing different progressions and practice conditions and players invest hours practicing various technical skills in different situations. Coaches also try to improve a player's movement through various open and closed agility and quickness drills. It is clear that only straight sprinting drills can make a player faster in a straight line, but will result in limited improvements in agility and quick reaction to the opponent's action. All coaches understand that speed and quickness training for soccer is fundamentally different from sprinting in track and field. The same training principles may apply, but motor control is totally different.

Strength training of most soccer players and teams however is still not really different from that of cyclic sports. The same principles apply to elicit neural and peripheral changes to enhance strength and power. In cyclic sports however, the strength and power enhancements only have to be transferred to a limited amount of motor patterns, while a soccer player has to be powerful in a variety of motor patterns. Principles of motor learning also need to be considered in strength training for soccer. Joint angles are different between acceleration and deceleration and kinematics vary between a change of direction with or without the ball.

4.1 Movement variability, movement mechanics, and body control

Strength training forms the foundation of correct, fluid movement. Improving and establishing correct movement quality starts from the weight room. Similar to technical soccer skills, the ability to generate force in a sporting activity is a skill (Jensen *et al.* 2005). On the pitch forces need to be generated with precision and strict timing (Jensen *et al.* 2005). How do we expect athletes to be able to quickly decelerate in the frontal plane (lateral) preparing them with a strength training that mainly focuses on the sagittal plane (flexion–extension)? How are players able to stabilize the tremendous rotational forces during high-speed changes of direction when their lower body strengthening does not sufficiently stress the transverse plane? Research showed that the majority of injuries occur during the deceleration phase of movement (Alentorn-Geli *et al.* 2009). Decelerating and concurrently controlling the ball will influence the knee position of the stance leg and deceleration mechanics. Adhering to monotonous strength training in which the movement of the knee is restricted will not prepare the knee for the angles and forces that have to be generated in soccer situations and puts the player at risk for injury. Good body control and deceleration mechanics start with correct motor pattern grooving during strength training. Due to the great movement variability in soccer, strength training variability is paramount. Strength training monotony will result in poor movement mechanics and body control. The principles of motor learning also apply when designing a strength training or rehabilitation program for the soccer player.

4.2 Generalized motor pattern

A soccer player executes many different movements and skills over the course of the game. These movements and skills are complex, with many degrees of freedom (force, speed, multiple joints and muscles) that need to be controlled (Turvey 1990). If the brain had a saved motor pattern for every separate movement, the catalogue of motor patterns would be so big it would be impossible to process, especially under the time pressure in sports.

Schmidt states in the generalized motor pattern theory that various similar movements are grouped together (Schmidt 1988). Some movement components are similar for the various related movements while other components are variable. During different step-up variations – step-up high bench, step-up low bench, lateral step-up, crossover step-up, step-off, step-up on unstable surface – some components remain the same regardless of the step-up variant (sagittal plane), while other components adapt to the demands of the environment (frontal, transverse plane). The body does not need a separate motor pattern for each variant. Related movements are grouped together by means of a generalized movement pattern. Evidence for the generalized motor patterns can be found in gait analysis. The relative timing of the four step cycles remains constant between different speeds of running or walking (Shapiro *et al.* 1981). Also during different breaststroke frequencies in swimming the relative timing of the different phases remains the same. Without the existence of generalized motor patterns any new movement would require extensive practice or could even be impossible because no motor pattern exists.

4.3 Repetition without repetition

These generalized movement patterns achieve increasing stability when more variations of a similar movement are trained. Through training variation a better differentiation between the invariable and variable movement components of a generalized motor pattern will transpire (Meijer and Roth 1988; Schmidt 1985). With the concept 'repetition without repetition' Bernstein described the importance of introducing variation in the training process to improve movement (Bernstein 1996). The goal of repetition is not to enable the player to perform nearly identical movements, but to consistently realize the goal of movement in changing environmental conditions (Bernstein 1996). A player with good body control does not only fluently execute movements that often occur in soccer (deceleration, change of direction, turn), but can also better handle perturbations of the optimal movement pattern as a consequence of an abrupt game situation or opponent's pressure.

Coordination training increases the corticospinal excitability to enable motor pattern formation (Jensen *et al.* 2005; Perez *et al.* 2004). An increase of the corticospinal excitability facilitates synaptogenesis (Weier and Kidgell 2012). Synaptogenesis is the process of formation of connections (synapses) between different neurons in the nervous system. The improved connective strength between neurons enables skill acquisition and refinement (Rosenkranz *et al.* 2007). Similar to skill training, single-leg squat and back squat training also result in significant increases of corticospinal excitability (Goodwill *et al.* 2012; Weier and Kidgell 2012; Weier *et al.* 2012). In contrast to these findings, no increase of corticospinal excitability was observed following four and eight weeks of strength training using the leg press (Latella *et al.* 2012). Monotonous strength training has even shown to decrease this excitability, which compromises the coordinative transfer of strength training (Carroll *et al.* 2002; Jensen *et al.* 2005). Stronger muscles will not expand their representation in the motor cortex, but stronger movement will (Jensen *et al.* 2005). A strength training routine that solely focuses on flexion–extension will not improve three-dimensional body control and coordination. For optimal performance enhancement and injury prevention, strength training for soccer has to be considered as skill training with increased resistance (Bosch 2012). A good balance between specificity, variation, and overload is paramount.

4.4 Importance of training organization for movement retention

Next to variation, also the organization of the training plays a role in increasing generalized motor pattern stability. Research shows that performing various movements in a random fashion results in better long-term retention of the motor pattern compared to blocked practice (Bortoli *et al.* 1992; Goode and Magill 1986; Hall *et al.* 1994; Smith and Davies 1995; Stevans and Hall 1998; Winstein 1991). The difference between both methods in number of times a motor pattern has to be recalled can explain the long-term superiority of random training (Lee and Magill 1983, 1985; Lee and Simon 2004). In random training the motor pattern has to be dumped from the working memory after each set in order to recall the motor pattern of the next movement (Lee and Magill 1983, 1985; Lee and Simon 2004). In blocked practice, the motor pattern only has to be recalled once. Although training volume is identical between both methods, the random training organization increases the number of times a motor pattern has to be recalled from the long-term memory, planned and executed (Lee and Magill 1983, 1985; Lee and Simon 2004). A circuit strength training, in which one set of each exercise is performed in an alternating fashion, is superior for motor pattern grooving. The strength training session performed in circuit will therefore contain a big variety of movements that comprise the three planes of motion.

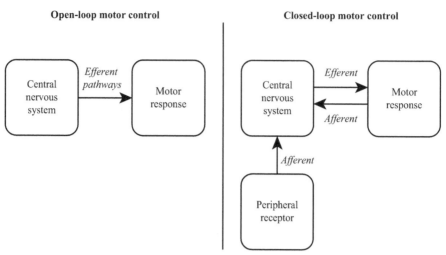

Open-loop motor control   **Closed-loop motor control**

FIGURE 4.1   Open–loop and closed–loop motor control

4.5 Open-loop and closed-loop motor control

When performing and controlling movement, both open–loop and closed–loop control systems are involved. An open–loop system is feedforward control of the movement. A feedback loop will take 50 ms or 100 ms, depending whether it is a spinal or longer loop reflex (Magill 2010). Quick ballistic movements, in which the movement ends before any feedback coupling is possible, depend on open–loop control. The motor pattern contains all the necessary information for the movement system. A closed–loop system involves feedback to accurately continue the movement. The feedback information can come from the proprioceptors (muscle spindle, Golgi-tendon organ, ligament and joint capsular receptors) as well as from the tactile, visual, and auditory receptors.

Most movements consist of both open- and closed-loop motor control (Adams 1976). Open-loop control is involved when the movement is initiated and closed-loop control will allow accurate termination of the movement (Adams 1976; Magill 2010; Figure 4.1).

4.6 Dynamic systems theory

An alternate approach to motor control is the dynamic systems theory (Turvey 1990). The dynamic systems theory de-emphasizes the role of the central command center and accentuates the role of the environment and the dynamic properties of the body and limbs. The dynamic systems theory emphasizes the flexible connection between the impulse of the central command center and the motor action. Motor impulse X will not always lead to movement X. The initial position of the body and the environmental constraints also influence the movement. Imagine a simple task like grasping a cup. In different starting positions of the arm and hand, identical nervous impulses will not result in the same end position. The same amount of neural stimulation will not always result in the same amount of force output, but depends also on the length of the muscle, etc. Rather than solely depending on a central command system, the nervous system can self-organize the motor pattern as a result of the interaction with the environment in which the movement is performed.

4.7 Perception–action coupling

The dynamic systems theory shows that afferent sensory information is not only used in a closed-loop situation, but also by the central nervous system in the open-loop system to prepare for the upcoming action (Ghez and Sainburg 1995; Magill 2010; Sjölander and Johansson 1997). This is called the perception–action coupling (Magill 2010). The central nervous system can use afferent information from previous experiences to preset joint stiffness and update motor patterns of feedforward muscle co-contraction (Johansson 1993). This will help improve joint stability in time-critical movements and increase the dynamic restraint to perturbations as a result of the opponent's pressure or unforeseen game situation. Plyometric training has been shown to alter feedforward motor strategies (Chimera *et al.* 2004). The increased preparatory adductor–abductor co-activation of the hip muscles results in a better lower body alignment at ground contact (Chimera *et al.* 2004).

4.8 Self-stabilization

Movement has a self-organizing aspect. The nervous system will self-organize the movement through the interaction with the environment. In running on an uneven surface the musculoskeletal system behaves like a spring. The leg stiffness will adjust to the stiffness of the underground, which will allow similar locomotion mechanics on a variety of terrains (Ferris and Farley 1997; Ferris *et al.* 1998). This is attributed to self-stabilization and does not require feedback control (Blickhan *et al.* 2007; Wagner and Blickhan 2003). Self-stability processes depend on the visco-elastic properties of the musculo-tendon unit, the force-velocity and force-length curve of the muscle (Blickhan *et al.* 2007; Wagner and Blickhan 2003; Figure 4.2). A muscle can produce more force when it contracts eccentrically. Lengthening of the muscle can also alter the working range and bring it closer to its optimal length. So when a muscle yields, the force output is automatically enhanced to compensate the sudden disturbance, which is crucial for the stabilizing effect of the muscle (Blickhan *et al.* 2007; Brown *et al.* 1996). These self-stabilization processes during agonist–antagonist co-contraction allow the individual to react immediately to movement perturbations without sensory feedback coupling. Feedforward control (co-contraction) in combination with self-stabilization does not require reaction time (0 ms) and increases the robustness of movement against perturbations from the environment

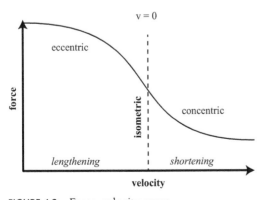

FIGURE 4.2 Force–velocity curve

(Bosch 2012). These self-stabilizing processes become more efficient with an increasing speed of movement (Blickhan *et al.* 2007). A well-designed strength training will also improve the self-stabilizing ability through a shift of the force–velocity and force–length curve and increased stiffness of the musculo-tendon unit (Blazevich *et al.* 2007; Jones *et al.* 2001; Kaneko *et al.* 1983; Kubo *et al.* 2010; McBride *et al.* 2002; Mahieu *et al.* 2008; Moss *et al.* 1997; O'Sullivan *et al.* 2012; Seynnes *et al.* 2007, 2009; Tillin *et al.* 2012; Wyon *et al.* 2013).

4.9 Motor control training and injury prevention

A feedback correction in response to an external postural perturbation takes 100 ms to occur (Magill 2010). Within this time the external force will have caused an injury (Milia *et al.* 1998). Anterior cruciate ligament (ACL) injuries for example have been estimated to occur between 17 and 50 ms after initial ground contact (Krosshaug *et al.* 2007). Closed-loop feedback control is not effective enough to prevent an injury in soccer. The aftermath feedback reaction will come too late in time-critical tasks. To effectively enhance joint stability and prevent injury in soccer, the task-dependent anticipatory feedforward control has to be trained (Ashton-Miller *et al.* 2001).

There is no research support to state that training can enhance the sensitivity of the proprioceptors (Ashton-Miller *et al.* 2001; Hughes and Rochester 2008; Kim *et al.* 2011; McKeon and Hertel 2008). The two classic modalities – joint position sense accuracy and the threshold for joint movement – seem not to be impaired following injury (Refshauge *et al.* 2000). Studies that reported proprioception was impaired following injury did measure the skill level of a motor task, such as balancing, which is not a true proprioception test (Ashton-Miller *et al.* 2001). Central nervous system adaptation through motor learning is the key factor to improve balance and reduce the risk of injuries (Kim *et al.* 2011).

4.10 Practical application

Research evidence supports both the generalized motor pattern theory and the dynamic systems theory (Kim *et al.* 2011). Where the generalized motor pattern theory emphasizes the role of motor pattern variability, the dynamic systems theory emphasizes the interaction with the environment. Ideal training should therefore train the variable and invariable components of a movement class and alter the environment to stimulate a dynamic pattern of movement.

Frans Bosch states that strength training is really suited to train and facilitate the motor learning of the attractors of movement (invariable movement component in generalized motor pattern theory). A well-designed strength training program will improve movement coordination, but the wrong training stimulus can also negatively affect movement coordination and performance (Bosch 2012).

From the theory of motor learning several practical applications can be derived for strength training:

1. Soccer is an acyclical, open sport in which various movements in all three planes of motion occur. Training variability consolidates the distinction between the variable and invariable components of movement and enhances movement efficiency and adaptability.
2. Integrating some circuit training sessions in which sets of different exercises and movements are alternated can facilitate motor pattern grooving. Integrating exercises that stress multiple planes of motion into the circuit training will further increase movement robustness.

3. During strength training with free weights the self-stabilizing processes correct small perturbations, facilitating proper balance and trajectory. In strength training with machines the trajectory of movement is predetermined and does not require balance. The movement is performed without interaction with the environment and hence transfer to athletic performance is limited.

4. In strength training with machines the movement is limited to one plane of motion and stability is provided by the machine. Only the prime movers are activated without proper firing of the stabilizers.

5. Limiting strength training particularly to flexion–extension training like in powerlifting will not enable a better differentiation between the variable and invariable components of movement to transpire. This compromises the adaptability and the application of force in soccer.

6. Machine strength training also limits the degrees of freedom. Strength training with free weights, pulley machines, and medicine balls is ground-based, is performed in multiple planes of motion, and uses multiple-joint movements.

7. Functional strength training and skill training elicit similar changes in cortical plasticity. In professional basketball teams, strength and skill training are often combined. Next to organizational advantages of concurrent strength and skill training, there is also a strong belief that shot accuracy is enhanced more when the shooting practice is preceded by a strength workout. The enhanced corticospinal excitability, intracortical facilitation, and decreased intracortical inhibition as a result of functional strength and skill training can explain this belief (Perez *et al.* 2004; Weier and Kidgell 2012). Functional strength and skill training both strengthen neural connections and may therefore positively interact.

8. Soccer players can start with strength training at a relatively young age. This does not mean high weights need to be lifted. The early stages of strength training can be performed using primarily body weight exercises. Incorporating exercises that comprise multiple joints and planes of motion and sufficient training variation will facilitate the strengthening of neural connections and differentiation between the variable and invariable movement components.

9. A well-designed strength and conditioning program will improve the dynamic restraint to perturbations from the environment through enhanced movement self-organization, perception–action coupling, and distinction of invariable and variable components of movement. Strength training is paramount to improve body control and athletic performance and reduce the risk of injury (Lauersen *et al.* 2014; McGeehan *et al.* 2012).

References

Adams JA. Issues for a closed-loop theory of motor learning. In: Stelmach GE, editor. *Motor control: issues and trends.* New York: Academic Press; 1976. pp. 87–101.

Alentorn-Geli E, Myer GD, Silvers HJ, Samitier G, Romero D, Lázaro-Haro C, Cugat R. Prevention of non-contact anterior cruciate ligament injuries in soccer players. Part 1: mechanisms of injury and underlying risk factors. *Knee Surg Sports Traumatol Arthrosc.* 2009 Jul;17(7):705–29.

Ashton-Miller JA, Wojtys EM, Huston LJ, Fry-Welch D. Can proprioception really be improved by exercises? *Knee Surg Sports Traumatol Arthrosc.* 2001 May;9(3):128–36.

Bernstein NA. On dexterity and its development. In: Latash ML, Turvey MT, editors. *Dexterity and its development (resources for ecological psychology).* New Jersey: Lawrence Erlbaum Associates; 1996. pp. 3–246.

Blazevich AJ, Cannavan D, Coleman DR, Horne S. Influence of concentric and eccentric resistance training on architectural adaptation in human quadriceps muscles. *J Appl Physiol (1985).* 2007 Nov;103(5):1565–75.

Blickhan R, Seyfarth A, Geyer H, Grimmer S, Wagner H, Günther M. Intelligence by mechanics. *Philos Trans A Math Phys Eng Sci.* 2007 Jan;365(1850):199–220.

Bortoli L, Robazza C, Durigon V, Carra C. Effects on contextual interference on learning technical sports skills. *Percept Mot Skills.* 1992 Oct;75:555–62.

Bosch F. *Krachttraining en coördinatie, een integratieve benadering.* Rotterdam: 2010 Uitgevers; 2012. 352 pp.

Brown IE, Scott SH, Loeb GE. Mechanics of feline soleus: II. Design and validation of a mathematical model. *J Muscle Res Cell Motil.* 1996 Apr;17(2):221–33.

Carroll TJ, Riek S, Carson RG. The sites of neural adaptation induced by resistance training in humans. *J Physiol.* 2002 Oct;544(Pt 2):641–52.

Chimera NJ, Swanik KA, Swanik CB, Straub SJ. Effects of plyometric training on muscle-activation strategies and performance in female athletes. *J Athl Train.* 2004 Mar;39(1):24–31.

Coyle D. *The talent code: Greatness isn't born. It's grown. Here's how.* New York: Bantam Dell; 2009. 256 pp.

Ferris DP, Farley CT. Interaction of leg stiffness and surfaces stiffness during human hopping. *J Appl Physiol (1985).* 1997 Jan;82(1):15–22; discussion 13–14.

Ferris DP, Louie M, Farley CT. Running in the real world: adjusting leg stiffness for different surfaces. *Proc Biol Sci.* 1998 Jun;265(1400):989–94.

Ghez C, Sainburg R. Proprioceptive control of interjoint coordination. *Can J Physiol Pharmacol.* 1995 Feb;73(2):273–84.

Goode S, Magill RA. Contextual interference effects in learning three badminton serves. *Res Q Exerc Sport.* 1986;57(4):308–14.

Goodwill AM, Pearce AJ, Kidgell DJ. Corticomotor plasticity following unilateral strength training. *Muscle Nerve.* 2012 Sep;46(3):384–93.

Hall KG, Domingues DA, Cavazos R. Contextual interference effects with skilled baseball players. *Percept Mot Skills.* 1994 Jun;78(3 Pt 1):835–41.

Hughes T, Rochester P. The effects of proprioceptive exercise and taping on proprioception in subjects with functional ankle instability: a review of the literature. *Phys Ther Sport.* 2008 Aug;9(3):136–47.

Jensen JL, Marstrand PC, Nielsen JB. Motor skill training and strength training are associated with different plastic changes in the central nervous system. *J Appl Physiol (1985).* 2005 Oct;99(4):1558–68.

Johansson H. Neurophysiology of joints. In: Wright V, Radin E, editors. *Mechanics of human joints, physiology, pathophysiology and treatment.* New York: Dekker; 1993. pp. 243–84.

Jones K, Bishop P, Hunter G, Fleisig G. The effects of varying resistance-training loads on intermediate- and high-velocity-specific adaptations. *J Strength Cond Res.* 2001 Aug;15(3):349–56.

Kaneko M, Fuchimoto T, Toji H, Suei K. Training effect of different loads on the force-velocity relationship and mechanical power output in human muscle. *Scand J Med Sci Sports.* 1983;5:50–5.

Kim D, Van Ryssegem G, Hong J. Overcoming the myth of proprioceptive training. *Clin kinesiol.* 2011;65(1):18–28.

Krosshaug T, Nakamae A, Boden BP, Engebretsen L, Smith G, Slauterbeck JR, Hewett TE, Bahr R. Mechanisms of anterior cruciate ligament injury in basketball: video analysis of 39 cases. *Am J Sports Med.* 2007 Mar;35(3):359–67.

Kubo K, Ikebukuro T, Yata H, Tsunoda N, Kanehisa H. Time course of changes in muscle and tendon properties during strength training and detraining. *J Strength Cond Res.* 2010 Feb;24(2):322–31.

Latella C, Kidgell DJ, Pearce AJ. Reduction in corticospinal inhibition in the trained and untrained limb following unilateral leg strength training. *Eur J Appl Physiol.* 2012 Aug;112(8):3097–107.

Lauersen JB, Bertelsen DM, Andersen LB. The effectiveness of exercise interventions to prevent sports injuries: a systematic review and meta-analysis of randomised controlled trials. *Br J Sports Med.* 2014 Jun;48(11):871–7.

Lee TD, Magill RA. The locus of contextual interference in motor-skill acquisition. *J Exp Psychol Learn Mem Cogn.* 1983;9:730–46.

Lee TD, Magill RA. Can forgetting facilitate skill acquisition? In: Goodman D, Wilberg RB, Franks IM, editors. *Differing perspectives in motor learning, memory, and control.* Amsterdam: Elsevier; 1985. pp. 3–22.

Lee TD, Simon D. Contextual interference. In: Williams AM, Hodges NJ, editors. *Skill acquisition in sport: research, theory and practice.* London: Routledge; 2004. pp. 29–44.

McBride JM, Triplett-McBride T, Davie A, Newton RU. The effect of heavy- vs. light-load jump squats on the development of strength, power, and speed. *J Strength Cond Res.* 2002 Feb;16(1):75–82.

McGeehan MR, Wright GA, Fleck SJ. Strength training for athletes: does it really help sports performance? *Int J Sports Physiol Perform.* 2012 Mar;7(1):2–5.

McKeon PO, Hertel J. Systematic review of postural control and lateral ankle instability, part II: is balance training clinically effective? *J Athl Train.* 2008 May–Jun;43(3):305–15.

Magill RA. *Motor learning and control: concepts and application.* 9th ed. New York: McGraw-Hill, 2010. 480 pp.

Mahieu NN, McNair P, Cools A, D'Haen C, Vandermeulen K, Witvrouw E. Effect of eccentric training on the plantar flexor muscle-tendon tissue properties. *Med Sci Sports Exerc.* 2008 Jan;40(1):117–23.

Meijer OG, Roth K. *Complex movement behaviour: the motor-action controversy (advances in psychology).* Amsterdam: Elsevier; 1988. 604 pp.

Milia M, Siskosky MJ, Wang YX, Boylan JP, Wojtys EM, Ashton-Miller JA. The role of the ankle evertor muscles in preventing inversion during a one-footed landing on a hard surface: an experimental study in healthy young males. Presented at the 24th annual meeting of American Orthopedic Society for Sports Medicine; 1998 Jul 12–15; Vancouver.

Moss BM, Refsnes PE, Abildgaard A, Nicolaysen K, Jensen J. Effects of maximal effort strength training with different loads on dynamic strength, cross-sectional area, load-power and load-velocity relationships. *Eur J Appl Physiol Occup Physiol.* 1997;75(3):193–9.

O'Sullivan K, McAuliffe S, Deburca N. The effects of eccentric training on lower limb flexibility: a systematic review. *Br J Sports Med.* 2012 Sep;46(12):838–45.

Perez MA, Lungholt BK, Nyborg K, Nielsen JB. Motor skill training induces changes in the excitability of the leg cortical area in healthy humans. *Exp Brain Res.* 2004 Nov;159(2):197–205.

Refshauge KM, Kilbreath SL, Raymond J. The effect of recurrent ankle inversion sprain and taping on proprioception at the ankle. *Med Sci Sports Exerc.* 2000 Jan;32(1):10–15.

Rosenkranz K, Kacar A, Rothwell JC. Differential modulation of motor cortical plasticity and excitability in early and late phases of human motor learning. *J Neurosci.* 2007 Oct;27(44):12058–66.

Schmidt RA. The search for invariance in skilled movement behaviour. *Res Q Exerc Sport.* 1985 Feb;56(2):188–200.

Schmidt RA. *Motor control and learning: a behavioral emphasis.* Champaign, IL: Human Kinetics; 1988. 578 pp.

Seynnes OR, de Boer M, Narici MV. Early skeletal muscle hypertrophy and architectural changes in response to high-intensity resistance training. *J Appl Physiol (1985).* 2007 Jan;102(1):368–73.

Seynnes OR, Erskine RM, Maganaris CN, Longo S, Simoneau EM, Grosset JF, Narici MV. Training-induced changes in structural and mechanical properties of the patellar tendon are related to muscle hypertrophy but not to strength gains. *J Appl Physiol (1985).* 2009 Aug;107(2):523–30.

Shapiro DC, Zernicke RF, Gregor RJ. Evidence for generalized motor programs using gait pattern analysis. *J Mot Behav.* 1981 Mar;13(1):33–47.

Sjölander P, Johansson H. Sensory endings in ligaments: response properties and effects on proprioception and motor control. In: Yahia L, editor. *Ligaments and ligamentoplastics.* New York: Springer; 1997. pp. 39–83.

Smith PJ, Davies M. Applying contextual interference to the Pawlata roll. *J Sports Sci.* 1995 Dec;13(6):455–62.

Stevans J, Hall KG. Motor skill acquisition strategies for rehabilitation of low back pain. *J Orthop Sports Phys Ther.* 1998 Sep;28(3):165–7.

Tillin NA, Pain MT, Folland JP. Short-term training for explosive strength causes neural and mechanical adaptations. *Exp Physiol.* 2012 May;97(5):630–41.

Turvey MT. Coordination. *Am Psychol.* 1990 Aug;45(8):938–53.

Wagner H, Blickhan R. Stabilizing function of antagonistic neuromusculoskeletal systems: an analytical investigation. *Biol Cybern.* 2003 Jul;89(1):71–9.

Weier AT, Kidgell DJ. Strength training with superimposed whole body vibration does not preferentially modulate cortical plasticity. *Scientific World Journal.* 2012;2012:876328.

Weier AT, Pearce AJ, Kidgell DJ. Strength training reduces intracortical inhibition. *Acta Physiol (Oxf).* 2012 Oct;206(2):109–19.

Winstein CJ. Designing practice for motor learning: clinical implications. In: Lister MJ, editor. *Contemporary management of motor control problems*: proceedings of the II step conference; 1991; Alexandria. Alexandria, VA: Foundation for Physical Therapy; 1991. pp. 65–76.

Wyon MA, Smith A, Koutedakis Y. A comparison of strength and stretch interventions on active and passive ranges of movement in dancers: a randomized controlled trial. *J Strength Cond Res.* 2013 Nov;27(11):3053–9.

PART II
Core training

5

CORE EXERCISES

The core is composed of the abdominal and lumbopelvic region of the body, including the abdominal and low back muscles, diaphragm, pelvic floor, and the gluteal muscles (Richardson et al. 1999). The core also comprises the shoulder and hip-girdle muscles as they are essential for the transfer of energy from the trunk to the extremities (Fig 2005). The core plays an important role in stabilizing the range of motion of the spine and maintaining optimal alignment and motion of the trunk over the pelvis (Kibler et al. 2006). The core is the link between the lower and upper body, transferring forces between the lower body and the upper body (Cholewicki and McGill 1996). For optimal performance the core needs to be solid, to avoid energy leaks within the kinetic chain. A dysfunctional core that ineffectively transfers forces will put more strain on the muscles of the extremities, increasing the risk of injury (Chumanov et al. 2007).

Core training is undertaken for the purpose of injury prevention and performance enhancement (Hibbs et al. 2008; Kibler et al. 2006). Core stability exercises are very popular in rehabilitation and also form an integral part of the training programs of athletes (Gamble 2013; Hibbs et al. 2008). The role of core training for the prevention and rehabilitation of injuries has been well established (Hibbs et al. 2008; Kankaanpää et al. 1998; Leetun et al. 2004; Vezina and Hubley-Kozey 2000). Although core stability and strength are believed to be critical for performance in most sports, research looking at the effect of core stability on athletic performance is more ambiguous (Lehman 2006; Roetert 2001). This ambiguity is probably due to the lack of functionality of the core training programs to induce improvements in performance (Hibbs et al. 2008). Low-threshold core exercise can positively affect core stability because only submaximal levels of activity are required to stabilize the spine (Barr et al. 2005; Lehman 2006). Core training programs that are intended to enhance performance however, require the implementation of higher-threshold exercises that challenge the core at a higher intensity to induce strength gains (Hibbs et al. 2006; Vezina and Hubley-Kozey 2000).

Core training is complex due to the many muscles involved and various core functions (Gamble 2013). The involvement of the different muscles of the core varies continuously according to the posture or movement (Juker et al. 1998; McGill et al. 2003; Martuscello et al. 2013).

A single core exercise that targets all core muscles does not exist (Martuscello *et al.* 2013). Developing total core stability requires a variety of exercises that address different planes of motion, force vectors, and challenge the core at different intensities/thresholds (Bergmark 1989).

5.1 Inner and outer unit

The core consists of local stabilizers (the inner unit) that provide segmental stabilization and global stabilizers and movers (the outer unit) that generate and keep tight control over the movement (Bergmark 1989; Comerford and Mottram 2001; Comerford *et al.* 2004). The inner and outer unit synergistically work together to stabilize the core and generate powerful movements of the extremities (Bergmark 1989; Comerford and Mottram 2001; Comerford *et al.* 2004).

The inner unit tonic muscles

The inner unit refers to the functional synergy between the deep muscles of the core.

The inner unit is composed of the transversus abdominis, the posterior fibers of the obliquus internus abdominis, the medial fibers of the obliquus externus abdominis, the diaphragm, the pelvic floor muscles, the multifidus, the medial fibers of the quadratus lumborum, and lumbar portions of the longissimus and iliocostalis (Faries and Greenwood 2007; Lee 2004; O'Sullivan 2000). These muscles have their origin or insertion at the vertebrae and generate little or no movement during activation (Bergmark 1989). Contraction of these deep core muscles provides segmental stabilization of the spine (Bergmark 1989).

The inner unit muscles are tonic muscles that function as stabilizers. They effectively stabilize the spine and sacroiliac joint at low levels of contraction with low susceptibility to fatigue. Coordination is critical for proper stabilization. The ability of the inner unit muscles to contract prior to force production of phasic muscles (geared toward movement) is more important than their strength (Cresswell *et al.* 1994; Hodges and Moseley 2003; Hodges and Richardson 1998; McGill 1998; Zattara *et al.* 1988). Prior to movement or perturbation of the body the inner unit is activated, contracting the transversus abdominis, obliquus internus and externus, rectus abdominis, and the multifidus (Cresswell *et al.* 1994; Hodges and Richardson 1998). The transversus abdominis is invariably the first muscle that is active (Cresswell *et al.* 1994; Hodges and Richardson 1997). Because the fibers of the transversus abdominis are horizontally orientated, the umbilicus is drawn in toward the spine on contraction (Cresswell *et al.* 1994). This drawing in of the abdominal wall compresses the internal organs. The up- and downward pressure generated by the compressed internal organs activates the diaphragm and the pelvic floor muscles. This simultaneous activation of the inner unit muscles stiffens the spine and provides segmental stabilization (Hodges and Richardson 1997; Richardson *et al.* 2004).

The outer unit phasic muscles

The outer unit consists of many muscles such as the obliquus externus, obliquus internus, erector spinae, latissimus dorsi, gluteus muscles, the quadratus lumborum, adductors, and hamstrings. Although the outer unit is a phasic system, with large muscles that are very well oriented to produce force and move the body, it also plays an important role in stabilization when the body is under load or during high-speed movements (Bergmark 1989; Comerford and Mottram 2001; Comerford *et al.* 2004). The outer unit consists of four myofascial systems that control the range of motion, generate movement, and provide gross stability.

The deep longitudinal system

In the deep longitudinal system (Figure 5.1) the biceps femoris is coupled with the spinal erectors through the sacrotuberous ligament (van Wingerden *et al.* 1993; Vleeming *et al.* 1989a). At the end of the swing phase the hamstrings eccentrically contract to control hip flexion and knee extension. The contraction of the biceps femoris strains the sacrotuberous ligament, assisting in stabilization of the sacroiliac joint (=force closure of the sacroiliac joint) (van Wingerden *et al.* 1993; Vleeming *et al.* 1989a, 1989b). Kinetic energy is dissipated by the erector spinae through rotary action on the spinal column.

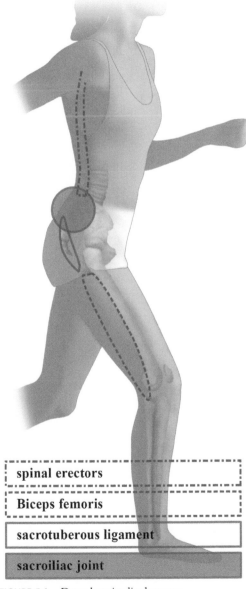

spinal erectors

Biceps femoris

sacrotuberous ligament

sacroiliac joint

FIGURE 5.1   Deep longitudinal system

The posterior oblique system

In the posterior oblique system (Figure 5.2) the gluteus maximus is connected to the latissimus dorsi of the opposite side through the thoracolumbar fascia (Bergmark 1989; Gracovetsky 1997; Greenman 1997; Vleeming *et al.* 1995). During walking or running, the gluteus maximus contracts on foot strike in concert with a contraction of the opposite latissimus dorsi (the latissimus dorsi extends the arm as a means of counter rotation) (Bergmark 1989; Gracovetsky

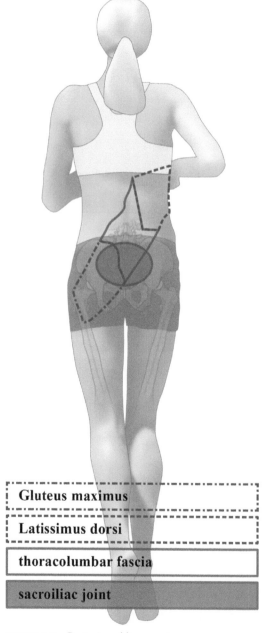

Gluteus maximus

Latissimus dorsi

thoracolumbar fascia

sacroiliac joint

FIGURE 5.2 Posterior oblique system

1997; Greenman 1997). This countered contraction creates tension on the thoracolumbar fascia, stabilizing the sacroiliac joint (force-closure) (Bergmark 1989; Gracovetsky 1997; Greenman 1997). The posterior oblique sling transfers power from the lower to the upper body, generates and stabilizes trunk rotation (Bergmark 1989; Gracovetsky 1997; Greenman 1997;Vleeming *et al.* 1995). Some authors described that the posterior oblique system may act like a smart spring (Gracovetsky 1997). The stored energy in the thoracolumbar fascia can be released with a subsequent contraction, minimizing muscle action and the metabolic cost of locomotion (Gracovetsky 1997).

The anterior oblique system

In the anterior oblique system (Figure 5.3) the thigh adductors are coupled with oblique abdominal muscles through the adductor-abdominal fascia. Rotational trunk movement first lengthens the muscles of the anterior oblique system and energy is stored (Logan and McKinney 1970). This energy is released during the subsequent concentric contraction of these muscles, allowing greater velocity. The anterior oblique system plays an important role during rotational ballistic motions such as throwing. Forces can also be transferred from the trunk and pelvis to the legs (Logan and McKinney 1970). A high amount of eccentric work is done by the hip adductors and obliques during the wind-up motion (loading phase) of the soccer kick (Borghuis *et al.* 2011; Charnock *et al.* 2009; Idoate *et al.* 2011). The stored energy is subsequently released during the swing phase to generate greater kicking velocities. This system also rotates the pelvis forward during the swing phase, playing an important role in locomotion.

The lateral system

The lateral system (Figure 5.4) stabilizes the body in the frontal plane. During a single-leg stance the hip abductors and adductors of the supporting leg work in concert with the opposite quadratus lumborum to stabilize the pelvis (Lyons *et al.* 1983; McGill *et al.* 1996). The oblique (both internal and external) musculature is also synergistic to secure a stable spine and pelvis (Andersen *et al.* 2014). Deficiency of the lateral system is a common source of injury in the back, sacroiliac joint, and supporting leg (Comfort *et al.* 2011; Ekstrom *et al.* 2007; Friel *et al.* 2006; Leetun *et al.* 2004; Zazulak *et al.* 2007). Soccer is single-leg dominant in nature. During running and sprinting the body is propelled forward through powerful single-leg actions. A strong and functional lateral system will help improve athletic performance, preserve energy, and prevent injuries (Butcher *et al.* 2007; Comfort *et al.* 2011; Ekstrom *et al.* 2007; Friel *et al.* 2006; Leetun *et al.* 2004; Zazulak *et al.* 2007).

5.2 High-threshold vs. low-threshold recruitment

Research shows that free weight, multiple-joint movements are optimal to elicit a strong activation of the core musculature (Martuscello *et al.* 2013). These free weight strength exercises are performed with additional weight, requiring greater recruitment of the trunk muscles to maintain proper posture (Hamlyn *et al.* 2007). Free weight, multiple-joint exercises train the different core functions simultaneously and the majority of these exercises are also performed standing, mimicking the core function patterns during sport activities or daily tasks (Tarnanen *et al.* 2012). It has been postulated that free weight strength exercises are sufficient

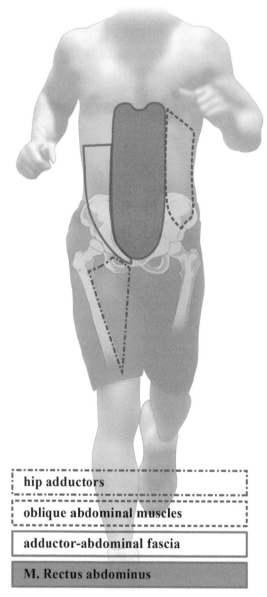

FIGURE 5.3   Anterior oblique system

to strengthen the core muscles and optimally develop core function and adding traditional core exercises is probably unnecessary (Martuscello *et al.* 2013; Tarnanen *et al.* 2012).

Core stability is as much about correct motor control and endurance capacity as it is about muscle stiffness and strength however (Hodges and Moseley 2003; McGill 1998; Zattara *et al.* 1988). The endurance capacity of the local core muscles is vital because these muscles are recruited at submaximal levels of activation for prolonged periods (Barr *et al.* 2005; Lehman 2006). A lot of back injuries occur as a result of incorrect motor control or insufficient endurance

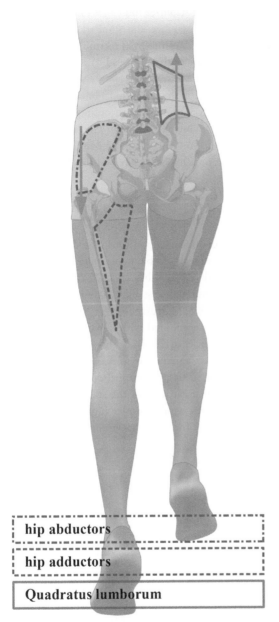

FIGURE 5.4   Lateral system

capacity (McGill 1998). The likelihood of motor control errors also increases with fatigue (McGill 1998). General free weight exercises are mainly high-load, low-repetition exercises. Low-load, higher-repetition exercises are also required to enhance endurance capacity of the global musculature (McGill 1998). Traditional core exercises are mainly body weight exercises and allow the performance of more repetitions and a longer time under tension to assist in the enhancement of the endurance capacity. Traditional core exercises are also crucial to improve the neuromuscular control of the local and global stabilizer muscles (Faries and Greenwood

2007). Low-threshold recruitment of the local and global stabilizer muscles is essential because minimal levels of muscle contraction are required to stabilize the spine (Lehman 2006). Incorporating traditional core exercises can enhance the low-threshold recruitment efficiency of the stabilizing muscles and avoid recruitment imbalances that can lead to movement dysfunction and an increased risk of injury (Comerford and Mottram 2001).

Multiple-joint exercises enhance the co-activation of the local and global system in a sport-specific, functional manner, while traditional core exercises are optimal to enhance the synchronization and endurance capacity of the stabilizing muscles. The lower load of traditional core exercises also allows their integration on a more regular basis into training. Performing exercises to activate the local stabilizing muscles on a daily basis has been shown to be more beneficial (McGill 1998).

5.3 Vector-specific core conditioning

The demands on the core during soccer occur in multiple positions and directions. To develop total core stability a range of different exercises should be incorporated that address the different planes of motion and vectors (Bergmark 1989; Hibbs *et al.* 2008). The activation level and combination of muscles that provide lumbopelvic stability have been shown to vary depending on the task and posture (Juker *et al.* 1998; Martuscello *et al.* 2013). Isometric exercises in which movement is prevented should be combined with dynamic exercises in which the range of motion has to be controlled (Hibbs *et al.* 2008). Both low-threshold and high-threshold training need to be included to emphasize neuromuscular control, endurance capacity, and strength (Comerford 2007; Hibbs *et al.* 2008). Traditional core exercises can enhance the low-threshold recruitment and endurance capacity of the stabilizing muscles, while free weight multiple-joint exercises can improve stability under high load or speed during functional positions and movement, specific to the demands imposed on the core during soccer (Leetun *et al.* 2004).

Core exercises can be categorized into four categories:

- anti-extension
- anti-rotation
- anti-lateral flexion
- anti-flexion.

5.4 Exercises

Anti-extension

Co-contraction of the abdominal muscles increases the anti-extension stiffness of the core to prevent hyperextension of the lumbar spine (Okubo *et al.* 2010). Anti-extension exercises therefore effectively target the abdominal muscles (Escamilla *et al.* 2006, 2010; Imai *et al.* 2010; Lehman *et al.* 2005; Martuscello *et al.* 2013; Okubo *et al.* 2010). The outer unit system that contributes to the anti-extension stability of the spine is the anterior oblique system.

Exercise variety is crucial to fully challenge the abdominal wall musculature, because the obliques consist of several neuromuscular compartments that are regionally activated (Badiuk *et al.* 2014; McGill 2007). Static anti-extension exercises such as the rollout, knee tuck, pike, and plank highly activate the abdominal muscles (Escamilla *et al.* 2006, 2010; Imai *et al.* 2010;

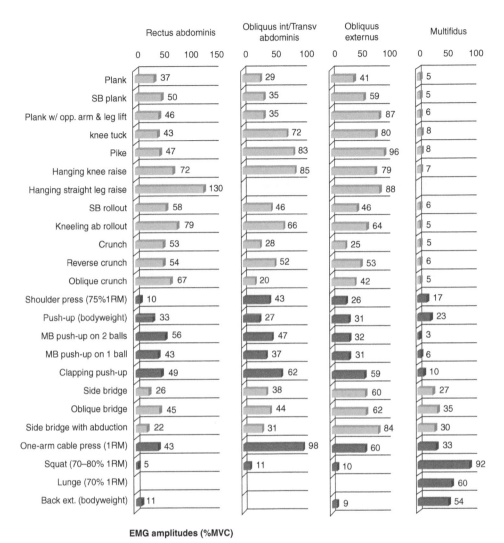

FIGURE 5.5 EMG signal amplitudes of the rectus abdominis, obliquus internus/transversus abdominis, obliquus externus, and lumbar multifidus (Colado *et al.* 2011; Czaprowski *et al.* 2014; Ekstrom *et al.* 2007; Escamilla *et al.* 2006, 2010; Freeman *et al.* 2006; Hamlyn *et al.* 2007; Imai *et al.* 2010; Kong *et al.* 2013; Konrad *et al.* 2001; Lehman *et al.* 2005; McGill 1998; McGill *et al.* 2014; Maeo *et al.* 2014; Nuzzo *et al.* 2008; Okubo *et al.* 2010; Santana *et al.* 2007; Willardson *et al.* 2009)

Lehman *et al.* 2005; Martuscello *et al.* 2013; Okubo *et al.* 2010). Pressing or holding a weight overhead (from a standing position or to a lesser extent from a seated position without back support) also requires a strong contraction of the anterior core to prevent lumbar hyper-extension (Willardson *et al.* 2009). And of course crunches can still makeup part of your core workout. When training for stability, emphasizing motor patterns that incorporate a co-contraction of many muscles is preferable over exercises that target just a few muscles (Kavcic *et al.* 2004). Although crunches mainly challenge the rectus abdominis and obliquus internus, there is a certain amount of carryover with enhanced anti-extension core stability as outcome (Sahrmann 2002; Wohlfart *et al.* 1993; Figure 5.5).

Multiple-joint anti-extension exercises

Push-up /push-up progression/plyometric push-up

Staggered-stance, one-arm cable press

Back lunge and one-arm press

Overhead press

Squat and press

Jerk

Power snatch (high hang power snatch/low hang power snatch/power snatch)

Plank progression

The plank exercise is a basic core stability exercise that targets the deep abdominal muscles (Lehman *et al.* 2005; Okubo *et al.* 2010). During these exercises the abdominal muscles co-contract isometrically to resist the torque produced by gravity to extend the spine. Although the plank is a basic exercise, the activation level of the deep abdominals seems sufficient to potentiate the motor pattern of abdominal co-contraction. The difficulty and intensity of the plank exercise can be increased through various progressions.

Plank

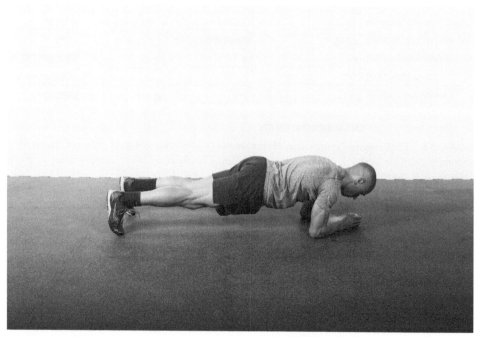

FIGURE 5.6   Plank

OBJECTIVE

The plank (Figure 5.6) is a beginner exercise to strengthen the motor engram of deep abdominal muscle activation and improve core stability.

STARTING POSITION

Place your forearms and toes on the floor.

Your feet are placed shoulder-width apart.

Keep the torso erect and the core tight. The knees and hips are extended and the spine is neutrally aligned.

EXECUTION

Hold the plank position for the prescribed amount of time.

COACHING KEYS

Keep your head in alignment with the body and look at the floor.

Place the elbows directly beneath the shoulders.

Stability ball plank

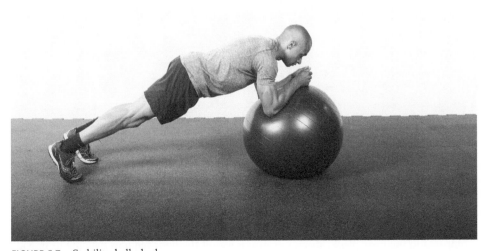

FIGURE 5.7   Stability ball plank

OBJECTIVE

Performing the plank (Figure 5.7) on a stability ball adds instability to the movement and increases the activity of the abdominal muscles (Czaprowski *et al*. 2014; Imai *et al*. 2010; Lehman *et al*. 2005; Martuscello *et al*. 2013).

STARTING POSITION

Place your forearms on a stability ball.

EXECUTION

Hold the plank position for the prescribed amount of time.

COACHING KEYS

Placing the feet on a box or bench will further increase the difficulty of the exercise.

Plank with arm/leg lift

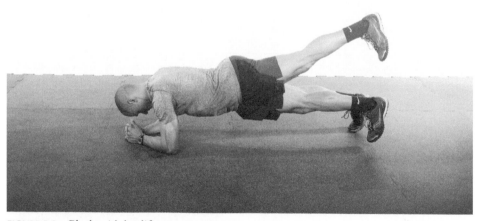

FIGURE 5.8   Plank with leg lift

OBJECTIVE

Compared to the basic plank, lifting the arm or leg off the floor requires the core to provide rotational stability (Figures 5.8 and 5.9).

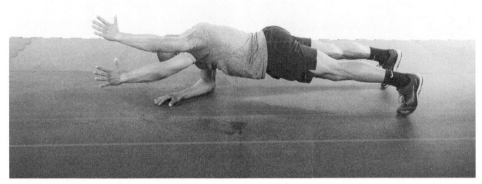

FIGURE 5.9   Plank with arm lift

STARTING POSITION

Assume a plank position with your feet shoulder-width apart.

Keep the torso erect and the core tight. The knees and hips are extended and the spine is neutrally aligned.

EXECUTION

Lift one arm or leg.

Hold for the prescribed amount of time and switch sides.

COACHING KEYS

Keep your weight evenly divided when lifting the toe or elbow off the floor.

Keep your trunk steady throughout the entire movement. Prevent spinal or hip rotation.

Plank with opposite arm and leg lift

OBJECTIVE

This advanced core strengthening exercise requires the trunk to be stabilized in all three planes of motion, eliciting a strong activation of the deep abdominal muscles (Okubo *et al.* 2010; Figure 5.10).

Lifting the opposite arm and leg requires very good rotational stability.

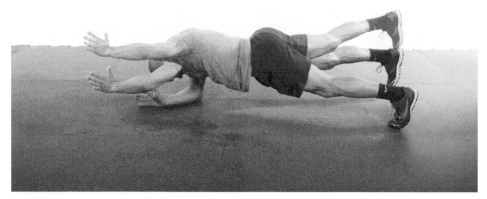

FIGURE 5.10   Plank with opposite arm and leg lift

STARTING POSITION

Assume a plank position.

EXECUTION

Lift one arm and raise the opposite leg.
   Hold the position for the prescribed amount of time and switch sides.

COACHING KEYS

Keep your trunk steady throughout the entire movement. Avoid swaying sideways and prevent spinal or hip rotation.

Knee tuck progression

OBJECTIVE

The knee tuck progression enhances core stability and strength (Figure 5.11). The knee tuck is a very effective exercise to activate the upper and lower rectus abdominis, external and internal obliques (Escamilla *et al.* 2006, 2010). The progression ranges in difficulty from beginner level to very challenging. The knee tuck and variations can be performed using a slide-board, TRX, or stability ball. The level of instability progressively increases from slide-board to TRX to stability ball. Adding instability will challenge the core to a greater extent (Behm *et al.* 2002).

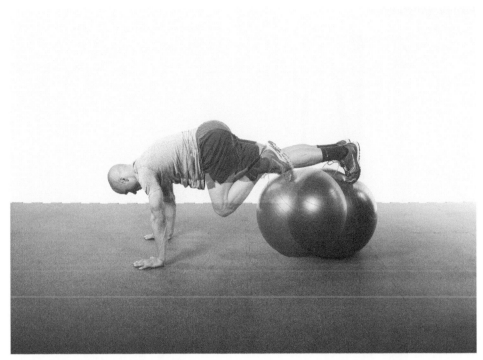

FIGURE 5.11   Stability ball knee tuck

More advanced variations, in which the knees are pulled up to the side (oblique knee-tuck) or one knee is pulled to the chest while the other leg is held up in the air (single-leg knee-tuck), can also be performed. All these different knee-tuck exercises give the trainer the possibility to progressively increase the intensity and add variety to the training.

STARTING POSITION

Assume a push-up position with your feet placed on the slide-board (wear slide-board booties), in the TRX straps, or the stability ball.

Keep the torso erect and the core tight. The knees and hips are extended and the spine is neutrally aligned.

EXECUTION

Pull your knees towards your chest.

Return to the starting position by extending both legs out again.

COACHING KEYS

Do not lower the hips while you pull the knees in. By keeping the hips up the core stays activated.

Pike progression

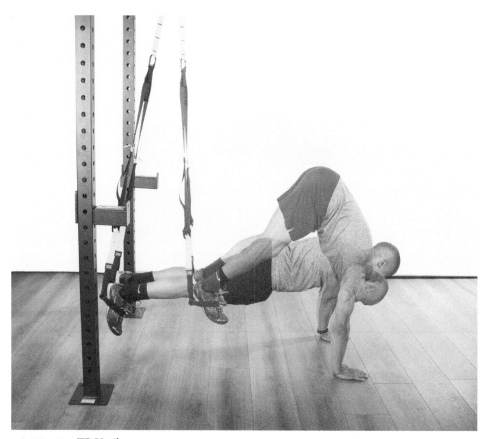

FIGURE 5.12 TRX pike

OBJECTIVE

The pike progression (Figure 5.12) elicits a stronger contraction of the anterior core muscles than most other core exercises (Escamilla *et al.* 2006, 2010; Martuscello *et al.* 2013). It is a very challenging core and abdominal exercise that also requires good upper body strength. By pulling your feet towards you, the hip flexors are heavily involved.

Identical to the knee-tuck progression, the degree of instability and the demand placed on the core can be increased by performing the exercise using a slide-board, a TRX, or a stability ball.

STARTING POSITION

Assume a push-up position with your feet placed on the slide-board (wear slide-board booties), in the TRX straps, or the stability ball.

Maintain the spine neutrally aligned and the core tight.

EXECUTION

Pull your feet towards your hands. Keep your knees extended.

Return to the starting position by extending both legs out again.

COACHING KEYS

Keep your knees extended.

Rollout progression

The rollouts (Figures 5.13–5.16) are core and abdominal strengthening exercises. Through various progressions the exercise intensity can be increased. The rollout can be performed using a stability ball or an ab wheel.

Stability ball rollout

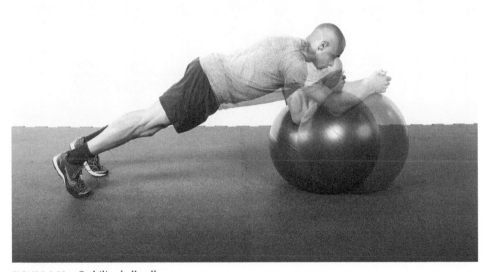

FIGURE 5.13   Stability ball rollout

OBJECTIVE

The stability ball rollout is the first step in the ab rollout progression. Placing the elbows on the ball reduces the lever arm and therefore the difficulty level of the exercise.

STARTING POSITION

Place your forearms on a stability ball.

Your feet are placed shoulder-width apart.

Keep the torso erect and the core tight. The knees and hips are extended and the spine is neutrally aligned.

EXECUTION

Roll the stability ball away from you.
Return to the initial position.

COACHING KEYS

In the starting position the elbows are placed directly beneath the shoulders. Do not roll the ball further towards you.

Kneeling straight-arm stability ball rollout

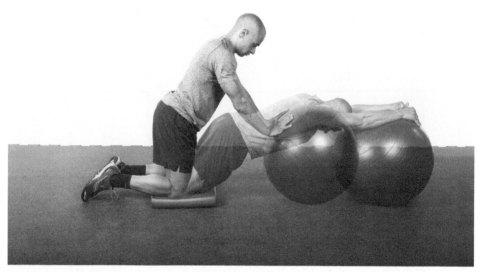

FIGURE 5.14 Kneeling straight-arm stability ball rollout

OBJECTIVE

The kneeling straight-arm stability ball rollout is a challenging exercise to strengthen the abs and core.

This exercise also elicits moderate pectoralis major and anterior deltoid activity and a strong contraction of the triceps brachii (Marshall and Desai 2010).

STARTING POSITION

Kneel in front of the stability ball, placing both hands on the ball. Maintain the arms extended.
Keep the core tight.

EXECUTION

Roll the stability ball out as far as possible.
   Lower your body to the floor by extending the arms forward.
   Return to the initial position.

COACHING KEYS

Squeeze your abs and prevent your back from arching when rolling the ball out.

Kneeling ab rollout

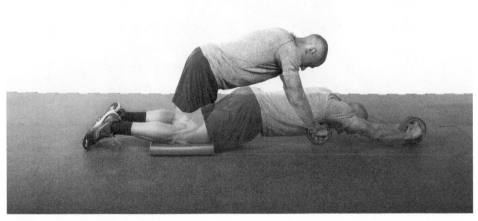

FIGURE 5.15   Kneeling ab rollout

OBJECTIVE

Performing the kneeling rollout with an ab wheel is more challenging compared with a stability ball. The kneeling ab rollout hence places a higher overload on the upper and lower rectus abdominis, internal and external obliques (Escamilla *et al.* 2006, 2010; Martuscello *et al.* 2013).

STARTING POSITION

Kneel down and grab the handles of the ab wheel.

EXECUTION

Roll the ab wheel out as far as possible.

Lower your body to the floor by extending the arms forward.
Return to the initial position.

COACHING KEYS

If you cannot maintain the spine neutrally aligned throughout the entire exercise, you should regress to perform the exercise with the stability ball.

Straight-arm stability ball rollout

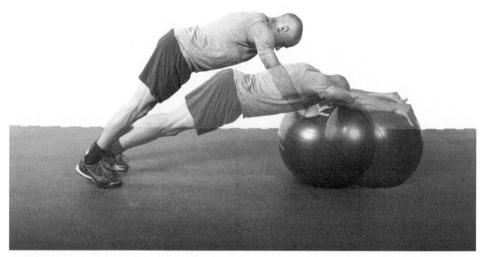

FIGURE 5.16   Straight–arm stability ball rollout

OBJECTIVE

The straight-arm stability ball rollout is the most challenging exercise of the rollout progression.

STARTING POSITION

Place your hands on the stability ball.
   Keep the core tight.
   The knees and arms are extended.

EXECUTION

Roll the stability ball out as far as possible.
   Lower your body to the floor by extending the arms forward.
   Return to the initial position.

COACHING KEYS

The narrower you place the feet, the higher will be the demand on the core to provide stability in the transverse plane of motion to prevent pelvic and spinal rotation while executing the exercise.

The hanging leg raise progression

This progression consists of exercises that produce very high levels of muscle activity in the abdominal wall (Escamilla *et al.* 2006; McGill *et al.* 2014; Martuscello *et al.* 2013). The abdominal muscles contract both isometrically and dynamically during these exercises. During the first phase of the movement the abdominals stabilize the pelvis to counteract the forces of the hip flexors. More towards the end of the movement the abdominal muscles contract dynamically to rotate the pelvis posteriorly and flatten the lumber spine (Escamilla *et al.* 2006).

Disc compression is higher however during hanging leg raises compared to most other core exercises. Spine loads during a regular bent-knee sit-up have been shown to be slightly higher than during the hanging leg raise (Escamilla *et al.* 2006; McGill *et al.* 2014). The rectus abdominis, internal and external oblique are significantly more activated during the hanging leg raise compared to the bent-knee sit-up (Escamilla *et al.* 2006; Martuscello *et al.* 2013). Although it is unclear whether long-term implementation of exercises that produce higher spine loads into training increases the injury risk in healthy people, the hanging leg raise progression may be inappropriate for some individuals with low back pathologies (Escamilla *et al.* 2006).

Hanging knee raise

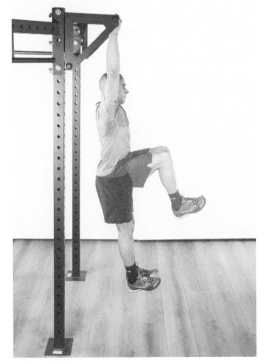

FIGURE 5.17   Hanging knee raise

OBJECTIVE

The hanging knee raise (Figure 5.17) is a challenging abdominal exercise that generates high levels of muscle activity in the upper and lower rectus abdominis, internal and external obliques (Escamilla *et al.* 2006). Through various progressions the intensity and difficulty of the exercise can be increased.

STARTING POSITION

Grasp the bar with an overhand grip (palms facing forward).
    The arms are straight.

EXECUTION

Pull your knees up towards your chest.
    Return to the starting position by lowering your legs in a controlled manner.

COACHING KEYS

Keep the core tight throughout the entire exercise.
    Lift your knees with a controlled motion. Do not swing your knees up.
    To add intensity, perform the exercise with a medicine ball or dumbbell squeezed between your knees or inner thighs.

Hanging oblique-knee raise

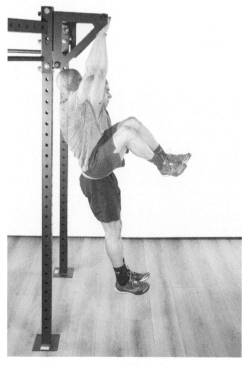

FIGURE 5.18   Hanging oblique-knee raise

OBJECTIVE

The rotation requires a stronger contraction of the obliques (Figure 5.18).

STARTING POSITION

Hang from a pull-up bar.

EXECUTION

Pull your knees up to one side as high as possible.
  Return to the starting position by lowering your legs in a controlled manner.
  Perform the prescribed number of repetitions alternating sides.

COACHING KEYS

Keep the knees squeezed together. Hip adductor contraction may facilitate abdominal muscle activity through the connection of the adductor longus with the distal rectus sheath (Norton-Old *et al.* 2013).

Hanging straight-leg raise

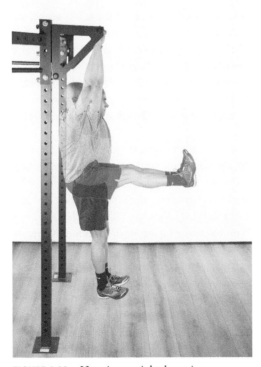

FIGURE 5.19   Hanging straight-leg raise

OBJECTIVE

Lifting the legs up straight increases the length of the lever arm and therefore the intensity of the exercise.

STARTING POSITION

Hang from a pull-up bar.

EXECUTION

Raise your legs up straight until they are parallel to the floor.

Return to the starting position by lowering your legs in a controlled manner.

COACHING KEYS

Keep your legs as straight as possible.

Anti-rotation

The anti-rotation function of the core stabilizes the trunk in the transverse plane of motion. In diagnosis and treatment of movement impairment syndromes Sahrmann (2002: 70) states: "A large percentage of low back problems occur because the abdominal muscles are not maintaining tight control over the rotation between the pelvis and the spine at the L5-S1 segment." The overall range of lumbar spine rotation is about 13 degrees. The rotation between each segment from T10 to L5 (thoracic 10th vertebra – lumbar 5th vertebra) is 2 degrees. The greatest rotational range is between L5 and S1, which is 5 degrees (Sahrmann 2002; White and Panjabi 1990). Increased rotational angles are possible when the spine is flexed (Pearcy 1993). Rotational ranges of 3½ degrees between segments have been shown to cause damage to the discs (Pearcy 1993). An overall range of lumbar spine rotation of 20–25 degrees is abnormal and unstable (White et al. 1990).

Most soccer players do not need to improve their lumbar rotational range of motion. The thoracic spine should be the site of greatest amount of rotation of the trunk. A solid range of motion in the hip is also important to avoid too much rotation at the lumbar spine. This is supported by a considerable amount of studies that show a correlation between a hip rotation deficit and low back pain (Chesworth et al. 1994; Ellison et al. 1990; Vad et al. 2004; Van Dillen et al. 2008).

Exercises to enhance rotational core stability emphasize the hip–spine dissociation (Moreside and McGill 2012). Poor dynamic control of the spine during rotation will result in a reactive tightening of the hip joints as a protective mechanism to avoid excessive low back rotation. Improved core stability means more hip movement can be produced without affecting the neutral lumbopelvic position. Enhancing the rotational stability and strength of the core will therefore facilitate hip range of motion and power (Kibler et al. 2006; Moreside and McGill 2012).

Rotational or anti-rotator spine stability is a big leap forward in sports training because lumbar spine rotation has been proven to be so damaging and yet most human movement is rotational in nature. Think of the counter-rotation of the pelvis and trunk during running or a soccer kick (Schache et al. 2002). Controlling and stabilizing the lumbar rotation is key to performance enhancement, and back health and exercises in which the core is forced to stabilize against rotary forces should form part of most workouts.

Two outer unit systems that play an important role in generating and stabilizing trunk rotation are the posterior oblique system and the anterior oblique system.

Multiple-joint anti-rotation exercises

Staggered-stance, one-arm press

Staggered-stance, one-arm row

Push–pull combination

Medicine ball crossover push-up

Slide-board front lever push-up

Back lunge and one-arm press

Front pull/resisted slide-board back lunge

Single-leg squat and pull

Single-leg Romanian deadlift and pull/single-leg Romanian deadlift

Single-leg back extension

Single-leg hamstring combination

One-arm dumbbell row

Battling ropes waves

Barbell torque

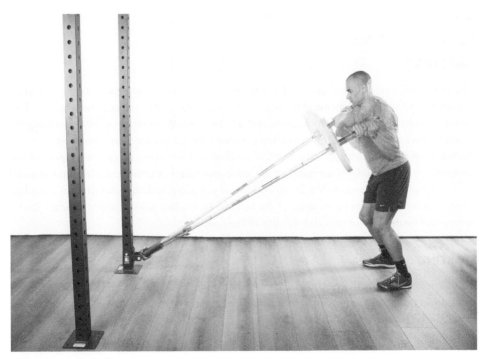

FIGURE 5.20   Barbell torque

OBJECTIVE

The barbell torque (Figure 5.20) trains the anti-rotator and anti-lateral flexion function of the core. Producing a large arc increases the demand on the core to stabilize against the rotational torque. The core has to stabilize and maintain proper alignment of the spine during movements of the arms. The core is trained to prevent movement in a standing position. It does not get more functional than this. Many back health specialists consider the ability to resist rotational forces as more important than the ability to create rotation.

STARTING POSITION

Place a barbell in a corner or in the center hole of a weight plate.
    The arms are extended at or slightly above shoulder height.
    Grasp the other end of the barbell with both hands.
    Stand shoulder-width apart with your knees and hips slightly bent.

EXECUTION

Rotate the bar to one side.
    On reaching the end of the range of motion, move the barbell back towards the center.
    Repeat the movement on the opposite side.
    Perform the prescribed number of repetitions.

COACHING KEYS

Keep the core tight and the torso erect throughout the entire movement.

Horizontal wood chop

OBJECTIVE

The horizontal wood chop (Figure 5.21) is an excellent exercise to improve rotational strength and stability of the core. During this exercise the core muscles have to generate rotation during the concentric part of the movement and actively control the range of motion during the eccentric part. Spinal rotation in a standing position (upright position combined with neutral alignment of the spine) is the safest form of rotation and has more carryover to sports. Axial compression locks the facet assembly of the spine and makes it more resistant to torsion and less susceptible to disc injury (Siff 2003). As long as you avoid end-range of motion and allow some rotation at the hips or pivoting of the feet, the horizontal wood chop is a great exercise to improve rotational strength and stability of the core.

STARTING POSITION

This exercise can be performed with elastic resistance or an adjustable cable column.
    Position the handle approximately at shoulder height.
    Grasp the handle with both hands.
    Assume a shoulder-width stance with the arms extended at shoulder height.

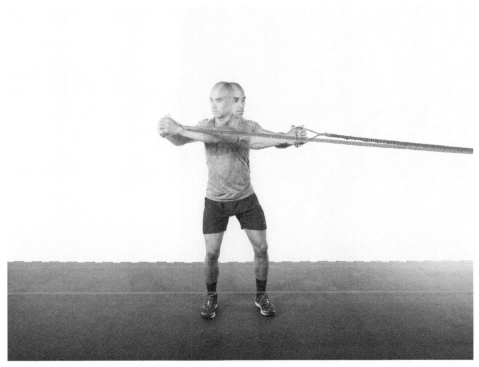

FIGURE 5.21 Horizontal wood chop

EXECUTION

Pull the handle all the way across the body by rotating the torso.
    Return to the starting position.
    Perform the prescribed number of repetitions and switch sides.

COACHING KEYS

Keep the core tight and the torso erect throughout the entire movement.
    Performing this exercise with some rotation at the hips can help enhance the spine–hip dissociation (strengthening of motor engrams in which hip rotation is the main driver of rotation).

Vertiball slam

OBJECTIVE

The vertiball slam exercise (Figure 5.22) requires the core to provide rotational stability during powerful upper body movements. This exercise will help improve the dynamic rotational stability and rotational strength of the core.

STARTING POSITION

Grasp the cords of the vertiball.
    Stand with your feet approximately shoulder-width apart.

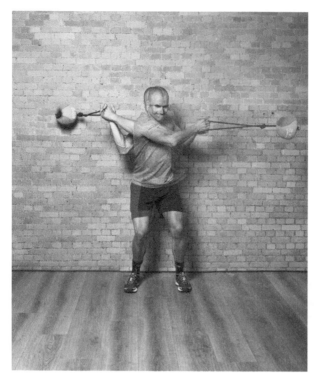

FIGURE 5.22 Vertiball slam

Stand with your back close to the wall, but leave enough space so you do not bump into the wall on rotation.

Assume the ready position.

Brace the core.

EXECUTION

Slam the ball from side to side into the wall, through powerful arm movements.

COACHING KEYS

Keep the arms extended.

Keep the spine neutrally aligned and the core tight throughout the entire exercise. Most of the movement should occur in the upper body while the lumbar spine transfers the momentum gained by the legs to the upper body. Allowing some hip rotation will avoid spinal end-range of motion.

Anti-lateral flexion

Anti-lateral flexion is the ability to stabilize the body in the frontal plane of motion. The pelvic stabilizers work in concert with the muscles of the core to resist a side-bending motion.

The lateral system plays an important role in anti-lateral flexion stability. Deficiency of the lateral system has implications all the way down the kinetic chain and is associated with increased incidence of lower extremity injuries and low back pain (Comfort *et al.* 2011; Ekstrom *et al.* 2007; Friel *et al.* 2006; Leetun *et al.* 2004; Zazulak *et al.* 2007).

These exercises may start with a basic side bridge and progress to exercises performed in a standing position that require more coordination and balance.

Multiple-joint anti-lateral flexion exercises

Single-leg knee dominant exercises (step-up/step-up variations, lunge/lunge variations, single-leg squat/single-leg squat progression/single-leg squat variations, slide-board exercises)

Single-leg Romanian deadlift/single-leg Romanian deadlift and pull

Slide-board front lever push-up

Battling ropes waves

Jerk

Staggered-stance one-arm press/staggered-stance one-arm pull/push–pull combinations

---

Side bridge progression

Like the plank, the side bridge (Figure 5.23) is a basic exercise to improve core stability through enhanced coordination and co-contraction of the local stabilizer muscles (Ekstrom *et al.* 2007; Lehman *et al.* 2005; McGill 1998; Okubo *et al.* 2010). Side bridge exercises also strengthen the lateral system, which plays an important role in lower body alignment and stabilization of the pelvis and spine (Ekstrom *et al.* 2007; McGill 1998; Youdas *et al.* 2014). Through various progressions the intensity and difficulty of the exercise can be increased.

Side bridge

OBJECTIVE

The side bridge is a beginner exercise to enhance the endurance, coordination, and motor control of the local system musculature (McGill 1998). The side bridge also provides strengthening benefits to the hip musculature (with especially a strong activation of the gluteus medius) on the weight-bearing side (Ekstrom *et al.* 2007; McGill 1998; Youdas *et al.* 2014).

STARTING POSITION

Lie on one side with your elbow directly beneath your shoulder and legs stacked.
    Push your body up until there is a straight line from head to feet.
    The elbow is positioned directly beneath the shoulder.

EXECUTION

Hold the side bridge for the prescribed amount of time.

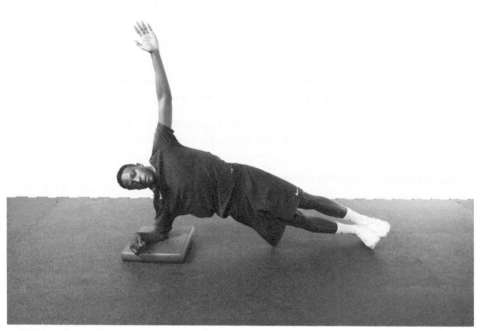

FIGURE 5.23 Side bridge

COACHING KEYS

Maintain a straight line from head to toe. Do not lower the hips.

Oblique bridge

OBJECTIVE

The oblique bridge (Figure 5.24) is the dynamic version of the side bridge. It is beneficial to strengthen the abdominal and hip muscles (Konrad *et al*. 2001; McGill 1998).

STARTING POSITION

Assume a side bridge position.

EXECUTION

Lower your body until the hips almost touch the floor.
   Return to the starting position.
   Perform the prescribed number of repetitions and switch sides.

COACHING KEYS

While lowering and raising your hips, ensure that the movement stays within the frontal plane of motion.

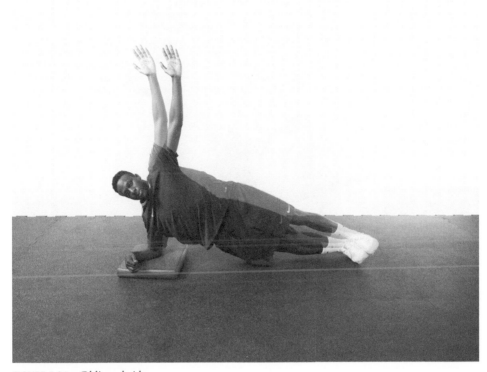

FIGURE 5.24   Oblique bridge

Side bridge with abduction

OBJECTIVE

This exercise is a more advanced side bridge variation. The side bridge with abduction (Figure 5.25) maximizes gluteus medius and maximus recruitment and is therefore also a very effective exercise to strengthen or (re-)activate the gluteal muscles (Boren *et al.* 2011).

STARTING POSITION

Assume a side bridge position.

EXECUTION

Lift the top leg as far up as you can.
  Return to the starting position.
  Perform the prescribed number of repetitions and switch sides.

COACHING KEYS

Keep the hip of the upper leg internally rotated to emphasize the posterior fibers of the gluteus medius. These posterior fibers are next to abduction also responsible for external rotation and frontal plane knee alignment during weight bearing.

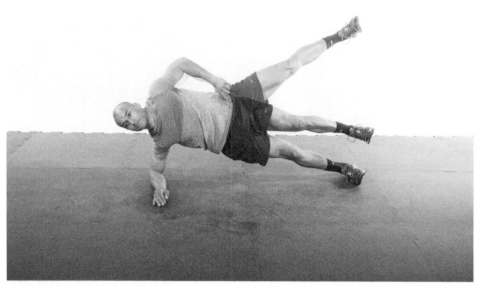

FIGURE 5.25 Side bridge with abduction

3D side bridge

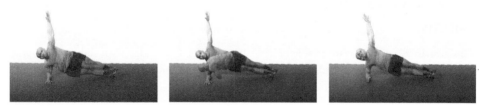

FIGURE 5.26 3D side bridge

OBJECTIVE

The 3D side bridge (Figure 5.26) consists of three dynamic side bridge exercises put in succession. Exercises that require stabilization of the lumbar spine while movement mainly occurs at the hip or chest region also emphasize the dissociation between the hips, lumbar and thoracic spine.

STARTING POSITION

Assume a side bridge position.

EXECUTION

Lower your body until the hips almost touch the floor.

Return to the starting position and perform this exercise for the prescribed number of repetitions.

Hold the side bridge position. Raise the upper arm directly above the shoulder so your body forms a T.

Rotate your upper body and reach with the hand of the upper arm underneath the body for the prescribed number of repetitions.

Hold the side bridge while moving your hips forward/backward.

Perform the prescribed number of repetitions and switch sides.

COACHING KEYS

The movement during these dynamic side bridges needs to occur mainly at hip or thoracic spine level.

Split stance core press

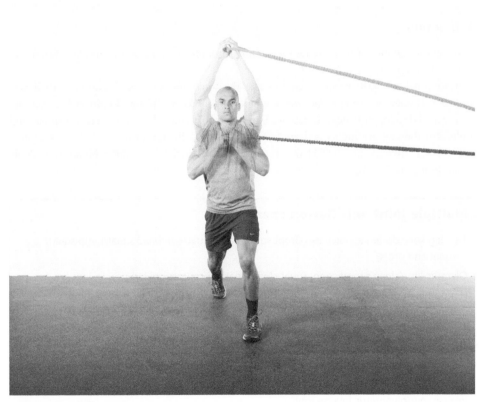

FIGURE 5.27   Split stance core press

OBJECTIVE

The split stance core press (Fig. 5.27) is beneficial to improve core stability and balance. This exercise allows you to train the anti-lateral flexion and anti-rotator stability of the core in a standing position.

STARTING POSITION

This exercise can be performed with elastic resistance or an adjustable cable column.
    Position the handle approximately at waist height.
    Grasp the handle with both hands.
    Stand perpendicular to the direction of the cable.
    Assume a split stance with the leg closest to the cable column forward.
    Hold the hands in front of the chest.

EXECUTION

Press the handle up overhead.
    Return to the starting position.
    Perform the prescribed number of repetitions and switch sides.

COACHING KEYS

Keep the core tight and the torso erect throughout the entire movement.

Anti-flexion

Anti-flexion stability of the core resists bending through the spine and counteracts the forces that tend to flex the trunk forward.

    Traditional strength training exercises like the squat, lunge, back extension, barbell row, inverse row, staggered-stance one-arm row, and various knee and hip dominant leg exercises are great to develop anti-flexion stability. During a squat and a deadlift the erector spinae and multifidus muscles are highly activated (Andersen *et al.* 2014; Colado *et al.* 2011; Comfort *et al.* 2011; Fenwick *et al.* 2009; Hamlyn *et al.* 2007; Martuscello *et al.* 2013; Nuzzo *et al.* 2008; Willardson *et al.* 2009).

Multiple-joint anti-flexion exercises

Two-leg knee dominant exercises (front squat/back squat/overhead squat/jump squat/ squat and press)

Olympic lifts (clean progression, squat clean, snatch progression, jerk)

Hip dominant leg exercises (Romanian deadlift/single-leg Romanian deadlift, Nordic hamstring exercise, assisted Nordic hamstring exercise, back extension/single-leg back extension, hamstring combination/single-leg hamstring combination)

Single-leg knee dominant exercises (step-up/step-up variations, lunge/lunge variations, single-leg squat/single-leg squat progression/single-leg squat variations, slide-board exercises

Inverse row/plyometric inverse row

Barbell row

Romanian deadlift and row

Staggered-stance one-arm row

Battling ropes waves

The deep longitudinal system and the posterior oblique system play an important role in pelvic and spinal anti-flexion. A contraction of the gluteus maximus and hamstring muscles stabilizes the sacroiliac joint (force-closure through the deep longitudinal and posterior oblique system) and will generate tension in the erector spinae muscles, providing stiffness to the spinal column (Snijders et al. 1993; van Wingerden et al. 1993; Vleeming et al. 1989b). Strong gluteus and hamstring muscles take pressure off the low back (Lafond et al. 1998; Wilson et al. 2005).

References

Andersen V, Fimland MS, Brennset O, Haslestad LR, Lundteigen MS, Skalleberg K, Saeterbakken AH. Muscle activation and strength in squat and Bulgarian squat on stable and unstable surface. *Int J Sports Med.* 2014 Sep 25. [Epub ahead of print]

Badiuk BW, Andersen JT, McGill SM. Exercises to activate the deeper abdominal wall muscles: the Lewit: a preliminary study. *J Strength Cond Res.* 2014 Mar;28(3):856–60.

Barr KP, Griggs M, Cadby T. Lumbar stabilization: core concepts and current literature, Part 1. *Am J Phys Med Rehabil.* 2005 Jun;84(6):473–80.

Behm DG, Anderson K, Curnew RS. Muscle force and activation under stable and unstable conditions. *J Strength Cond Res.* 2002 Aug;16(3):416–22.

Bergmark A. Stability of the lumbar spine. A study in mechanical engineering. *Acta Orthop Scand Suppl.* 1989;230:1–54.

Boren K, Conrey C, Le Coguic J, Paprocki L, Voight M, Robinson TK. Electromyographic analysis of gluteus medius and gluteus maximus during rehabilitation exercises. *Int J Sports Phys Ther.* 2011 Sep;6(3):206–23.

Borghuis AJ, Lemmink KA, Hof AL. Core muscle response times and postural reactions in soccer players and nonplayers. *Med Sci Sports Exerc.* 2011 Jan;43(1):108–14.

Butcher SJ, Craven BR, Chilibeck PD, Spink KS, Grona SL, Sprigings EJ. The effect of trunk stability training on vertical takeoff velocity. *J Orthop Sports Phys Ther.* 2007 May;37(5):223–31.

Charnock BL, Lewis CL, Garrett WE Jr, Queen RM. Adductor longus mechanics during the maximal effort soccer kick. *Sports Biomech.* 2009 Sep;8(3):223–34.

Chesworth BM, Padfield BJ, Helewa A, Stitt LW. A comparison of hip mobility in patients with low back pain and matched healthy subjects. *Physiother Can.* 1994;46:267–74.

Cholewicki J, McGill SM. Mechanical stability of the in vivo lumbar spine: implications for injury and chronic low back pain. *Clin Biomech (Bristol, Avon).* 1996 Jan;11(1):1–15.

Chumanov ES, Heiderscheit BC, Thelen DG. The effect of speed and influence of individual muscles on hamstring mechanics during the swing phase of sprinting. *J Biomech.* 2007;40(16):3555–62.

Colado JC, Pablos C, Chulvi-Medrano I, Garcia-Masso X, Flandez J, Behm DG. The progression of paraspinal muscle recruitment intensity in localized and global strength training exercises is not based on instability alone. *Arch Phys Med Rehabil.* 2011 Nov;92(11):1875–83.

Comerford MJ. Performance stability, module 1: stability for performance. Course 1: core stability concepts. Ludlow: Comerford & Performance Stability; 2007.

Comerford MJ, Mottram SL. Movement and stability dysfunction–contemporary developments. *Man Ther.* 2001 Feb;6(1):15–26.

Comerford MJ, Mottram SL, Gibbons SG. Understanding movement and function 'concepts'. Kinetic control movement dysfunction course. Southampton: Kinetic Control; 2004.

Comfort P, Pearson SJ, Mather D. An electromyographical comparison of trunk muscle activity during isometric trunk and dynamic strengthening exercises. *J Strength Cond Res.* 2011 Jan;25(1):149–54.

Cresswell AG, Oddsson L, Thorstensson A. The influence of sudden perturbations on trunk muscle activity and intra-abdominal pressure while standing. *Exp Brain Res.* 1994;98(2):336–41.

Czaprowski D, Afeltowicz A, Gębicka A, Pawłowska P, Kędra A, Barrios C, Hadała M. Abdominal muscle EMG-activity during bridge exercises on stable and unstable surfaces. *Phys Ther Sport.* 2014 Aug;15(3):162–8.

Ekstrom RA, Donatelli RA, Carp KC. Electromyographic analysis of core trunk, hip, and thigh muscles during 9 rehabilitation exercises. *J Orthop Sports Phys Ther*. 2007 Dec;37(12):754–62.

Ellison, JB, Rose SJ, Sahrmann SA. Patterns of hip rotation range of motion: a comparison between healthy subjects and patients with low back pain. *Phys Ther*. 1990 Sep;70(9):537–41.

Escamilla RF, Babb E, DeWitt R, Jew P, Kelleher P, Burnham T, Busch J, D'Anna K, Mowbray R, Imamura RT. Electromyographic analysis of traditional and nontraditional abdominal exercises: implications for rehabilitation and training. *Phys Ther*. 2006 May;86(5):656–71.

Escamilla RF, Lewis C, Bell D, Bramblet G, Daffron J, Lambert S, Pecson A, Imamura R, Paulos L, Andrews JR. Core muscle activation during Swiss ball and traditional abdominal exercises. *J Orthop Sports Phys Ther*. 2010 May;40(5):265–76.

Faries MD, Greenwood M. Core training: stabilizing the confusion. *Strength Cond J*. 2007 Apr;29(2):10–25.

Fenwick CM, Brown SH, McGill SM. Comparison of different rowing exercises: trunk muscle activation and lumbar spine motion, load, and stiffness. *J Strength Cond Res*. 2009 Aug;23(5):1408–17.

Fig G. Strength training for swimmers: training the core. *Strength Cond J*. 2005 Feb;27(2):40–2.

Freeman S, Karpowicz A, Gray J, McGill S. Quantifying muscle patterns and spine load during various forms of the push-up. *Med Sci Sports Exerc*. 2006 Mar;38(3):570–7.

Friel K, McLean N, Myers C, Caceres M. Ipsilateral hip abductor weakness after inversion ankle sprain. *J Athl Train*. 2006 Mar;41(1):74–8.

Gamble P. *Strength and conditioning for team sports: sport-specific physical preparation for high performance*. 2nd ed. New York: Routledge; 2013. 304 pp.

Gracovetsky S. Linking the spinal engine with the legs: A theory of human gait. In: Vleeming A, Mooney V, Dorman T, Snijders C, Stoeckart R, editors. *Movement, stability and low back pain*. New York: Churchill Livingstone; 1997. pp. 243.

Greenman PE. Clinical aspects of sacroiliac joint in walking. In: Vleeming A, Mooney V, Dorman T, Snijders C, Stoeckart R, editors. *Movement, stability and low back pain*. New York: Churchill Livingstone; 1997. pp. 243–51.

Hamlyn N, Behm DG, Young WB. Trunk muscle activation during dynamic weight-training exercises and isometric instability activities. *J Strength Cond Res*. 2007 Nov;21(4):1108–12.

Hibbs AE, Thompson KG, French D, Wrigley A, Spears I. Optimizing performance by improving core stability and core strength. *Sports Med*. 2008;38(12):995–1008.

Hodges PW, Moseley GL. Pain and motor control of the lumbopelvic region: effect and possible mechanisms. *J Electromyogr Kinesiol*. 2003 Aug;13(4):361–70.

Hodges PW, Richardson CA. Contraction of the abdominal muscles associated with movement of the lower limb. *Phys Ther*. 1997 Feb;77(2):132–44.

Hodges PW, Richardson CA. Delayed postural contraction of transversus abdominis in low back pain associated with movement of the lower limb. *J Spinal Disord*. 1998 Feb;11(1):46–56.

Idoate F, Calbert JA, Izquierdo M, Sanchis-Moysi J. Soccer attenuates the asymmetry of rectus abdominis muscle observed in non-athletes. *PLoS One*. 2011 Apr;6(4):e19022.

Imai A, Kaneoka K, Okubo Y, Shiina I, Tatsumura M, Izumi S, Shiraki H. Trunk muscle activity during lumbar stabilization exercises on both a stable and unstable surface. *J Orthop Sports Phys Ther*. 2010 Jun;40(6):369–75.

Juker D, McGill S, Kropf P, Steffen T. Quantitative intramuscular myoelectric activity of lumbar portions of psoas and the abdominal wall during a wide variety of tasks. *Med Sci Sports Exerc*. 1998 Feb;30(2):301–10.

Kankaanpää M, Taimela S, Laaksonen D, Hänninen O, Airaksinen O. Back and hip extensor fatigability in chronic low back pain patients and controls. *Arch Phys Med Rehabil*. 1998 Apr;79(4):412–7.

Kavcic N, Grenier S, McGill SM. Determining the stabilizing role of individual torso muscles during rehabilitation exercises. *Spine (Phila Pa 1976)*. 2004 Jun;29(11):1254–65.

Kibler WB, Press J, Sciascia A. The role of core stability in athletic function. *Sports Med*. 2006;36(3):189–98.

Kong YS, Cho YH, Park JW. Changes in the activities of the trunk muscles in different kinds of bridging exercises. *J Phys Ther Sci*. 2013 Dec;25(12):1609–12.

Konrad P, Schmitz K, Denner A. Neuromuscular evaluation of trunk-training exercises. *J Athl Train*. 2001 Jun;36(2):109–18.

Lafond D, Normand MC, Gosselin G. Rapport force. *J Can Chiropr Assoc*. 1998 Jun;42(2):90–100.

Lee D. *The pelvic girdle: an approach to the examination and treatment of the thoracolumbar-hip region*. 3rd ed. Edinburgh: Churchill Livingstone; 2004. 267 pp.

Leetun DT, Ireland ML, Willson JD, Ballantyne BT, Davis IM. Core stability measures as risk factors for lower extremity injury in athletes. *Med Sci Sports Exerc*. 2004 Jun;36(6):926–34.

Lehman GJ. Resistance training for performance and injury prevention in golf. *J Can Chiropr Assoc*. 2006 Mar;50(1):27–42.

Lehman GJ, Hoda W, Oliver S. Trunk muscle activity during bridging exercises on and off a Swiss ball. *Chiropr Osteopat*. 2005 Jul 30;13:14.

Logan G, McKinney W. The serape effect. In: Lockhart A, editor. *Anatomic kinesiology*. 3rd ed. Dubuque, IA: Wm C Brown Company Publishers; 1970. pp. 287–302.

Lyons K, Perry J, Gronley JK, Barnes L, Antonelli D. Timing and relative intensity of hip extensor and abductor muscle action during level and stair ambulation. An EMG study. *Phys Ther*. 1983 Oct;63(10):1597–605.

McGill SM. Low back exercises: evidence for improving exercise regimens. *Phys Ther*. 1998 Jul;78(7):754–65.

McGill SM. *Low back disorders: evidence-based prevention and rehabilitation*. 2nd ed. Champaign, IL: Human Kinetics; 2007. 328 pp.

McGill S, Juker D, Kropf P. Quantitative intramuscular myoelectric activity of quadratus lumborum during a wide variety of tasks. *Clin Biomech (Bristol, Avon)*. 1996 Apr;11(3):170–2.

McGill SM, Grenier S, Kavcic N, Cholewicki J. Coordination of muscle activity to assure stability of the lumbar spine. *J Electromyogr Kinesiol*. 2003 Aug;13(4):353–9.

McGill S, Andersen J, Cannon J. Muscle activity and spine load during anterior chain whole body linkage exercises: the body saw, hanging leg raise and walkout from a push-up. *J Sports Sci*. 2014 Aug 11:1–8. [Epub ahead of print]

Maeo S, Chou T, Yamamoto M, Kanehisa H. Muscular activities during sling- and ground-based push-up exercise. *BMC Res Notes*. 2014 Mar;7:192.

Marshall PW, Desai I. Electromyographic analysis of upper body, lower body, and abdominal muscles during advanced Swiss ball exercises. *J Strength Cond Res*. 2010 Jun;24(6):1537–45.

Martuscello JM, Nuzzo JL, Ashley CD, Campbell BI, Orriola JJ, Mayer JM. Systematic review of core muscle activity during physical fitness exercises. *J Strength Cond Res*. 2013 Jun;27(6):1684–98.

Moreside JM, McGill SM. Hip joint range of motion improvements using three different interventions. *J Strength Cond Res*. 2012 May;26(5):1265–73.

Norton-Old KJ, Schache AG, Barker PJ, Clark RA, Harrison SM, Briggs CA. Anatomical and mechanical relationship between the proximal attachment of adductor longus and the distal rectus sheath. *Clin Anat*. 2013 May;26(4):522–30.

Nuzzo JL, McCaulley GO, Cormie P, Cavill MJ, McBride JM. Trunk muscle activity during stability ball and free weight exercises. *J Strength Cond Res*. 2008 Jan;22(1):95–102.

Okubo Y, Kaneoka K, Imai A, Shiina I, Tatsumura M, Izumi S, Miyakawa S. Electromyographic analysis of transversus abdominis and lumbar multifidus using wire electrodes during lumbar stabilization exercises. *J Orthop Sports Phys Ther*. 2010 Nov;40(11):743–50.

O'Sullivan PB. Lumbar segmental 'instability': clinical presentation and specific stabilizing exercise management. *Man Ther*. 2000 Feb;5(1):2–12.

Pearcy MJ, Twisting mobility of the human back in flexed postures. *Spine (Phila Pa 1976)*. 1993 Jan;18(1):114–19.

Richardson C, Jull G, Hodges P, Hides J. *Therapeutic exercise for spinal segmental stabilization in low back pain: scientific basis and clinical approach*. Edinburgh: Churchill Livingstone; 1999. 192 pp.

Richardson C, Hodges PW, Hides J. *Therapeutic exercise for lumbopelvic stabilization: a motor control approach for the treatment and prevention of low back pain*. 2nd ed. Edinburgh: Churchill Livingstone; 2004. 280 pp.

Roetert PE. 3D balance and core stability. In: Foran B, editor. *High-performance sports conditioning: modern training for ultimate athletic development.* Champaign, IL: Human Kinetics; 2001. pp. 119–38.

Sahrmann S. *Diagnosis and treatment of movement impairment syndromes.* St Louis, MO: Mosby; 2002. 384 pp.

Santana JC, Vera-Garcia FJ, McGill SM. A kinetic and electromyographic comparison of the standing cable press and bench press. *J Strength Cond Res.* 2007 Nov;21(4):1271–7.

Schache AG, Blanch P, Rath D, Wrigley T, Bennell K. Three-dimensional angular kinematics of the lumbar spine and pelvis during running. *Hum Mov Sci.* 2002 Jul;21(2):273–93.

Siff MC. *Facts and fallacies of fitness.* 6th ed. West Warwick: Perform Better; 2003. 319 pp.

Snijders CJ, Vleeming A, Stoeckart R. Transfer of lumbosacral load to iliac bones and legs. Part 1: biomechanics of self-bracing of the sacroiliac joints and its significance for treatment and exercise. *Clin Biomech (Bristol, Avon).* 1993 Nov;8(6):285–94.

Tarnanen SP, Siekkinen KM, Häkkinen AH, Mälkiä EA, Kautiainen HJ, Ylinen JJ. Core muscle activation during dynamic upper limb exercises in women. *J Strength Cond Res.* 2012 Dec;26(12):3217–24.

Vad VB, Bhat AL, Basrai D, Gebeh A, Aspergren DD, Andrews JR, Low back pain in professional golfers: the role of associated hip and low back range-of-motion deficits. *Am J Sports Med.* 2004 Mar;32(2):494–7.

Van Dillen LR, Bloom NJ, Gombatto SP, Susco TM. Hip rotation range of motion in people with and without low back pain who participate in rotation-related sports. *Phys Ther Sport.* 2008 May;9(2):72–81.

van Wingerden JP, Vleeming A, Stam HJ, Stoeckart R. Interaction of the spine and legs: influence of the hamstring tension on lumbopelvic rhythm. Second Interdisciplinary World Congress on Low Back Pain. San Diego, CA 1993; Nov 9–11.

Vezina MJ, Hubley-Kozey CL. Muscle activation in therapeutic exercises to improve trunk stability. *Arch Phys Med Rehabil.* 2000 Oct;81(10):1370–9.

Vleeming A, Pool-Goudzwaard AL, Stoeckart R, van Wingerden JP, Snijders CJ. The posterior layer of the thoracolumbar fascia. Its function in load transfer from spine to legs. *Spine (Phila Pa 1976).* 1995 Apr;20(7):753–8.

Vleeming A, Stoeckart R, Snijders CJ. The sacrotuberous ligament: a conceptual approach to its dynamic role in stabilizing the sacroiliac joint. *Clin Biomech.* 1989a;4(4):201–3.

Vleeming A, Van Wingerden JP, Snijders CJ, Stoeckart R and Stijnen T. Load application to the sacrotuberous ligament; influences on sacroiliac joint mechanics. *Clin Biomech.* 1989b;4(4):204–9.

White AA, Panjabi MM. *Clinical biomechanics of the spine.* 2nd ed. Philadelphia: Lippincott Williams & Wilkins; 1990. 752 pp.

Willardson JM, Fontana FE, Bressel E. Effect of surface stability on core muscle activity for dynamic resistance exercises. *Int J Sports Physiol Perform.* 2009 Mar;4(1):97–109.

Wilson J, Ferris E, Heckler A, Maitland L, Taylor C. A structured review of the role of gluteus maximus in rehabilitation. *N Z J Physiother.* 2005 Nov;33(3):95–100.

Wohlfart D, Jull G, Richardson C. The relationship between dynamic and static function of the abdominal muscles. *Aust J Phys.* 1993;39(1):9–13.

Youdas JW, Boor MM, Darfler AL, Koenig MK, Mills KM, Hollman JH. Surface electromyographic analysis of core trunk and hip muscles during selected rehabilitation exercises in the side-bridge to neutral spine position. *Sports Health.* 2014 Sep;6(5):416–21.

Zattara M, Bouisset S. Posturo-kinetic organisation during the early phase of voluntary upper limb movement. 1. Normal subjects. *J Neurol Neurosurg Psychiatry.* 1988 Jul;51(7):956–65.

Zazulak BT, Hewett TE, Reeves NP, Goldberg B, Cholewicki J. Deficits in neuromuscular control of the trunk predict knee injury risk: a prospective biomechanical-epidemiologic study. *Am J Sports Med.* 2007 Jul;35(7):1123–30.

PART III
Strength training

6

TWO-LEG KNEE DOMINANT EXERCISES

The squat strengthens the knee and hip extensor muscles, which are the prime movers of sprinting and jumping and nearly every other type of athletic movement, as well as the muscles of the lower back to stabilize the torso. Because of the sport-specific character, the squat has an excellent transfer to athletic performance.

The squat is a closed kinetic chain exercise (exercise where the foot is the base of support). Like athletic movement, the force during the squat is applied into the ground, which makes it functional.

Research shows that a clear relationship exists between free weight squat strength and a variety of performance parameters such as sprinting, accelerating, and jumping (Comfort et al. 2012; Cunningham et al. 2013; López-Segovia et al. 2011, 2014; McBride et al. 2009; Wisløff et al. 2004). Also in elite and recreational soccer players strong correlations have been reported between squat strength and 10 and 30 m sprints as well as agility performance and jumping height (López-Segovia et al. 2011, 2014; Wisløff et al. 2004). This can be explained by the fact that accelerations and jumps start from zero or slow velocities, and strength is important during this initial movement phase to overcome the inertia of the body mass (Comfort et al. 2012). Peak ground contact force and impulse are strong determinants of sprint performance (Comfort et al. 2012; Hunter et al. 2005; Weyand et al. 2000). Applying greater forces to the ground during sprinting provides greater forward propulsion (Weyand et al. 2000).

Improving squat strength will not only benefit performance, but also seems to reduce the risk of injury (McCurdy et al. 2014). A relationship exists between the level of squat strength and knee and hip mechanics during landing (McCurdy et al. 2014). Athletes with higher levels of squat strength show better frontal plane control during landing (less knee valgus) (McCurdy et al. 2014). Improving squat strength should be considered as an important part of a training routine to reduce the risk of anterior cruciate ligament (ACL) injury (McCurdy et al. 2014).

Its functionality, the ability to overload the muscles during the exercise, and the reported impact of squat training on various athletic performance parameters explain the broad use of the squat in strength training programs for athletes in various sports (Clark et al. 2012; Cormie et al. 2010).

6.1 Full versus partial squats

Different ranges of motion are used and recommended for squat training. Quarter squats consist of squatting down only a quarter of the trajectory to an approximate knee angle of 120 degrees. Parallel squats are carried out until the top of the thighs are parallel to the floor, while during deep squats the hips pass well below knee height.

Muscle activation during the squat exercise is dependent on both training load and squat depth (Bryanton *et al.* 2012; Gorsuch *et al.* 2013). Activation of both the hip and knee extensors increases with greater squat depth, while heavier loads only augment hip extensor activity (Bryanton *et al.* 2012). Deep squats seem to be required to maximize knee extensor activation (Bryanton *et al.* 2012). This is in accordance with research findings that observed deep squat training elicits superior increments in strength and thigh hypertrophy compared to partial squat training (Bloomquist *et al.* 2013; Hartmann *et al.* 2012; Raastad *et al.* 2008; Weiss *et al.* 2000). Deep squat training also results in a superior increase in jump performance compared to quarter squat training (Bloomquist *et al.* 2013; Hartmann *et al.* 2012). Despite lower training loads, deep and parallel squats induce higher levels of knee extensor activation and tension for the improvement of hypertrophy and strength (Bloomquist *et al.* 2013; Bryanton *et al.* 2012; Gorsuch *et al.* 2013; Hartmann *et al.* 2012; Raastad *et al.* 2008; Weiss *et al.* 2000).

The confusion that deep squats would be detrimental for knee health has also been cleared. This confusion originated with a publication of Klein in 1961, stating that deep squats could increase the laxity of the knee ligaments (Klein 1961). Contrary to the hypothesis of Klein, ACL and PCL forces peak at 30 and 90 degrees respectively and decrease significantly with higher knee flexion angles (Li *et al.* 2004). The highest patellofemoral compressive forces occur at 90 degrees (Hartmann *et al.* 2013). With increasing knee flexion the retropatellar articular surface enlarges, which diminishes the patellofemoral stress (Hartmann *et al.* 2013). The contact between the soft tissues of the back of the thigh and calf also limits the tibial translation and enhances force distribution and the load tolerance in higher angles of knee flexion (Hartmann *et al.* 2013). Deep squats can be considered safe in terms of not causing permanent stretching of the knee ligaments, nor do they increase the risk of passive tissue injury (Chandler *et al.* 1989; Hartmann *et al.* 2013; Steiner *et al.* 1986). Powerlifters and weightlifters that incorporate deep squats into their training routine have even been shown to have higher knee stability compared to controls (Chandler *et al.* 1989). Provided that deep squats can be performed with proper form, they are not contraindicated for soccer players that have no existing knee pathology.

Deep and parallel squats may even reduce the risk of injury by using lighter weights. During quarter squats excessive weight has to be lifted to provide a training stimulus. These high loads increase the axial loading and compressive forces on the lumbar spine, which increases shear forces and intradiscal pressure (Cappozzo *et al.* 1985; Hartmann *et al.* 2012; Schmidt *et al.* 2007). Even novice lifters can handle loads of up to four times their body weight during quarter squats (Hartmann *et al.* 2012). Such a high load places an extremely high demand on the lower back extensors to stabilize the spine. Rather than the legs, the lower back would limit performance during the quarter squat (Hartmann *et al.* 2012). The overload and training effect for the legs is therefore limited during quarter squats (Hartmann *et al.* 2012). Strict partial-range squat training does not provide an adequate lower body hypertrophy and strength stimulus and compromises the transfer to athletic performance (Bloomquist *et al.* 2013; Hartmann *et al.* 2012; Raastad *et al.* 2008; Weiss *et al.* 2000).

To maximize the speed-strength ability and athletic performance deep or parallel squats need to be included into training (Bloomquist *et al.* 2013; Hartmann *et al.* 2012). The better transfer to athletic performance with deep squat compared to quarter squat training is in contrast with the concept of superior angle-specific transfer, which states that strength training performed in the range of motion of competition enhances sport-specific power gains (Hartmann *et al.* 2012).

Deep and parallel squats provide better neural and tension stimuli to the knee and hip extensors, which results in greater hypertrophy, strength, and power gains (Bloomquist *et al.* 2013; Bryanton *et al.* 2012; Gorsuch *et al.* 2013; Hartmann *et al.* 2012; Raastad *et al.* 2008; Weiss *et al.* 2000). The higher movement velocities and activation level of the leg extensor muscles during deep squats compared to partial squats result in an enhanced fast-twitch muscle fiber recruitment (Bryanton *et al.* 2012; Drinkwater *et al.* 2012; Gorsuch *et al.* 2013; Wakeling *et al.* 2006). Architectural changes induced by deep squat training could also explain the higher transfer into speed-strength performance. Full range-of-motion training results in the addition of sarcomeres in series (Blazevich *et al.* 2007; McMahon *et al.* 2014; Seynnes *et al.* 2007). Muscles with longer fascicle lengths can contract faster because a greater number of contractile elements can shorten simultaneously, which will benefit the rate of force development (Huijbregts and Clarijs 1995; Jones and Round 1990).

The higher muscle activation and excitation during parallel squats also induce a greater post-activation potentiation effect compared to partial squats (Esformes *et al.* 2013). Parallel squats enhance subsequent jumping performance to a greater extent than partial squats (Esformes *et al.* 2013). When strength training incorporates ballistic or plyometric exercises, deep or parallel squats should be favored because they enhance the subsequent power performance more than partial squats (Esformes *et al.* 2013).

6.2 Jump, athletic, and power-lifting stance

Squats can be performed using various stance widths and foot positions. The lifter can choose between a jump stance (feet between hip- and shoulder-width apart and toes pointing forward), an athletic stance (feet slightly wider than shoulder-width and toes pointing forward), and a power-lifting stance (feet wider than shoulder-width apart and toes pointing outward). Gluteus maximus and hip adductor activity progressively increase with an increasing stance width (McCaw and Melrose 1999; Paoli *et al.* 2009). Contrary to what is commonly believed, a narrower stance does not enhance quadriceps activity (McCaw and Melrose 1999). The relative contribution of the hip adductors during the squat progressively increases by externally rotating the hips (pointing feet outward) (Pereira *et al.* 2010).

Squatting with a power-lifting stance is less specific to sports, but assures a more upright trunk position and requires less mobility at the ankle joint (Escamilla *et al.* 2001; Swinton *et al.* 2012). The power-lifting stance favors more activity from the gluteus maximus and hip adductors while the jump and athletic stance resemble frequently encountered positions during soccer and can therefore maximize the transfer to athletic performance.

6.3 Exercises

Back squat

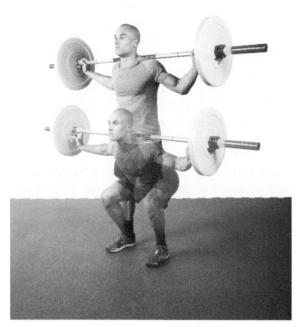

FIGURE 6.1   Back squat

OBJECTIVE

The back squat (Figure 6.1) promotes lower body and posterior core strength and develops the foundation for more sport-specific training. A good strength level in the squat exercise contributes significantly to athletic performance.

STARTING POSITION

Position a bar on the back of the shoulders. Grab the bar with a pronated grip and raise the elbows to provide a secure location for the bar.

Choose between a jump stance, an athletic stance, or a power-lifting stance.

Keep the torso erect and the core tight. Look straight ahead.

EXECUTION

Descend with control. Keep the body weight centered over the heel and mid-foot. Keep the heels in contact with the floor throughout the descent.

Squat back up by extending the knees and hips.

COACHING KEYS

Descend in a controlled manner when squatting. Prevent bouncing out of the bottom position.

The knees should point in the same direction as the feet throughout the movement. Do not let the knees sway in.

Let the knees move slightly in front of the toes during the descent. Keep the heels in contact with the floor. Restricting the knees to move in front of the toes results in a more anterior lean of the trunk to maintain the center of gravity within the foot base (Fry *et al.* 2003). This may minimize the stress on the knees, but forces are inappropriately transferred to the hip and lower back region (Fry *et al.* 2003). Excessive forward lean of the trunk during the back squat is a common error for novice lifters. Performing the back squat in a power-lifting stance can be a good alternative to assure proper positioning of the trunk when there is restricted mobility at the ankles.

Front squat

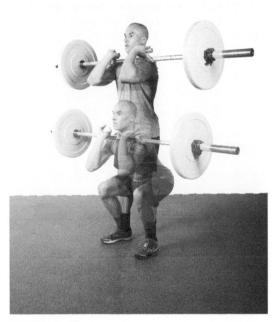

FIGURE 6.2 Front squat

OBJECTIVE

Compared with the back squat, the front squat (Figure 6.2) is performed with less hip flexion and forward inclination of the trunk (Fry *et al.* 1993). Less weight can be lifted during the front squat, due to a less favorable moment arm (Gullett *et al.* 2009; Hartmann *et al.* 2012). Due to the reduced training load in combination with a more erect trunk position, the front squat places less compressive and shear forces on the spine compared to the back squat (Cappozzo *et al.* 1985;

Escamilla *et al.* 2000). Muscle activity is not different however between the front and back squat. The front squat is an excellent alternative to the more frequently used back squat, to maximally challenge the leg extensor muscles while decreasing joint loads (Gullett *et al.* 2009).

STARTING POSITION

Set up a bar at chest level in a squat or power rack.

Grab the bar slightly wider than shoulder-width. Rotate the elbows around the bar and lift the elbows up and forward to position the bar on front of the shoulders.

Assume a jump stance.

EXECUTION

Squat down, keeping the body weight centered over the heel and mid-foot. Keep the heels in contact with the floor throughout the descent.

Squat back up.

COACHING KEYS

Keep the trunk as erect as possible and the elbows high throughout the entire movement.

When you have limited flexibility at the wrists you can opt to use a cross-arm grip. Another option is to loop lifting straps around the bar.

Overhead squat

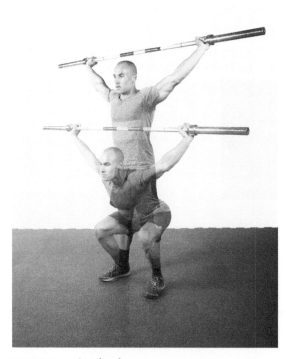

FIGURE 6.3 Overhead squat

OBJECTIVE

Incorporating the overhead squat (Figure 6.3) in your training or warm-up will promote core strength, stability, balance, and flexibility. It requires good dynamic flexibility in the upper and lower back, hips, ankles, and shoulders and optimal stability throughout the spine.

STARTING POSITION

The exercise can be performed with a dowel or a barbell.

To determine the appropriate grip width, measure the distance from the outside edge of the shoulder to the knuckles of the opposite arm, which is abducted parallel to the floor. Assume an athletic or jump stance.

Snatch the bar overhead or press it overhead to get into the starting position.

Keep the torso erect and the core tight. Look straight ahead.

EXECUTION

Keep the body weight centered over the heel and mid-foot and keep the heels in contact with the floor throughout the descent.

Squat back up by pushing through the heel and mid-foot.

COACHING KEYS

Maintain the bar aligned over the ankle joint throughout the entire movement.

Good ankle, hip, back, and shoulder flexibility and a correct squat and overhead press technique will facilitate to perform the overhead squat with proper form.

Jump squat

OBJECTIVE

The jump squat (Figure 6.4) is a ballistic squat exercise to improve lower body power and movement velocity (Jones *et al.* 2001; McBride *et al.* 2002). At the end of the range of motion the body is projected. Jumping out allows greater force and power production later during the squat movement because the load can be accelerated over a larger trajectory compared to a traditional squat (Newton *et al.* 1996). Low-to-moderate load squat jump training improves power production and movement velocity through an enhanced recruitment of high-threshold motor units and synchronization of peak muscle activation (Cormie *et al.* 2007; Cronin and Sleivert 2005; Harris *et al.* 2007; Jones *et al.* 2001; McBride *et al.* 2002; Sale 1992). Athletes with adequate strength levels show poor improvement in speed-strength ability as a response to traditional weight training. The principle of velocity specificity dictates that low-load/high-speed movements are required to further improve the velocity component of power (Jones *et al.* 2001; Kaneko *et al.* 1983; McBride *et al.* 2002; Morrissey *et al.* 1995; Wilson *et al.* 1993).

STARTING POSITION

Position a bar on the back of the shoulders.

Assume a jump stance.

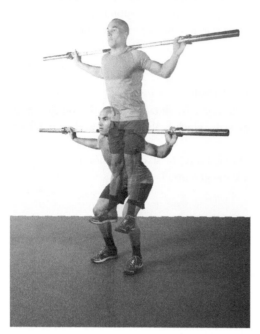

FIGURE 6.4   Jump squat

EXECUTION

Squat down to a knee angle between 110 and 150 degrees. Keep the body weight centered over the heel and mid-foot. Keep the heels in contact with the floor throughout the descent. Quickly turn around the movement at the bottom position to squat back up as explosively as possible and jump out.

On landing, lower your body back into the squat position.

COACHING KEYS

The highest power outputs for the jump squat are seen with loads between 10 percent and 45 percent of a 1RM squat (Jones *et al.* 2001; Stone *et al.* 2003; Wilson *et al.* 1993). The percentage of 1RM at which peak power occurs seems to depend on the maximal strength level of the athlete (Stone *et al.* 2003). Stronger athletes produce peak power output at higher percentages of 1RM compared to athletes with a less developed strength base (Stone *et al.* 2003).

References

Blazevich AJ, Cannavan D, Coleman DR, Horne S. Influence of concentric and eccentric resistance training on architectural adaptation in human quadriceps muscles. *J Appl Physiol (1985)*. 2007 Nov;103(5):1565–75.

Bloomquist K, Langberg H, Karlsen S, Madsgaard S, Boesen M, Raastad T. Effect of range of motion in heavy load squatting on muscle and tendon adaptations. *Eur J Appl Physiol.* 2013 Aug;113(8):2133–42.

Bryanton MA, Kennedy MD, Carey JP, Chiu LZ. Effect of squat depth and barbell load on relative muscular effort in squatting. *J Strength Cond Res.* 2012 Oct;26(10):2820–8.

Cappozzo A, Felici F, Figura F, Gazzani F. Lumbar spine loading during half-squat exercises. *Med Sci Sports Exerc.* 1985 Oct;17(5):613–20.

Chandler TJ, Wilson GD, Stone MH. The effect of the squat exercise on knee stability. *Med Sci Sports Exerc.* 1989 Jun;21(3):299–303.

Clark DR, Lambert MI, Hunter AM. Muscle activation in the loaded free barbell squat: a brief review. *J Strength Cond Res.* 2012 Apr;26(4):1169–78.

Comfort P, Bullock N, Pearson SJ. A comparison of maximal squat strength and 5-, 10-, and 20-meter sprint times, in athletes and recreationally trained men. *J Strength Cond Res.* 2012 Apr;26(4):937–40.

Cormie P, Deane R, McBride JM. Methodological concerns for determining power output in the jump squat. *J Strength Cond Res.* 2007 May;21(2):424–30.

Cormie P, McGuigan MR, Newton RU. Adaptations in athletic performance after ballistic power versus strength training. *Med Sci Sports Exerc.* 2010 Aug;42(8):1582–98.

Cronin J, Sleivert G. Challenges in understanding the influence of maximal power training on improving athletic performance. *Sports Med.* 2005;35(3):213–34.

Cunningham DJ, West DJ, Owen NJ, Shearer DA, Finn CV, Bracken RM, Crewther BT, Scott P, Cook CJ, Kilduff LP. Strength and power predictors of sprinting performance in professional rugby players. *J Sports Med Phys Fitness.* 2013 Apr;53(2):105–11.

Drinkwater EJ, Moore NR, Bird SP. Effects of changing from full range of motion to partial range of motion on squat kinetics. *J Strength Cond Res.* 2012 Apr;26(4):890–6.

Escamilla RF, Lander JE, Garhammer J. Biomechanics of powerlifting and weightlifting exercises. In: Garrett WE, Kirkendall DT, editors. *Exercise and sport science.* Philadelphia: Lippincott, Williams & Wilkins; 2000. pp. 585–615.

Escamilla RF, Fleisig GS, Zheng N, Lander JE, Barrentine SW, Andrews JR, Bergemann BW, Moorman CT 3rd ed. Effects of technique variations on knee biomechanics during the squat and leg press. *Med Sci Sports Exerc.* 2001 Sep;33(9):1552–66.

Esformes JI, Bampouras TM. Effect of back squat depth on lower-body postactivation potentiation. *J Strength Cond Res.* 2013 Nov;27(11):2997–3000.

Fry AC, Aro TA, Bauer JA, Kraemer WJ. A comparison of methods for determining kinematic properties of three barbell squat exercises. *J Hum Move Stud.* 1993;24:83–95.

Fry AC, Smith JC, Schilling BK. Effect of knee position on hip and knee torques during the barbell squat. *J Strength Cond Res.* 2003 Nov;17(4):629–33.

Gorsuch J, Long J, Miller K, Primeau K, Rutledge S, Sossong A, Durocher JJ. The effect of squat depth on multiarticular muscle activation in collegiate cross-country runners. *J Strength Cond Res.* 2013 Sep;27(9):2619–25.

Gullett JC, Tillman MD, Gutierrez GM, Chow JW. A biomechanical comparison of back and front squats in healthy trained individuals. *J Strength Cond Res.* 2009 Jan;23(1):284–92.

Harris NK, Cronin JB, Hopkins WG. Power outputs of a machine squat-jump across a spectrum of loads. *J Strength Cond Res.* 2007 Nov;21(4):1260–4.

Hartmann H, Wirth K, Klusemann M, Dalic J, Matuschek C, Schmidtbleicher D. Influence of squatting depth on jumping performance. *J Strength Cond Res.* 2012 Dec;26(12):3243–61.

Hartmann H, Wirth K, Klusemann M. Analysis of the load on the knee joint and vertebral column with changes in squatting depth and weight load. *Sports Med.* 2013 Oct;43(10):993–1008.

Huijbregts PA, Clarijs JP. *Krachttraining in revalidatie en sport.* Utrecht: De Tijdstroom; 1995. 175 pp.

Hunter JP, Marshall RN, McNair PJ. Relationships between ground reaction force impulse and kinematics of sprint-running acceleration. *J Appl Biomech.* 2005 Feb;21(1):31–43.

Jones D, Round D. *Skeletal muscle in health and disease.* Manchester: Manchester University Press; 1990. 224 pp.

Jones K, Bishop P, Hunter G, Fleisig G. The effects of varying resistance-training loads on intermediate- and high-velocity-specific adaptations. *J Strength Cond Res.* 2001 Aug;15(3):349–56.

Kaneko M, Fuchimoto T, Toji H, Suei K. Training effect of different loads on the force-velocity relationship and mechanical power output in human muscle. *Scand J Med Sci Sports.* 1983;5:50–5.

Klein K. The deep squat exercise as utilized in weight training for athletes and its effects on the ligaments of the knee. *J Assoc Phys Ment Rehabil.* 1961;15:6–11.

Li G, Zayontz S, Most E, DeFrate LE, Suggs JF, Rubash HE. In situ forces of the anterior and posterior cruciate ligaments in high knee flexion: an in vitro investigation. *J Orthop Res.* 2004 Mar;22(2):293–7.

López-Segovia M, Marques MC, van den Tillaar R, González-Badillo JJ. Relationships between vertical jump and full squat power outputs with sprint times in u21 soccer players. *J Hum Kinet.* 2011 Dec;30:135–44.

López-Segovia M, Dellal A, Chamari K, González-Badillo JJ. Importance of muscle power variables in repeated and single sprint performance in soccer players. *J Hum Kinet.* 2014 Apr;40:201–11.

McBride JM, Triplett-McBride T, Davie A, Newton RU. The effect of heavy- vs. light-load jump squats on the development of strength, power, and speed. *J Strength Cond Res.* 2002 Feb;16(1):75–82.

McBride JM, Blow D, Kirby TJ, Haines TL, Dayne AM, Triplett NT. Relationship between maximal squat strength and five, ten, and forty yard sprint times. *J Strength Cond Res.* 2009 Sep;23(6):1633–6.

McCaw ST, Melrose DR. Stance width and bar load effects on leg muscle activity during the parallel squat. *Med Sci Sports Exerc.* 1999 Mar;31(3):428–36.

McCurdy K, Walker J, Armstrong R, Langford G. The relationship between selected measures of strength and hip and knee excursion during unilateral and bilateral landings in females. *J Strength Cond Res.* 2014 Jun 17. [Epub ahead of print]

McMahon GE, Morse CI, Burden A, Winwood K, Onambélé GL. Impact of range of motion during ecologically valid resistance training protocols on muscle size, subcutaneous fat, and strength. *J Strength Cond Res.* 2014 Jan;28(1):245–55.

Morrissey MC, Harman EA, Johnson MJ. Resistance training modes: specificity and effectiveness. *Med Sci Sports Exerc.* 1995 May;27(5):648–60.

Newton RU, Kraemer WJ, Hakkinen K, Humphries BJ, Murphy AJ. Kinematics, kinetics, muscle activation during explosive upper body movements: implications for power development. *J Appl Biomech.* 1996 Feb;12(1):31–43.

Paoli A, Marcolin G, Petrone N. The effect of stance width on the electromyographical activity of eight superficial thigh muscles during back squat with different bar loads. *J Strength Cond Res.* 2009 Jan;23(1):246–50.

Pereira GR, Leporace G, Chagas Dd, Furtado LF, Praxedes J, Batista LA. Influence of hip external rotation on hip adductor and rectus femoris myoelectric activity during a dynamic parallel squat. *J Strength Cond Res.* 2010 Oct;24(10):2749–54.

Raastad T, Karlsen S, Madsgaard S, Boesen M, Langberg H. Effects of heavy strength training with deep or shallow squats on muscle cross sectional area and muscle function. In: Cabri J, Alves F, Araújo D, Barreiros J, Diniz J, Veloso A, editors. *Proceedings of the 13th Annual Congress of the European College of Sport Science*; 2008 July 9–12; Estoril, Portugal. Cologne, Germany: European College of Sport Science; 2008. p. 515. [The training period comprised 12 weeks: personal communication from Prof. Dr. Raastad on Jan 18 2009.]

Sale DG. Neural adaptations to strength training. In: Komi PV, editor. *Strength and power in sport.* Oxford: Blackwell Scientific; 1992. pp. 249–60.

Schmidt H, Kettler A, Heuer F, Simon U, Claes L, Wilke HJ. Intradiscal pressure, shear strain, and fiber strain in the intervertebral disc under combined loading. *Spine (Phila Pa 1976).* 2007 Apr;32(7):748–55.

Seynnes OR, de Boer M, Narici MV. Early skeletal muscle hypertrophy and architectural changes in response to high-intensity resistance training. *J Appl Physiol (1985).* 2007 Jan;102(1):368–73.

Steiner ME, Grana WA, Chillag K, Schelberg-Karnes E. The effect of exercise on anterior-posterior knee laxity. *Am J Sports Med.* 1986 Jan–Feb;14(1):24–9.

Stone MH, O'Bryant HS, McCoy L, Coglianese R, Lehmkuhl M, Schilling B. Power and maximum strength relationships during performance of dynamic and static weighted jumps. *J Strength Cond Res.* 2003 Feb;17(1):140–7.

Swinton PA, Lloyd R, Keogh JW, Agouris I, Stewart AD. A biomechanical comparison of the traditional squat, powerlifting squat, and box squat. *J Strength Cond Res.* 2012 Jul;26(7):1805–16.

Wakeling JM, Uehli K, Rozitis AI. Muscle fiber recruitment can respond to the mechanics of the muscle contraction. *J R Soc Interface.* 2006 Aug 22;3(9):533–44.

Weiss LW, Fry AC, Wood LE, Relyea GE, Melton C. Comparative effects of deep versus shallow squat and leg-press training on vertical jumping ability and related factors. *J Strength Cond Res.* 2000 Aug;14(3):241–7.

Weyand PG, Sternlight DB, Bellizzi MJ, Wright S. Faster top running speeds are achieved with greater ground forces not more rapid leg movements. *J Appl Physiol (1985).* 2000 Nov;89(5):1991–9.

Wilson GJ, Newton RU, Murphy AJ, Humphries BJ. The optimal training load for the development of dynamic athletic performance. *Med Sci Sports Exerc.* 1993 Nov;25(11):1279–86.

Wisløff U, Castagna C, Helgerud J, Jones R, Hoff J. Strong correlation of maximal squat strength with sprint performance and vertical jump height in elite soccer players. *Br J Sports Med.* 2004 Jun;38(3):285–8.

7

SINGLE-LEG KNEE DOMINANT EXERCISES

The squat has a high carry-over to jumping and sprinting and improves athletic performance. Sports however are single-leg dominant in nature. During running and sprinting the body is propelled forward through powerful single-leg actions. Single-leg exercises that involve simultaneous knee and hip extension are therefore even more sport-specific than bilateral squats.

The single-leg stance places a high demand on the quadratus lumborum of the opposite side and on the hip abductors, hip external rotators, and vastus medialis obliquus of the supporting leg to stabilize the pelvis and knee. Weakness of any of these muscles causes the pelvis to tilt and the knee of the supporting leg to drift inward during single-leg support, creating an overload on the lumbar spine, sacroiliac joint, and increasing the knee valgus angle and torque.

The generated forces during sprinting, single-leg landings, and jumps multiply body weight several times, placing a very high demand on stabilization. Single-leg exercises are therefore an important part of the program to enhance athletic performance and prevent injuries. Unilateral ground-based exercises improve single-leg stability and balance and assure balanced leg strength development.

The category of single-leg knee dominant movements consists of exercises that require movement at the knee joint through a big range of motion. Although the range of motion may be greater at the knee compared to the hip joint, the joint moments at the hip may be far greater than those at the knee. From a kinetic point of view, exercises such as the lunge and single-leg squat can therefore be considered as hip dominant movements.

7.1 The step-up

The step-up exercise is an effective exercise to strengthen the knee extensors, hip extensors, and abductors (Lubahn *et al.* 2011). Step-ups are a good way to start with single-leg training, to develop single-leg strength and balance.

A combination of lateral and crossover step-ups adds a lateral and rotational component to the movement, increasing strength and balance in all three planes of motion.

The lateral step-up places a greater demand on the knee extensors and ankle plantar flexors, while the forward step-up loads the hip extensors more (Simenz *et al.* 2012; Wang *et al.*

2003). While the forward step-up requires greater gluteus maximus activation, the lateral and crossover step-up elicit greater gluteus medius activation (Mercer *et al.* 2009; Simenz *et al.* 2012). The gluteus medius is considered to play an important role to stabilize the pelvis and prevent hip adduction and maintaining proper thigh alignment during functional activity (Hamstra-Wright and Huxel Bliven 2012).

Forward step-up

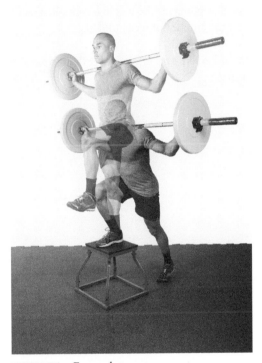

FIGURE 7.1 Forward step-up

OBJECTIVE

The forward step-up (Figure 7.1) is a good beginner exercise to start with unilateral strength training and to strengthen the lateral system.

STARTING POSITION

Stand facing a box.

The height of the box should be approximately knee height, so your thigh is parallel to the floor in the starting position.

Keep your back upright in neutral alignment.

EXECUTION

The exercise can be performed with a barbell or dumbbells.

Step up placing the whole foot on the box.

Ascend by fully extending the lead leg. Avoid hyperextension.

In the top position balance on the lead leg. Do not let the foot of the trail leg touch the box.

Descend with a controlled eccentric contraction.

Keep the lead foot on the box until you complete the desired number of repetitions, then switch sides.

COACHING KEYS

Descend with a controlled eccentric contraction. If stepping off the box in a controlled manner is not possible, lower the height of the box or the amount of weight lifted.

Do not cheat by pushing off with the foot on the ground.

Do not let the knee of the front leg move inward. Make sure it tracks over the second and third toe, staying well aligned between hip and ankle.

Lateral step-up

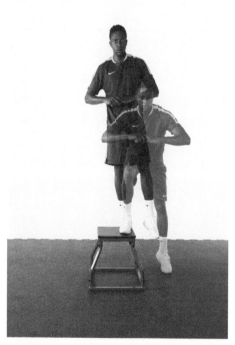

FIGURE 7.2   Lateral step–up

OBJECTIVE

Compared to the forward step–up, the lateral step–up (Figure 7.2) places a greater demand on the knee extensors and ankle plantar flexors. The range of motion at the ankle joint is greater during the lateral step–up compared to the forward step–up.

STARTING POSITION

Stand to the left-hand side of the box.

EXECUTION

Step up laterally with the right foot onto the box.
   Ascend by fully extending the right leg.
   Balance on the right leg in the top position.
   Step back off the box with the left leg, maintaining the right foot on the box.
   Keep the right foot on the box until you complete the desired number of repetitions, then switch sides.

COACHING KEYS

Make sure the heel of the lead foot stays on the box.

Crossover and lateral step-up

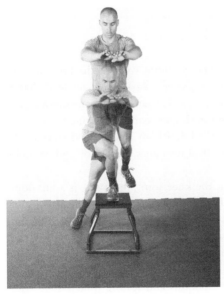 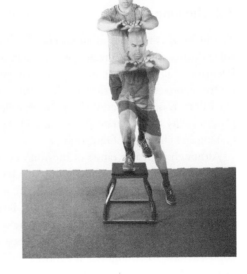

FIGURE 7.3   Crossover and lateral step-up

OBJECTIVE

A combination of lateral and crossover step-ups (Figure 7.3) adds a rotational component to the movement. The movement addresses all three planes of movement and is biomechanically very similar to the lateral movements so frequently seen in soccer.

STARTING POSITION

Stand to the left-hand side of a box.

The height of the box should be approximately knee height, so your thigh is parallel to the floor in the starting position. You can also choose to use a lower box, so joint angles approximate the angles worked at in soccer.

EXECUTION

Step across the body with the left foot up onto a box.

Ascend by fully extending the left leg.

In the top position balance on the left leg. Do not let the right foot touch the box.

Step laterally off the box with the right leg.

Repeat the movement in the opposite direction, leading with the left foot, for the desired number of repetitions.

COACHING KEYS

Other variations in which the lead leg is alternated are also possible: lateral step-up and crossover step-off, lateral step-up and lateral step-off, crossover step-up and crossover step-off. With all these variations the athlete crosses over the box from one side to the other on each repetition.

7.2 The lunge

The lunge is considered as an eccentric exercise. The eccentric work at the knee and the ankle during a lunge is greater than the amount of concentric work (Jönhagen *et al.* 2009b; Riemann *et al.* 2012). The negative movement has to be decelerated and turned into a concentric contraction to return to the starting position. Implementing the lunge into training will increase the energy-absorbing capacity of the lower body muscles and enhance the player's ability to decelerate movements. This is excellent for injury prevention and promotes braking and changing of direction.

Although a greater range of motion occurs at the knee joint, the lunge is a hip dominant exercise from a kinetic point of view (Dwyer *et al.* 2010; Farrokhi *et al.* 2008; Flanagan *et al.* 2004; Riemann *et al.* 2012). Joint moments are far greater at the hip compared to the knee (Flanagan *et al.* 2004; Riemann *et al.* 2012). Performing lunges with additional weight will further increase the relative contribution of the hip extensors and ankle plantar flexors compared to the knee extensors (Riemann *et al.* 2012). It is also a good exercise to strengthen the vastus medialis obliquus and restore preferential vastus medialis obliquus/vastus lateralis ratio (Ekstrom *et al.* 2007; Irish *et al.* 2010). The load on the anterior cruciate ligament is neglectable while performing the lunge. It is therefore a safe exercise to strengthen the lower body following anterior cruciate ligament replacement surgery. The lunge is also an effective exercise to load the long head of the biceps femoris, which is the affected muscle during the majority of hamstring strain-type injuries (Mendiguchia *et al.* 2013). Hamstring injury is often associated with inhibition and atrophy of the long head of the biceps femoris (Croisier *et al.* 2002; Silder *et al.* 2008). To counter this inhibition and selective atrophy of the biceps femoris, the lunge should form part of the training protocol for the prevention and rehabilitation of hamstring injuries (Mendiguchia *et al.* 2013).

To address more planes of motion the lunge can be performed in different directions. The lateral lunge is more difficult to perform than the forward lunge. It requires good ankle and hip adductor flexibility (Riemann *et al.* 2013). The contribution of the ankle plantar flexors and knee extensors is also greater during the lateral lunge, while the forward lunge places higher demands on the hip extensors (Riemann *et al.* 2013).

The incorporation of different lunge variations into training has been shown to increase hamstring strength and sprinting speed of young soccer players (Jönhagen *et al.* 2009a). The lunge variations are also a valuable tool to enhance ankle, hip flexor, and adductor flexibility.

Forward lunge

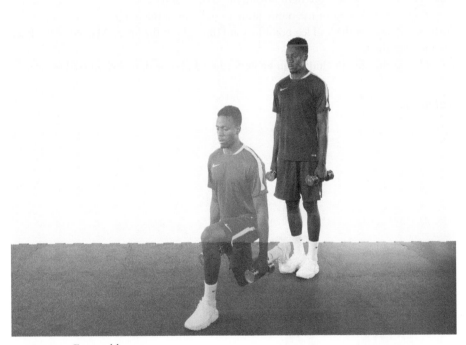

FIGURE 7.4   Forward lunge

OBJECTIVE

Increase the energy-absorbing capacity of the lower body muscles and enhance the player's ability to decelerate movements.

The forward lunge (Figure 7.4) can also be integrated in the dynamic warm-up to develop dynamic flexibility in the hip flexor muscles. Combining the lunge with trunk rotation over the lead leg or an overhead position of the arms will increase the pull on the fascial chain and will enhance the effectiveness of the stretch.

STARTING POSITION

The exercise can be performed with a barbell or dumbbells.

The feet should be hip-width apart and pointing forward.

The torso should remain erect.

EXECUTION

Take an elongated step straight forward with the lead leg.

Lower the body by flexing the knee and hip of front leg until the knee of the rear leg is almost in contact with the floor.

Return to the original standing position by forcefully pushing off the floor with the lead leg.

COACHING KEYS

Keep the torso erect and the core tight during the whole exercise.

Do not hinge at the waist or use momentum to pull out of the lunge.

The foot and knee of the lead leg point forward throughout the lunge. Make sure the knee stays in line with the foot.

To emphasize the core the lunge can be performed with one dumbbell instead of two.

Lateral lunge

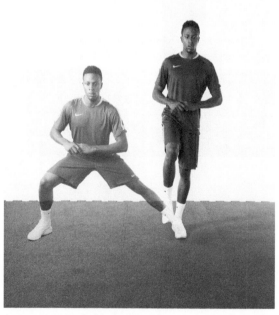

FIGURE 7.5   Lateral lunge

OBJECTIVE

Implementing the lateral lunge (Figure 7.5) into training will improve the player's cutting ability and lateral movement.

The lateral lunge is more difficult to perform than the forward lunge. The contribution of the ankle plantar flexors and knee extensors is greater during the lateral lunge compared to the forward lunge.

Development of dynamic flexibility in the adductor muscles of the hip. The lateral lunge also requires good ankle mobility.

STARTING POSITION

The lateral lunge is a challenging exercise, also without adding extra weight. The exercise can be performed with a barbell or dumbbells to add extra weight.

EXECUTION

Take an elongated step to one side with the lead leg.

The toe of the lead leg is pointing forward or is turned slightly out.

Lower the body by flexing the knee and hip of the lead leg, while keeping the other leg straight.

Return to the original standing position by forcefully pushing off the floor with the lead leg.

COACHING KEYS

Keep the foot and knee of the lead leg pointed in the same direction throughout the lunge.

Other lunge variations

RESISTED LUNGE

The ground reaction forces during the resisted lunge (Figure 7.6) are more horizontally oriented compared to the forward lunge, which will challenge the player more to brake the forward movement. The resisted lunge is highly reflective of decelerations and forward–backward changes of direction seen during soccer.

Set the cable column height to the lowest setting to enhance both horizontal and vertical ground reaction forces. Strap a belt around the waist and attach the cable of the cable column to the front of the belt. Because the resistance is applied directly to the waist, the resisted lunge requires a strong core to perform the exercise with correct technique.

WALKING LUNGE

Compared to the regular lunge, the walking lunge (Figure 7.7) has a more accelerative character, mimicking the muscle actions of acceleration during a sprint.

THREE-SPOT LUNGE

The three-spot lunge (Figure 7.8) combines a forward, transverse, and lateral lunge to enhance lower extremity strength and balance in all three planes of motion. The weight that can be handled

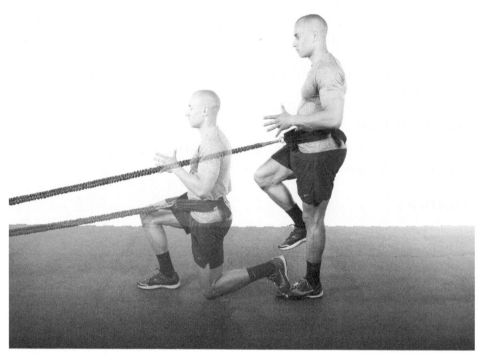

FIGURE 7.6 Resisted lunge

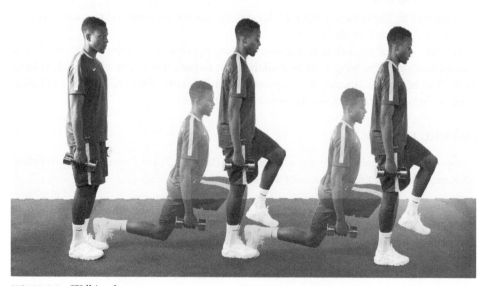

FIGURE 7.7 Walking lunge

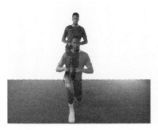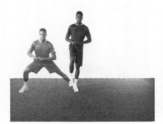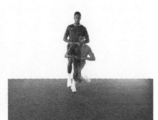

FIGURE 7.8   Three-spot lunge

during the forward lunge is significantly higher compared to the transverse and especially lateral lunge. The three-spot lunge may therefore be difficult to implement during the strength training, but can be perfectly incorporated into a dynamic warm-up to enhance overall hip mobility.

7.3 Single-leg squat progression

The single-leg squat is one of the most challenging lower body strengthening exercises. This exercise elicits a higher level of gluteus maximus and medius activation than the double-leg squat, lunge, or step-up (Ayotte *et al.* 2007; Boren *et al.* 2011; Boudreau *et al.* 2009; Lubahn *et al.* 2011). The hamstring/quadriceps co-activation ratio is also higher in the single-leg squat compared to the double-leg squat or lunge (Begalle *et al.* 2012; McCurdy *et al.* 2010).

It has been shown that subjects with weak hip and thigh muscles demonstrate higher knee valgus angles during running or single-leg landings, which is a potential source of lower extremity injury (Hamstra-Wright and Huxel Bliven 2012; Heinert *et al.* 2008; Leetun *et al.* 2004; McCurdy *et al.* 2014). Weight-bearing exercises are favored to strengthen these hip and thigh muscles due to the neuromuscular similarity to athletic movement (Hall and Brody 2004; Lubahn *et al.* 2011). Due to the unilateral base of support, the high activation levels of the hip and thigh muscles and sport-specific character, the single-leg squat is a key strengthening exercise to enhance performance and prevent injury. Executing the single-leg squat with proper form may improve recruitment and force production of the hip muscles during functional and sport-specific movements (Hall and Brody 2004; Lubahn *et al.* 2011). It has been shown that performance of the single-leg squat is related to performance of tasks such as running and cutting (Alenezi *et al.* 2014; Atkin *et al.* 2014). If a player shows poor motion during the single-leg squat, it is probable he also has increased knee valgus angles across other athletic movements such as running, cutting, and single-leg landings (Alenezi *et al.* 2014; Atkin *et al.* 2014).

The single-leg squat is a more advanced exercise, but can be mastered through the single-leg squat progression, in which each subsequent exercise places a higher demand on the lateral system in order to control pelvic positioning and alignment of the stance-leg.

Split squat

OBJECTIVE

The split squat (Figure 7.9) is a beginner exercise to develop single-leg strength and balance.

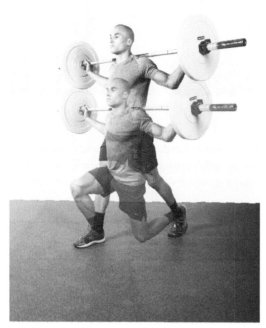

FIGURE 7.9   Split squat

STARTING POSITION

The exercise can be performed with a barbell or dumbbells.
   Keep your back upright in neutral alignment.
   For a good balance distribute the weight as evenly as possible over both feet.
   Toes are pointing forward.

EXECUTION

Squat down.
   Keep the torso erect during the whole exercise.

COACHING KEYS

Squat straight down. Avoid driving the hips forward.
   While squatting down make sure the front knee doesn't go over the toes, and avoid touching the floor with the back knee.
   Avoid the knee of the supporting leg moving inward. Make sure it tracks over the second and third toe, staying well aligned between hip and ankle.

Bulgarian split squat

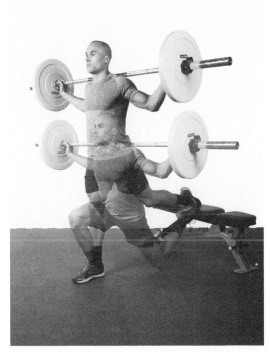

FIGURE 7.10   Bulgarian split squat

OBJECTIVE

Compared to the split squat, there is only one stable point of support. This makes it harder to perform the exercise in good balance.

The Bulgarian split squat (Figure 7.10) can also contribute to an enhanced range of motion of the hip flexors.

STARTING POSITION

Stand facing away from a bench. Extend your leg back and place your foot on the bench. The exercise can be performed with a barbell or dumbbells.

EXECUTION

Squat down by flexing the knee and hip of the front leg until the rear knee almost touches the floor or the thigh is parallel to the floor.

Keep the torso erect during the whole exercise.

COACHING KEYS

Make sure the knee does not move beyond the toes when squatting down and up. Minimize the movement at the ankle.

Single-leg squat

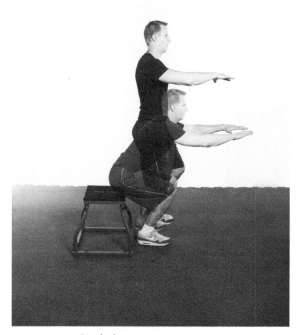

FIGURE 7.11 Single-leg squat

OBJECTIVE

The single-leg squat (Figure 7.11) is an intermediate exercise to develop single-leg strength. The exercise is performed on one leg, without the assistance of the second leg for stability and balance. The single-leg squat places a high proprioceptive demand on the body.

STARTING POSITION

Stand facing away from a bench or a wall.
    Lift one foot from the floor.

EXECUTION

Squat down and back.
    When squatting down keep the heel on the floor. Minimize the movement at the ankle.

Make contact with the bench or box and squat back up using only the leg you are balancing on.

COACHING KEYS

Make contact with the bench or box. Do not sit down, so you hold the contraction.

Single-leg box squat

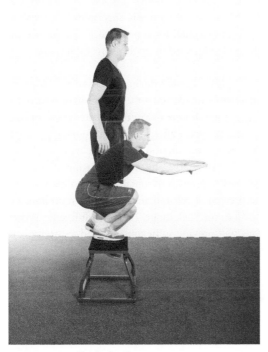

FIGURE 7.12 Single-leg box squat

OBJECTIVE

The single-leg box squat (Figure 7.12) is an advanced exercise. Because of the bigger range of motion compared to the single-leg squat, more strength and balance are required to be able to perform this exercise.

STARTING POSITION

Assume a single-leg stance on a box.

EXECUTION

Squat down by flexing the knee. Keep the heel on the bench.

As you squat down, raise your arms to shoulder height as a counterbalance.

Squat down until the thigh is parallel to the floor. Then squat back up using only the leg you are balancing on.

COACHING KEYS

Keep the knee of the supporting leg well aligned between the hip and toes.

7.4 Resisted slide-board back lunge or front pull

Due to the unilateral base of support and the forceful simultaneous hip and knee extension, the resisted slide-board back lunge (Figure 7.13) is biomechanically similar to locomotion. The resisted slide-board back lunge also requires horizontal force production. Similar to the leg action during sprinting, the body has to be pulled forward through a forceful simultaneous hip and knee extension.

The biceps femoris and gluteal muscles are highly recruited during this exercise (Hopkins *et al.* 1999). Biceps femoris inhibition is often a consequence and/or a root cause of hamstring injury. Inhibition of the gluteus maximus can change muscle recruitment patterns and place a higher load on the hamstrings. Upon returning to soccer after hamstring injury, players are slower and show reduced horizontal force and power production (Mendiguchia *et al.* 2014). The resisted slide-board back lunge targets the biceps femoris, improves intermuscular coordination between the glutes and hamstrings, and requires horizontal force production and should therefore form part of any program to prevent or rehabilitate hamstring strain injuries. The movement during the front pull is identical to the back lunge. The only difference is that the resistance is applied to the swing leg. This will provide sufficient overload to strengthen the hip flexors and also places a higher demand on the core muscles to counteract the forces of the hip flexors.

The resisted back lunge is identical to the resisted slide-board back lunge. Because it is harder to maintain balance during the resisted back lunge it is more difficult to provide sufficient overload.

Resisted slide-board back lunge

OBJECTIVE

The resisted slide-board back lunge has a high carry-over to sprinting.

Implementing the resisted slide-board back lunge into training will help strengthen the biceps femoris and gluteal muscles and can enhance the intermuscular coordination between the glutes and hamstrings to improve performance and prevent injury.

STARTING POSITION

Wear a slide-board bootie on the back foot and position it on the slide-board.

Strap the belt around the waist.

Set the cable column height to the lowest setting.

Attach the cable of the cable column to the back of the belt.

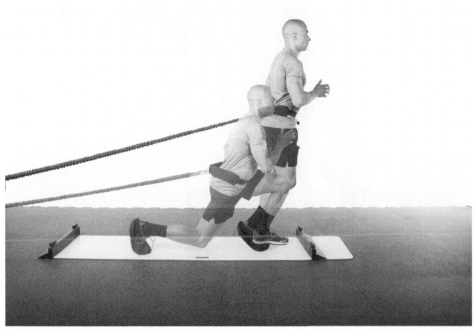

FIGURE 7.13   Resisted slide-board back lunge

EXECUTION

Slide the back foot backwards until the back knee almost touches the slide-board.

Return to the starting position by performing a single-leg squat movement with the front leg.

COACHING KEYS

Keep the torso erect and the core tight during the whole exercise.

If a slide-board is not available, the exercise can be performed with the back foot on a towel. The towel will minimize the friction with the gym floor.

The resisted slide-board back lunge can also be performed with the front foot elevated on a step for a bigger range of motion.

Front pull

OBJECTIVE

The front pull (Figure 7.14) requires good anti-rotation and anti-extension core function. While the slide-board back lunge places a higher load on the lower body, exercise pull exercises requires a stronger activation of the hip flexor and core muscles.

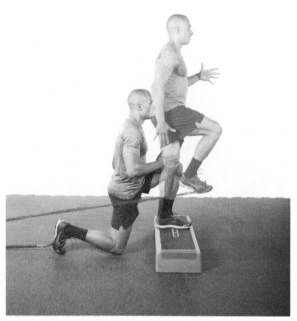

FIGURE 7.14   Front pull

STARTING POSITION

Wrap an ankle strap around the right ankle.

Set the cable column height to the lowest setting and attach the cable of the cable column to the ankle strap.

Face away from the cable column. Assume a split stance, with the forward foot (left foot) placed on a step or low box.

EXECUTION

Step up onto the box while raising the right knee to hip height.

Descend with a controlled eccentric contraction and repeat for the prescribed number of repetitions.

COACHING KEYS

Place the whole foot on the step or box.

In the top position balance on the lead leg. Do not let the foot of the trail leg touch the box.

7.5 Single-leg squat variations

Performing the single-leg squat with increased forward inclination of the trunk at mid-point may enhance the activity of the hip and back extensor muscles.

Single-leg squat and reach

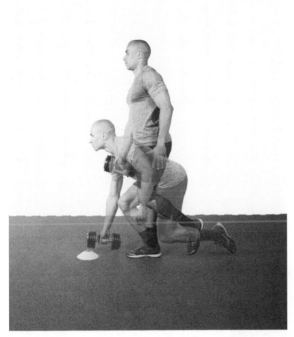

FIGURE 7.15 Single-leg squat and reach

OBJECTIVE

Compared to the single-leg squat, the single-leg squat and reach (Figure 7.15) has a bigger range of motion at the hip.

STARTING POSITION

Assume a single-leg stance.
  Hold a dumbbell in the opposite hand.

EXECUTION

Squat down and touch the floor or cone in front of you.
  If you perform the exercise without a dumbbell, touch the cone or floor with the opposite hand.

COACHING KEYS

Try to keep your back as neutrally aligned as possible. Focus on keeping your shoulders as high as possible. The emphasis has to be more on squatting than on leaning forward.

Avoid the knee of the supporting leg moving inward. Make sure the knee stays well aligned between hip and ankle.

Single-leg squat and reach around the clock

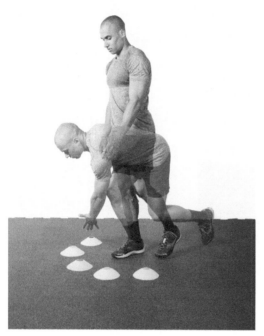

FIGURE 7.16 Single-leg squat and reach around the clock

OBJECTIVE

This exercise (Figure 7.16) incorporates rotation of the trunk over the femur. The hip rotation makes the exercise more multi-planar in nature compared to the single-leg squat and reach.

STARTING POSITION

Assume a single-leg stance, facing four or five cones or marks on the floor.

Hold a dumbbell in the opposite hand.

EXECUTION

Squat down and touch the first cone or mark on the floor.

Squat back up to the starting position.

Repeat the squat and reach at different points from 9 o'clock to 3 o'clock, making sure to come back to the starting position before touching another cone or mark.

COACHING KEYS

Focus on rotating the trunk toward the cone you have to touch. Rotating the torso toward the direction of travel is an important biomechanical factor related to cutting ability and should therefore if possible be emphasized during multiplanar strength exercises (Marshall *et al.* 2014).

7.6 Bulgarian split deadlift

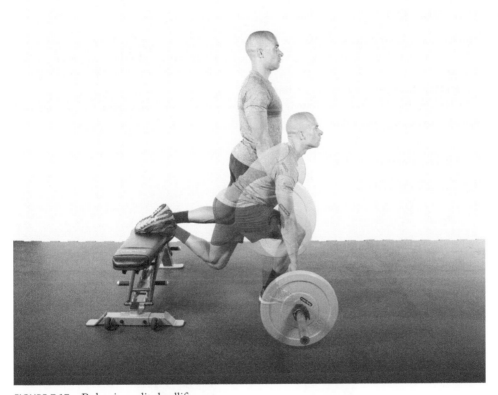

FIGURE 7.17   Bulgarian split deadlift

OBJECTIVE

The Bulgarian split deadlift (Figure 7.17) looks identical to the Bulgarian split squat, but the feeling on performing both exercises is different. The same load will probably seem heavier when performing the Bulgarian split deadlift. Compared to the Bulgarian split squat, the hip and back extensors are more engaged when performing the Bulgarian split deadlift.

STARTING POSITION

Stand facing away from a bench.

Place a barbell on the ground in front of you.

Extend your leg back and put your foot on the bench.

Grasp the barbell slightly wider than shoulder-width.

Stand tall with the back slightly arched and the shoulder blades retracted.

EXECUTION

Squat up by extending the knee and hip of the front leg.

Lower the barbell, to return to the starting position, by dropping the hip and flexing the knee.

COACHING KEYS

Simultaneously extend the knee and the hip.

Keep your chest up, your back slightly arched, and the core tight throughout the whole exercise.

Avoid any lateral movement at the hips.

Make sure the knee of the front leg tracks over the second and third toe, staying well aligned between hip and ankle.

7.7 Slide-board exercises

Slide-board lateral slide

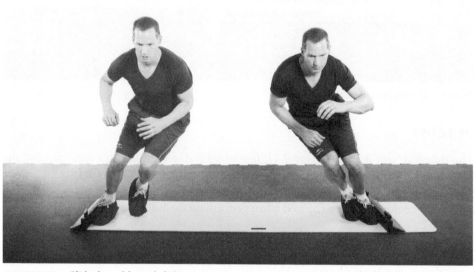

FIGURE 7.18 Slide–board lateral slide

OBJECTIVE

The slide-board lateral slide (Figure 7.18) is an excellent exercise to strengthen the hip extensors and abductors.

Besides the hip abductors and extensors, the hip adductors also play an important role during skating movements. The slide-board lateral slide requires a substantial eccentric contraction of the hip adductor muscles (Chang *et al.* 2009).

The slide-board lateral slide promotes lateral change of direction strength and power.

Including lateral slides into the rehabilitation program following ACL reconstruction has also been shown to boost knee extension strength gains (Blanpied *et al.* 2000).

STARTING POSITION

Put the slide-board booties on both feet.

Stand on one end of the slide-board with the outside of the foot against the block.

EXECUTION

Push off explosively and slide to the opposite side until the other foot hits the block.

Repeat for the prescribed number of repetitions or amount of time.

COACHING KEYS

Push off with a powerful extension of the hip, knee, and ankle.

Perform a fluid skating motion. Do not pause when hitting the block.

Slide-board lateral lunge

OBJECTIVE

The slide-board lateral lunge (Figure 7.19) is a single-leg squat variation that places a high eccentric emphasis on the hip adductors to decelerate the movement. It is an excellent ground-based exercise to eccentrically strengthen the hip adductor muscles and prevent groin injuries.

Development of dynamic flexibility in the adductor muscles of the hip.

STARTING POSITION

Stand with your feet hip-width apart, toes pointing forward. Wear a slide-board bootie on the left foot and position it on the slide-board.

EXECUTION

Lower the body by flexing the knee and hip of the right leg. Slide the left foot to the side. Keep the left leg straight.

Lower the body until the thigh of the supporting leg is parallel to the floor.

Return to the starting position by performing a single-leg squat movement with the right leg.

Perform the prescribed number of repetitions and then switch sides.

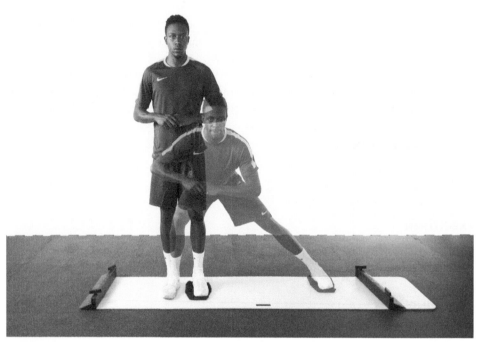

FIGURE 7.19   Slide-board lateral lunge

COACHING KEYS

Keep the torso erect and the core tight during the whole exercise.

If a slide-board is not available, the exercise can be performed with one foot on a towel. This will minimize the friction with the gym floor.

References

Alenezi F, Herrington L, Jones P, Jones R. Relationship between lower limb biomechanics during single leg squat with running and cutting tasks: a preliminary investigation. *Br J Sports Med*. 2014;48:560–1.

Atkin K, Herrington L, Alenezi F, Jones P, Jones R. The relationship between 2D knee valgus angle during single leg squat (SLS), single leg landing (SLL), and forward running. *Br J Sports Med*. 2014;48:563.

Ayotte NW, Stetts DM, Keenan G, Greenway EH. Electromyographical analysis of selected lower extremity muscles during 5 unilateral weight-bearing exercises. *J Orthop Sports Phys Ther*. 2007 Feb;37(2):48–55.

Begalle RL, Distefano LJ, Blackburn T, Padua DA. Quadriceps and hamstrings coactivation during common therapeutic exercises. *J Athl Train*. 2012 Jul–Aug;47(4):396–405.

Blanpied P, Carroll R, Douglas T, Lyons M, Macalisang R, Pires L. Effectiveness of lateral slide exercise in an anterior cruciate ligament reconstruction rehabilitation home exercise program. *J Orthop Sports Phys Ther*. 2000 Oct;30(10):602–8; discussion 609–11.

Boren K, Conrey C, Le Coguic J, Paprocki L, Voight M, Robinson TK. Electromyographic analysis of gluteus medius and gluteus maximus during rehabilitation exercises. *Int J Sports Phys Ther*. 2011 Sep;6(3):206–23.

Boudreau SN, Dwyer MK, Mattacola CG, Lattermann C, Uhl TL, McKeon JM. Hip-muscle activation during the lunge, single-leg squat, and step-up-and-over exercises. *J Sport Rehabil.* 2009 Feb;18(1):91–103.

Chang R, Turcotte R, Pearsall D. Hip adductor muscle function in forward skating. *Sports Biomech.* 2009 Sep;8(3):212–22.

Croisier J, Forthomme B, Namurois M, Vanderthommen M, Crielaard J. Hamstring muscle strain recurrence and strength performance disorders. *Am J Sports Med.* 2002 Mar–Apr;30(2):199–203.

Dwyer MK, Boudreau SN, Mattacola CG, Uhl TL, Lattermann C. Comparison of lower extremity kinematics and hip muscle activation during rehabilitation tasks between sexes. *J Athl Train.* 2010 Mar–Apr;45(2):181–90.

Ekstrom RA, Donatelli RA, Carp KC. Electromyographic analysis of core trunk, hip, and thigh muscles during 9 rehabilitation exercises. *J Orthop Sports Phys Ther.* 2007 Dec;37(12):754–62.

Farrokhi S, Pollard CD, Souza RB, Chen YJ, Reischl S, Powers CM. Trunk position influences the kinematics, kinetics, and muscle activity of the lead lower extremity during the forward lunge exercise. *J Orthop Sports Phys Ther.* 2008 Jul;38(7):403–9.

Flanagan SP, Wang MY, Greendale GA, Azen SP, Salem GJ. Biomechanical attributes of lunging activities for older adults. *J Strength Cond Res.* 2004 Aug;18(3):599–605.

Hall CM, Brody LT. *Therapeutic exercise: moving toward function.* 2nd ed. Philadelphia, PA: Lippincott Williams & Wilkins; 2004. 488 pp.

Hamstra-Wright KL, Huxel Bliven K. Effective exercises for targeting the gluteus medius. *J Sport Rehabil.* 2012 Aug;21(3):296–300.

Heinert BL, Kernozek TW, Greany JF, Fater DC. Hip abductor weakness and lower extremity kinematics during running. *J Sport Rehabil.* 2008 Aug;17(3):243–56.

Hopkins JT, Ingersoll CD, Sandrey MA, Bleggi SD. An electromyographic comparison of 4 closed chain exercises. *J Athl Train.* 1999 Oct;34(4):353–7.

Irish SE, Millward AJ, Wride J, Haas BM, Shum GL. The effect of closed-kinetic chain exercises and open-kinetic chain exercise on the muscle activity of vastus medialis oblique and vastus lateralis. *J Strength Cond Res.* 2010 May;24(5):1256–62.

Jönhagen S, Ackermann P, Saartok T. Forward lunge: a training study of eccentric exercises of the lower limbs. *J Strength Cond Res.* 2009a May;23(3):972–8.

Jönhagen S, Halvorsen K, Benoit DL. Muscle activation and length changes during two lunge exercises: implications for rehabilitation. *Scand J Med Sci Sports.* 2009b Aug;19(4):561–8.

Leetun DT, Ireland ML, Willson JD, Ballantyne BT, Davis IM. Core stability measures as risk factors for lower extremity injury in athletes. *Med Sci Sports Exerc.* 2004 Jun;36(6):926–34.

Lubahn AJ, Kernozek TW, Tyson TL, Merkitch KW, Reutemann P, Chestnut JM. Hip muscle activation and knee frontal plane motion during weight bearing therapeutic exercises. *Int J Sports Phys Ther.* 2011 Jun;6(2):92–103.

McCurdy K, O'Kelley E, Kutz M, Langford G, Ernest J, Torres M. Comparison of lower extremity EMG between the 2-leg squat and modified single-leg squat in female athletes. *J Sport Rehabil.* 2010 Feb;19(1):57–70.

McCurdy K, Walker J, Armstrong R, Langford G. The relationship between selected measures of strength and hip and knee excursion during unilateral and bilateral landings in females. *J Strength Cond Res.* 2014 Jun 17. [Epub ahead of print]

Marshall BM, Franklyn-Miller AD, King EA, Moran KA, Strike SC, Falvey ÉC. Biomechanical factors associated with time to complete a change of direction cutting maneuver. *J Strength Cond Res.* 2014 Oct;28(10):2845–51.

Mendiguchia J, Garrues MA, Cronin JB, Contreras B, Los Arcos A, Malliaropoulos N, Maffulli N, Idoate F. Nonuniform changes in MRI measurements of the thigh muscles after two hamstring strengthening exercises. *J Strength Cond Res.* 2013 Mar;27(3):574–81.

Mendiguchia J, Samozino P, Martinez-Ruiz E, Brughelli M, Schmikli S, Morin JB, Mendez-Villanueva A. Progression of mechanical properties during on-field sprint running after returning to sports from a hamstring muscle injury in soccer players. *Int J Sports Med.* 2014 Jul;35(8):690–5.

MercerVS, Gross MT, Sharma S,Weeks E. Comparison of gluteus medius muscle electromyographic activity during forward and lateral step-up exercises in older adults. *Phys Ther.* 2009 Nov;89(11):1205–14.

Riemann BL, Lapinski S, Smith L, Davies G. Biomechanical analysis of the anterior lunge during 4 external-load conditions. *J Athl Train.* 2012 Jul–Aug;47(4):372–8.

Riemann B, Congleton A,Ward R, Davies GJ. Biomechanical comparison of forward and lateral lunges at varying step lengths. *J Sports Med Phys Fitness.* 2013 Apr;53(2):130–8.

Silder A, Heiderscheit BC,Thelen DG, Enright T,Tuite MJ. MR observations of long-term musculotendon remodeling following a hamstring strain injury. *Skeletal Radiol.* 2008;37:1101–9.

Simenz CJ, Garceau LR, Lutsch BN, Suchomel TJ, Ebben WP. Electromyographical analysis of lower extremity muscle activation during variations of the loaded step-up exercise. *J Strength Cond Res.* 2012 Dec;26(12):3398–405.

Wang MY, Flanagan S, Song JE, Greendale GA, Salem GJ. Lower-extremity biomechanics during forward and lateral stepping activities in older adults. *Clin Biomech (Bristol, Avon).* 2003 Mar;18(3):214–21.

8

HIP DOMINANT LEG EXERCISES

The hip dominant exercises strengthen the posterior chain. The posterior chain consists of the hamstrings, gluteal, and lower back muscles. A strong posterior chain will help maintain proper lower body alignment, stabilize the knee, pelvis, and lower back, and can prevent many injuries of the lower extremities and lower back.

The hip dominant exercise group also comprises exercises that target the hip adductor muscles. The hip adductor muscles are stressed substantially in soccer, especially during cutting, changing of direction, and kicking actions (Charnock *et al.* 2009).

8.1 Romanian deadlift

OBJECTIVE

The Romanian deadlift (Figure 8.1) strengthens the posterior chain. The gluteus muscles, hamstrings, and adductor magnus are strengthened dynamically while synergistically working together to extend the hips.

The Romanian deadlift is a very effective exercise to strengthen the hamstring muscle group. The activity of the different hamstring muscles is maximized during the Romanian deadlift (McAllister *et al.* 2014; Wright *et al.* 1999; Zebis *et al.* 2013).

The lower back extensors are strengthened isometrically. Rounding the back during the Romanian deadlift puts the lower back at risk for injuries. The weight that has to be lifted, to properly stress the hamstrings and gluteus, is too high to be handled safely with a rounded back. By maintaining an arched back throughout the entire movement, the extensor muscles of the back function as stabilizers. Performing this exercise with good technique will make the lower back stronger.

Development of dynamic flexibility in the hamstring muscles.

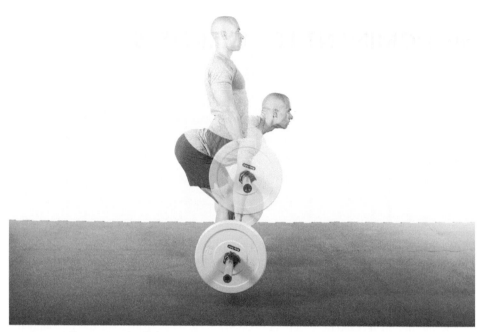

FIGURE 8.1   Romanian deadlift

STARTING POSITION

Hold a barbell in an overhand grip in front of the thighs. Keep the elbows straight.
   Stand with the feet hip-width apart.
   Keep the back straight and the torso tight. Look straight ahead.
   The shoulder blades are retracted.

EXECUTION

Lower the upper body by bending at the hips. Keep the back straight.
   Slide the bar down the thighs and shins. Push the hips back and slightly bend the knees during the descent.
   Lower the bar until a mild stretch is felt in the hamstrings.
   Return to the starting position.

COACHING KEYS

Focus on pushing the hips back and not on bending at the hips.
   The movement occurs at hip level. Keep the spine neutrally aligned throughout the entire exercise. By flexing the knees to about 20° the back can be maintained in an arched position while the trunk is lowered until it is almost parallel to the floor.

8.2 Single-leg Romanian deadlift

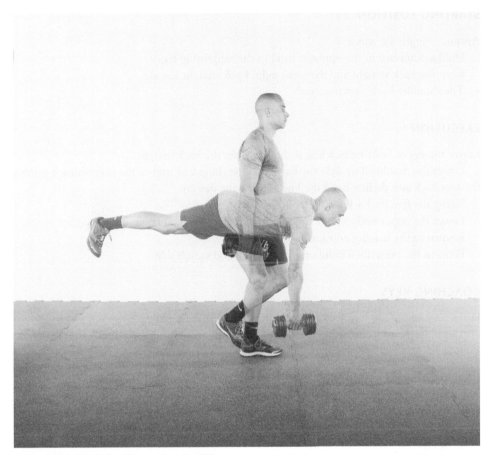

FIGURE 8.2   Single-leg Romanian deadlift

OBJECTIVE

The single-leg Romanian deadlift (Figure 8.2) strengthens the posterior chain. The gluteus maximus, medius, and hamstring muscles are highly active during this exercise (Begalle *et al.* 2012; Boren *et al.* 2011; Distefano *et al.* 2009; Ebben 2009).

Opar *et al.* (2012) suggested that the single-leg Romanian deadlift promotes eccentric hamstring strength at longer muscle lengths. This seems a coherent conclusion because the exercise is more challenging towards the end range of motion as momentum increases. The eccentric activity of the different hamstring muscles has also been shown to be higher in the Romanian deadlift compared to other hamstring exercises (McAllister *et al.* 2014).

The single-leg stance requires greater stability and balance and makes the exercise more sport-specific. The hip abductors and external rotators together with the vastus medialis obliquus and medial hamstrings are required to stabilize the pelvis and the knee of the supporting leg while the movement is performed.

Development of dynamic flexibility in the hamstring muscles.

STARTING POSITION

Assume a single-leg stance.
  Hold a dumbbell in the opposite hand of the supporting leg.
  Keep the back straight and the torso tight. Look straight ahead.
  The shoulder blades are retracted.

EXECUTION

Lower the upper body by bending at the hip. Keep the back straight.
  Lower the dumbbell or slide the bar down the thigh and shin of the supporting leg. Push the hips back and slightly bend the knee during the descent.
  Swing the free leg back so it stays in line with the torso.
  Lower the upper body until a mild stretch is felt in the hamstrings.
  Return to the starting position.
  Perform the prescribed number of repetitions and switch sides.

COACHING KEYS

Focus on pushing the hips back and not on bending at the hips.
  The movement occurs at hip level. Keep the spine neutrally aligned throughout the entire exercise.

8.3 Nordic hamstring exercise

OBJECTIVE

The Nordic hamstring exercise (Figure 8.3) is very effective to eccentrically strengthen the hamstring muscles. This exercise has been shown to elicit a strong activation of the short and long head of the biceps femoris muscle, which is the main muscle affected during hamstring strain injuries (Ditroilo et al. 2013; Ebben 2009; Koulouris and Connell 2003; Mendiguchia et al. 2013; Woods et al. 2004). A lack of eccentric hamstring strength, inhibition and atrophy of the long head of the biceps femoris predispose the player to hamstring injury and recurrence (Brockett et al. 2004; Brughelli et al. 2009; Croisier et al. 2002; Sanfilippo et al. 2013; Silder et al. 2008; Sole et al. 2011). The two heads of the biceps femoris are innervated separately (Williams and Warwick 1980). A lack of coordination between the two heads of the biceps femoris reduces the strength and energy-absorbing capacity of the muscle and increases the risk of injury (Sutton 1984; Woods et al. 2004; Zuluaga et al. 1995). The Nordic hamstring exercise can improve the intermuscular coordination between both heads of the biceps femoris and enhance the energy-absorbing capacity of the hamstring muscles.
  The Nordic hamstring exercise also changes the optimal length of the hamstrings, so they can produce greater forces at longer muscle lengths, reducing the susceptibility to strain injury (Brockett et al. 2001, 2004; Brughelli et al. 2009, 2010; Seynnes et al. 2007). The hamstrings function at long lengths during sprinting (Chumanov et al. 2012; Petersen and Hölmich

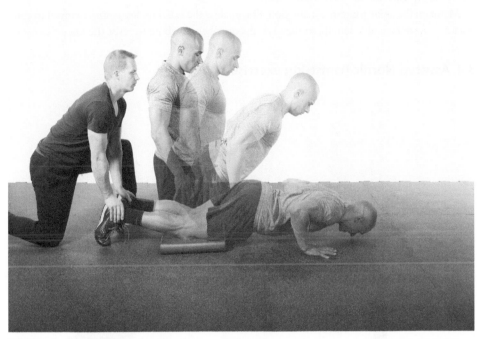

FIGURE 8.3   Nordic hamstring exercise

2005). Shifting the length-tension curve and increasing the end-range strength of the hamstrings prevents fibers from reaching a length where they are susceptible to tearing (Brughelli *et al.* 2010).

Implementing the Nordic hamstring exercise into the training program has been shown to substantially reduce the incidence (60 percent) and recurrence (85 percent) of hamstring injuries of soccer players (Thorborg 2012).

STARTING POSITION

Kneel tall, placing the knees on a balance pad or other soft surface.

Anchor the ankles under a stable object.

Keep the back straight and the torso tight. Look straight ahead.

EXECUTION

Lower yourself through a controlled extension of the knees.

When the chest touches the floor, forcefully extend the arms to return to the starting position.

COACHING KEYS

Keep the hips extended throughout the entire exercise.

Lower the body in a controlled manner throughout the entire range of motion. Try to avoid a sharp increase in downward velocity.

Maintain the ankle joint in dorsiflexion. This enables the calf muscles (gastrocnemius) to contract at a more favorable length, so they can maximally contribute to resist the knee extension.

8.4 Assisted Nordic hamstring exercise

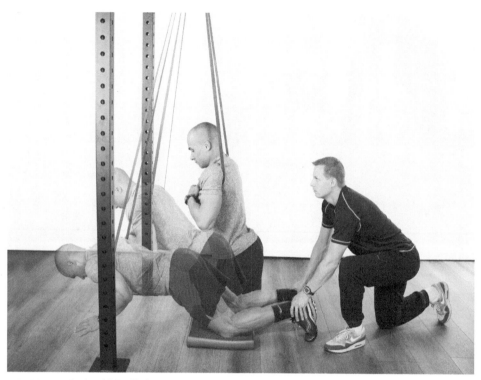

FIGURE 8.4 Assisted Nordic hamstring exercise

OBJECTIVE

The Nordic hamstring exercise is effective to reduce the risk of hamstring strain injury because it increases the end-range eccentric hamstring strength. Muscle activity is highest during the mid-phase of the movement (60–31°) and remains elevated towards a more extended knee position (0–30°) (Iga *et al.* 2012). The difficulty level of the Nordic hamstring exercise is more advanced however. Players with poor eccentric hamstring strength may therefore be unable to lower the body in a controlled manner during the Nordic hamstring exercise. The higher the speed at which the body is lowered, the lower will be the activation level of the hamstring muscles (Ditroilo *et al.* 2013). If the player has poor eccentric hamstring strength, the sharp increase in velocity will also occur earlier in the movement trajectory. Performing the exercise with a high movement speed may therefore be ineffective to enhance the eccentric hamstring strength at longer muscle lengths. The assisted Nordic hamstring exercise (Figure 8.4) enables a more progressive increment of the exercise intensity. The slower movement speed during the assistant Nordic hamstring exercise probably also results in increased hamstring activation at elongated muscle lengths, facilitating a shift in optimal muscle length.

STARTING POSITION

Kneel tall, placing the knees on a balance pad or other soft surface.

Anchor the ankles under a stable object.

Attach an elastic band to a stable object above (or above and behind) you. Strap the band around the chest.

Keep the back straight and the torso tight. Look straight ahead.

EXECUTION

Lower yourself through a controlled extension of the knees.

When the chest touches the floor, forcefully extend the arms to return to the starting position.

COACHING KEYS

Once you are able to perform 12–15 repetitions, with a controlled speed throughout the entire range of motion, progress to the Nordic hamstring exercise.

8.5 Back extension

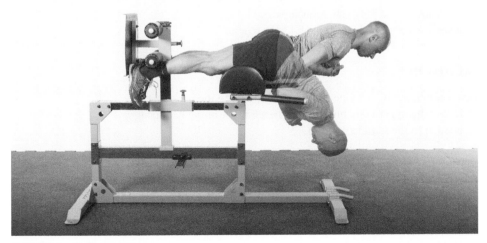

FIGURE 8.5 Back extension

OBJECTIVE

The back extension (Figure 8.5) strengthens the entire posterior chain. To strongly engage all posterior chain muscles, the exercise should be performed with the upper thigh on the edge of the couch. If the movement during the back extension occurs at the hip joint and the torso remains stable, the force output from gluteus maximus and hamstring muscles is far greater compared to executing the back extension with the pelvis stabilized and movement taking place at the back (Graves *et al.* 1994; Mayer *et al.* 2003; Pollock *et al.* 1989). Paraspinal muscle activation is also high when the exercise is performed with the spine maintained in neutral alignment throughout the entire exercise (Arokoski *et al.* 1999; Clark *et al.* 2002). This will emphasize the postural role of the paraspinal muscles and the coupling between the biceps femoris, gluteus maximus, and paraspinal muscles. The deeper low back muscles are better adapted to fulfill a specific stabilizing role (Clark *et al.* 2002; De Ridder *et al.* 2013; Macintosh and Bogduk 1987; Panjabi *et al.* 1989).

By increasing the exercise intensity during the back extension, the force production of the gluteus maximus and hamstring muscles augments to a greater extend compared to the paraspinal muscles (Clark *et al.* 2002; Ploutz-Snyder *et al.* 2001). Due to the high relative percentage of type I fibers, the deep lumbar extensors accommodate less to an increasing load (Clark *et al.* 2002; Mannion *et al.* 1997; Thorstensson and Carlson 1987). To specifically address the deep lumbar muscles, increasing the number of repetitions may be more effective than increasing the load (Clark *et al.* 2002). Performing the exercise with the legs fixed in a horizontal position or with an accentuated lumbar lordosis will further increase activation of the lumbar extensors (Mayer *et al.* 1999, 2002).

Stabilizing the pelvis during the back extension will isolate the lumbar area and can further increase the potential to strengthen the back extensor muscles (Graves *et al.* 1994; Pollock *et al.* 1989). This will however minimize the hip–spine coupling and train the back extensors as prime movers.

STARTING POSITION

Lie face down on a back extension apparatus.
    Raise the upper body until the body is straight.

EXECUTION

Lower the upper body by bending at the hips. Keep the back straight.
    Lower the upper body until a mild stretch is felt in the hamstrings.
    Return to the starting position.

COACHING KEYS

The movement occurs at hip level. Keep the spine neutrally aligned throughout the entire exercise.
    Keep the head neutrally aligned with the spine.
    Hold a weight plate behind the head or in front of the chest to add difficulty.

8.6 Single-leg back extension

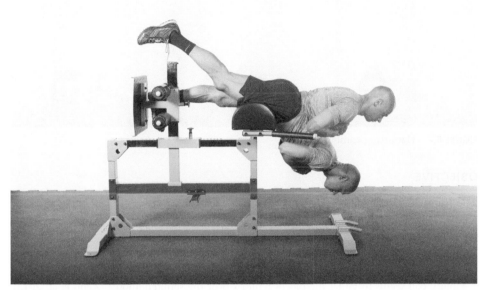

FIGURE 8.6   Single-leg back extension

OBJECTIVE

During the single-leg back extension (Figure 8.6) the body's center of gravity is located medially from the axis of rotation. The posterior core does not only have to generate movement
but also has to stabilize the pelvis and trunk in the transverse plane of motion to resist the
gravitational torque. This need to stabilize against rotation elicits a strong multifidus contraction and a more appropriate stability pattern (Richardson *et al.* 1990; Sahrmann 2002; Valencia
and Munro 1985).

STARTING POSITION

Fix one leg under the heel pad.

EXECUTION

Lower the upper body by bending at the hips until a stretch is felt in the hamstrings. Keep
the back straight.

Return to the starting position.

Perform the required number of repetitions and switch sides.

COACHING KEYS

Keep the spine neutrally aligned throughout the entire exercise.
Avoid rotation at the hip or spine.

8.7 Hamstring combination

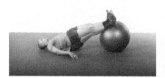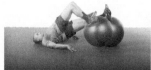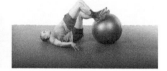

FIGURE 8.7   Hamstring combination

OBJECTIVE

The hamstring combination (Figure 8.7) consists of three hamstring strengthening exercises, which are performed in succession: the straight-leg hip extension, the leg curl, and the bent-knee hip extension.

During a machine leg curl the semitendinosus is loaded more than the biceps femoris (McAllister *et al.* 2014; Mendiguchia *et al.* 2013; Ono *et al.* 2010). Performing the leg curl using a stability ball seems to target the biceps femoris over the semitendinosus (Zebis *et al.* 2013). The machine leg curl isolates the hamstrings by only involving movement at the knee joint, while the stability ball leg curl incorporates the gluteus maximus to maintain the hip bridge position. The gluteus maximus and the long head of the biceps femoris are connected through the sacrotuberous ligament (Vleeming *et al.* 1989). The activity of the gluteus maximus during this exercise may facilitate a stronger biceps femoris contraction during the stability ball leg curl.

STARTING POSITION

Put your heels on the ball, keeping your legs straight.

EXECUTION

Lift the hips from the floor to a straight-body position. Lower your hips until the butt almost touches the floor. Repeat this first exercise for the prescribed number of repetitions.

Hold the end position of the first exercise. Curl the ball while the body is held straight. Repeat for the prescribed number of repetitions.

Hold the end position from the second exercise where the ball is curled. Lift your hips until extension. Perform the prescribed number of repetitions.

COACHING KEYS

Start with five repetitions for each exercise. Every week you can add two repetitions to each exercise.

8.8 Single-leg hamstring combination

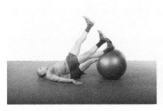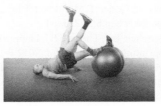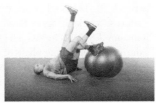

FIGURE 8.8   Single-leg hamstring combination

OBJECTIVE

The single-leg hamstring combination (Figure 8.8) strengthens the hamstrings and posterior core.

Performing the hamstring combination with only one leg doubles the hamstring load. The greater instability and need to resist the rotation from the pelvis and trunk also place a higher demand on the posterior core muscles.

STARTING POSITION

Put one heel on the ball, keeping your leg straight. Lift the other foot off the floor by bending at the hip and knee.

EXECUTION

Perform the three movements consecutively for the prescribed number of reps and switch legs.

COACHING KEYS

Start with five reps for each exercise. Every week you can add two reps to each exercise. When you reach fifteen reps for each exercise, the exercise can be performed with a weight plate on the chest.

References

Arokoski JP, Kankaanpää M, Valta T, Juvonen I, Partanen J, Taimela S, Lindgren KA, Airaksinen O. Back and hip extensor muscle function during therapeutic exercises. *Arch Phys Med Rehabil.* 1999 Jul;80(7):842–50.

Begalle RL, Distefano LJ, Blackburn T, Padua DA. Quadriceps and hamstrings coactivation during common therapeutic exercises. *J Athl Train.* 2012 Jul–Aug;47(4):396–405.

Boren K, Conrey C, Le Coguic J, Paprocki L, Voight M, Robinson TK. Electromyographic analysis of gluteus medius and gluteus maximus during rehabilitation exercises. *Int J Sports Phys Ther.* 2011 Sep;6(3):206–23.

Brockett CL, Morgan DL, Proske U. Human hamstring muscles adapt to eccentric exercise by changing optimum length. *Med Sci Sports Exerc.* 2001 May;33:783–90.

Brockett CL, Morgan DL, Porske U. Predicting hamstring strain injury in elite athletes. *Med Sci Sports Exerc.* 2004 Mar;36(3):379–87.

Brughelli M, Nosaka K, Cronin J. Application of eccentric exercise on an Australian rules football player with recurrent hamstring injuries. *Phys Ther Sport.* 2009 May;10(2):75–80.

Brughelli M, Cronin J, Mendiguchia J, Kinsella D, Nosaka K. Contralateral leg deficits in kinetic and kinematic variables during running in Australian rules football players with previous hamstring injuries. *J Strength Cond Res.* 2010 Sep;24(9):2539–44.

Charnock BL, Lewis CL, Garrett WE Jr, Queen RM. Adductor longus mechanics during the maximal effort soccer kick. *Sports Biomech.* 2009 Sep;8(3):223–34.

Chumanov ES, Schache AG, Heiderscheit BC, Thelen DG. Hamstrings are most susceptible to injury during the late swing phase of sprinting. *Br J Sports Med.* 2012 Feb;46(2):90.

Clark BC, Manini TM, Mayer JM, Ploutz-Snyder LL, Graves JE. Electromyographic activity of the lumbar and hip extensors during dynamic trunk extension exercise. *Arch Phys Med Rehabil.* 2002 Nov;83(11):1547–52.

Croisier J, Forthomme B, Namurois M, Vanderthommen M, Crielaard J. Hamstring muscle strain recurrence and strength performance disorders. *Am J Sports Med.* 2002 Mar–Apr;30(2):199–203.

De Ridder EM, Van Oosterwijck JO, Vleeming A, Vanderstraeten GG, Danneels LA. Posterior muscle chain activity during various extension exercises: an observational study. *BMC Musculoskelet Disord.* 2013 Jul 9;14(1):204.

Distefano LJ, Blackburn JT, Marshall SW, Padua DA. Gluteal muscle activation during common therapeutic exercises. *J Orthop Sports Phys Ther.* 2009 Jul;39(7):532–40.

Ditroilo M, De Vito G, Delahunt E. Kinematic and electromyographic analysis of the Nordic hamstring exercise. *J Electromyogr Kinesiol.* 2013 Oct;23(5):1111–18.

Ebben WP. Hamstring activation during lower body resistance training exercises. *Int J Sports Physiol Perform.* 2009 Mar;4(1):84–96.

Graves JE, Webb DC, Pollock ML, Matkozich J, Leggett SH, Carpenter DM, Foster DN, Cirulli J. Pelvic stabilization during resistance training: its effect on the development of lumbar extension strength. *Arch Phys Med Rehabil.* 1994 Feb;75(2):210–15.

Iga J, Fruer CS, Deighan M, Croix MD, James DV. 'Nordic' hamstrings exercise – engagement characteristics and training responses. *Int J Sports Med.* 2012 Dec;33(12):1000–4.

Koulouris G, Connell D. Evaluation of the hamstring muscle complex following acute injury. *Skeletal Radiol.* 2003 Oct;32(10):582–9.

McAllister MJ, Hammond KG, Schilling BK, Ferreria LC, Reed JP, Weiss LW. Muscle activation during various hamstring exercises. *J Strength Cond Res.* 2014 Jun;28(6):1573–80.

Macintosh JE, Bogduk N. The morphology of the lumbar erector spinae. *Spine (Phila Pa 1976).* 1987 Sep;12(7):658–68.

Mannion AF, Dumas GA, Cooper RG, Espinosa FJ, Faris MW, Stevenson JM. Muscle fibre size and type distribution in thoracic and lumbar regions of erector spinae in healthy subjects without low back pain: normal values and sex differences. *J Anat.* 1997 May;190 (Pt 4):505–13.

Mayer JM, Graves JE, Robertson VL, Pierra EA, Verna JL, Ploutz-Snyder LL. Electromyographic activity of the lumbar extensor muscles: effect of angle and hand position during Roman chair exercise. *Arch Phys Med Rehabil.* 1999 Jul;80(7):751–5.

Mayer JM, Verna JL, Manini TM, Mooney V, Graves JE. Electromyographic activity of the trunk extensor muscles: effect of varying hip position and lumbar posture during Roman chair exercise. *Arch Phys Med Rehabil.* 2002 Nov;83(11):1543–6.

Mayer JM, Udermann BE, Graves JE, Ploutz-Snyder LL. Effect of Roman chair exercise training on the development of lumbar extension strength. *J Strength Cond Res.* 2003 May;17(2):356–61.

Mendiguchia J, Arcos AL, Garrues MA, Myer GD, Yanci J, Idoate F. The use of MRI to evaluate posterior thigh muscle activity and damage during Nordic hamstring exercise. *J Strength Cond Res.* 2013 Dec;27(12):3426–35.

Ono T, Okuwaki T, Fukubayashi T. Differences in activation patterns of knee flexor muscles during concentric and eccentric exercises. *Res Sports Med.* 2010 Jul;18(3):188–98.

Opar DA, Williams MD, Shield AJ. Hamstring strain injuries: factors that lead to injury and re-injury. *Sports Med.* 2012 Mar;42(3):209–26.

Panjabi M, Abumi K, Duranceau J, Oxland T. Spinal stability and intersegmental muscle forces. A biomechanical model. *Spine (Phila Pa 1976).* 1989 Feb;14(2):194–200.

Petersen J, Hölmich P. Evidence based prevention of hamstring injuries in sport. *Br J Sports Med.* 2005 Jun;39(6):319–23.

Ploutz-Snyder LL, Mayer JM, Caruso R, Formikell M, Graves JE. The use of magnetic resonance imaging to evaluate lumbar muscle function during Roman chair trunk extension exercise. *Med Sci Sports Exerc.* 2001;33(5):S2351.

Pollock ML, Leggett SH, Graves JE, Jones A, Fulton M, Cirulli J. Effect of resistance training on lumbar extension strength. *Am J Sports Med.* 1989 Sep–Oct;17(5):624–9.

Richardson C, Toppenberg R, Jull G. An initial evaluation of eight abdominal exercises for their ability to provide stabilisation for the lumbar spine. *Aust J Physiother.* 1990;36(1):6–11.

Sahrmann S. *Diagnosis and treatment of movement impairment syndromes.* St Louis, MO: Mosby; 2002. 384 pp.

Sanfilippo JL, Silder A, Sherry MA, Tuite MJ, Heiderscheit BC. Hamstring strength and morphology progression after return to sport from injury. *Med Sci Sports Exerc.* 2013;45(3):448–54.

Seynnes OR, de Boer M, Narici MV. Early skeletal muscle hypertrophy and architectural changes in response to high-intensity resistance training. *J Appl Physiol (1985).* 2007 Jan;102(1):368–73.

Silder A, Heiderscheit BC, Thelen DG, Enright T, Tuite MJ. MR observations of long-term musculotendon remodeling following a hamstring strain injury. *Skeletal Radiol.* 2008 Dec;37(12):1101–9.

Sole G, Milosavljevic S, Nicholson HD, Sullivan SJ. Selective strength loss and decreased muscle activity in hamstring injury. *J Orthop Sports Phys Ther.* 2011 May;41(5):354–63.

Sutton G. Hamstrung by hamstring strains: a review of the literature. *J Orthop Sports Phys Ther.* 1984;5(4):184–95.

Thorborg K. Why hamstring eccentrics are hamstring essentials. *Br J Sports Med.* 2012 Jun;46(7):463–5.

Thorstensson A, Carlson H. Fibre types in human lumbar back muscles. *Acta Physiol Scand.* 1987 Oct;131(2):195–202.

Valencia FP, Munro RR. An electromyographic study of the lumbar multifidus in man. *Electromyogr Clin Neurophysiol.* 1985 May–Jun;25(4):205–21.

Vleeming A, Stoeckart R, Snijders CJ. The sacrotuberous ligament: a conceptual approach to its dynamic role in stabilizing the sacroiliac joint. *Clin Biomech.* 1989 Nov;4(4):201–3.

Williams PL, Warwick R. *Gray's anatomy.* 36th ed. Edinburgh: Churchill Livingstone; 1980. 1578 pp.

Woods C, Hawkins RD, Maltby S, Hulse M, Thomas A, Hodson A. The Football Association Medical Research Programme: an audit of injuries in professional football – analysis of hamstring injuries. *Br J Sports Med.* 2004 Feb;38(1):36–41.

Wright GA, Delong TH, Gehlsen G. Electromyographic activity of the hamstrings during performance of the leg curl, stiff-leg deadlift, and back squat movements. *J Strength Cond Res.* 1999 May;13(2):168–74.

Zebis MK, Skotte J, Andersen CH, Mortensen P, Petersen HH, Viskaer TC, Jensen TL, Bencke J, Andersen LL. Kettlebell swing targets semitendinosus and supine leg curl targets biceps femoris: an EMG study with rehabilitation implications. *Br J Sports Med.* 2013 Dec;47(18):1192–8.

Zuluaga M, Briggs C, Carlisle J, McDonald V. *Sports physiotherapy: applied science and practice.* 1st ed. Edinburgh: Churchill Livingstone; 1995. 544 pp.

9

UPPER BODY PRESS EXERCISES

The upper body pressing exercises include horizontal and vertical pressing. The horizontal pressing exercises strengthen the pectoralis major, triceps brachii, and anterior deltoid muscles. The vertical pressing exercises develop shoulder strength. Additionally the core and legs are engaged to stabilize the body when lifting overhead (Saeterbakken and Fimland 2012).

The horizontal pressing exercises can be further divided into three categories: bench press and variations, push-up and variations, and standing chest press exercises.

The bench press is the upper body exercise in which the highest amount of weight can be lifted. It is probably the most used exercise to evaluate and develop upper body strength (Padulo *et al.* 2014; Welsch *et al.* 2005). The bench press and variations are excellent exercises to create an overload on the upper body muscles to improve strength. Adding extra resistance to the push-up can induce similar levels of muscle activity and strength gains as the bench press exercise however (Calatayud *et al.* 2014). The push-up exercise also targets the abdominal muscles and can be used to considerably enhance the strength and function of the scapular and rotator cuff muscles (Andersen *et al.* 2012; Decker *et al.* 2003; Escamilla *et al.* 2009; Howarth *et al.* 2008; Ludewig *et al.* 2004). This advocates the use of push-ups in addition the bench press and its variations.

9.1 Bench press (barbell)

OBJECTIVE

The bench press (Figure 9.1) is the upper body exercise in which the highest amount of weight can be lifted. It is therefore an excellent exercise to create an overload on the upper body muscles to develop hypertrophy and strength (Santana *et al.* 2007).

STARTING POSITION

Lie supine on a bench, grasping a barbell slightly wider then shoulder-width.

Position your feet on the floor.

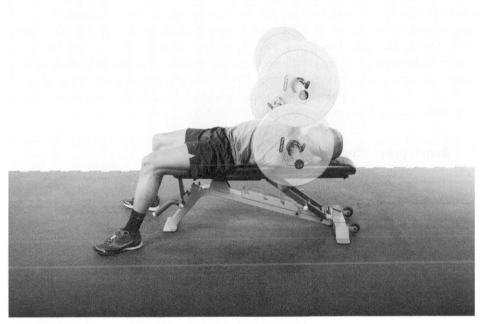

FIGURE 9.1 Bench press (barbell)

EXECUTION

Lift the barbell from the rack.

Lower the barbell to the middle of the chest.

Press the barbell back up until the elbows are fully extended.

On completing the prescribed number of repetitions return the barbell to the rack.

COACHING KEYS

Do not arch your back or lift the hips from the bench while pressing up.

Do not bounce the barbell off the chest at the bottom position.

The bench press can be performed with various inclination angles and hand positions. With a regular bench press grip the lifter grasps the bar with the upper arms abducted 90° relative to the trunk and a 90° angle at the elbows (Clemons and Aaron 1997). This grip width places the pectoralis major in favorable mechanical position to generate greater muscle force, while the triceps is also highly active (Clemons and Aaron 1997; Madsen and McLaughlin 1984). Wider grips should not be used for soccer or sports training. With increasing grip width the vertical distance from the chest to the bar reduces, decreasing the range of motion at the shoulder and elbow joints and compromising the optimal development of upper body pushing strength and explosiveness (Clemons and Aaron 1997; Lander *et al.* 1985). A closer grip is advisable for players with shoulder problems (Green and Comfort 2007). Reducing the grip width from a regular grip to a shoulder-width grip does not significantly affect the recruitment of the pectoralis major or anterior deltoid, but decreases the peak torque and stress occurring at the shoulder joint (Clemons and Aaron 1997; Fees *et al.* 1998; Green and Comfort 2007; Haupt 2001). For the close-grip bench press, grasp the barbell with a shoulder-width grip. This exercise emphasizes the clavicular head of the pectoralis major, the anterior deltoid, and the triceps muscles more compared to the regular bench press (barbell) (Barnett *et al.* 1995; Lehman 2005). During the incline bench press the activity of the anterior deltoid increases while the activity of the sternocostal head of the pectoralis major decreases, compared to the horizontal bench press (Barnett *et al.* 1995; Trebs *et al.* 2010). Greater angles of bench incline (45–60°) are required to enhance the recruitment of the clavicular head of the pectoralis major (Barnett *et al.* 1995; Glass and Armstrong 1997; Trebs *et al.* 2010).

9.2 Bench press (dumbbells)

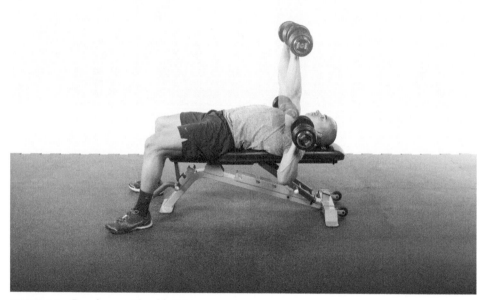

FIGURE 9.2   Bench press (dumbbells)

OBJECTIVE

Because the arms are used independently, training with dumbbells requires more coordination and stabilization (Saeterbakken *et al.* 2011). This means the shoulder-stabilizing muscles are more active during the dumbbell bench press (Figure 9.2) compared to the barbell bench press (Welsch *et al.* 2005). Due to the higher load that can be lifted, the barbell bench press is considered as the best exercise to develop upper body pushing strength and power (Welsch *et al.* 2005). The peak activation levels of the pectoralis major and anterior deltoid during the dumbbell bench press are equivalent to the levels observed during the barbell bench press however (Lander *et al.* 1985; Saeterbakken *et al.* 2011; Welsch *et al.* 2005). In a periodized training program, the dumbbell bench press can be used as an alternative to the barbell bench press to add training variation and challenge the upper body with a range of movements.

STARTING POSITION

Lie supine on a bench, holding dumbbells at the lateral sides of the chest, near the armpit.
Position your feet on the floor.

EXECUTION

Press the dumbbells up until the arms are fully extended.
Return to the starting position by lowering the dumbbells.

COACHING KEYS

Do not arch your back or lift the hips from the bench while pressing up.
Keep the forearms perpendicular to the floor throughout the movement.
Do not bounce the dumbbells off the chest at the bottom position.

9.3 Push-up

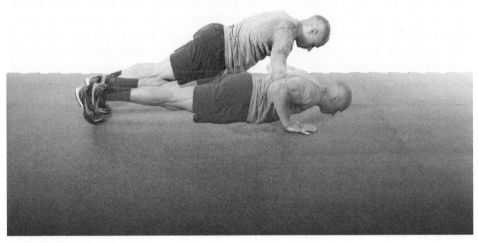

FIGURE 9.3 Push-up

OBJECTIVE

The push-up (Figure 9.3) is a great exercise to develop upper body pressing strength. In addition to loading the pectoralis major, anterior deltoid, and triceps brachii, it is also a valuable exercise to enhance core and shoulder stability (Beneka *et al*. 2002; Giannakopoulos *et al*. 2004; Howarth *et al*. 2008; Malliou *et al*. 2004). The rectus abdominis is the major contributor during the push-up to prevent hip sagging while the obliquus internus and externus prevent twisting and lateral bending (Howarth *et al.* 2008). The rotator cuff and scapular stabilizing muscles also exhibit higher activity levels during the push-up compared to other exercises (Andersen *et al.* 2012; Chulvi-Medrano *et al.* 2012; Decker *et al.* 2003; Escamilla *et al.* 2009). The push-up is unfairly considered by many however as an auxiliary exercise. More experienced lifters think too quickly that they have outgrown the push-up. The push-up however has multiple variations and progressions through which the intensity and difficulty of the exercise can be increased. The push-up can also be effectively loaded by placing a weight plate on the back or using elastic bands or a weight vest. It has been shown that a loaded push-up elicits similar levels of muscle activity and strength gains as the bench press exercise (Calatayud *et al.* 2014).

The push-up can also improve shoulder function and is commonly used in shoulder reha-bilitation (Beneka *et al.* 2002; Blievernicht 2000; Chulvi-Medrano *et al.* 2012; Giannakopoulos *et al.* 2004; Malliou *et al.* 2004). The push-up is a closed kinetic chain exercise (hands are fixed during the movement). The fixed position of the hands stimulates co-contraction of the mus-cles that act on the shoulder, which results in a greater joint stabilization capability (Dillman *et al.* 1994; Escamilla *et al.* 2009). Closed kinetic chain exercises also stimulate proprioception, favor joint congruence, and reduce shear forces (Kibler 2000; Tucci *et al.* 2011). People with shoulder pain or instability are associated with imbalances of the muscles that attach to the scapula (Cools *et al.* 2003; Page 2011). These muscle imbalances can alter the normal upward motion of the scapula and cause the compression of the supraspinatus tendon against the acromion during shoulder flexion and abduction (Cools *et al.* 2003; Page 2011). A common imbalance in people with shoulder instability is a strong upper part of the trapezius, compared to a weaker middle and lower part of the trapezius (Cools *et al.* 2003). Weakness of the serratus anterior is also often accompanied by overactivity of the upper trapezius due to compensa-tory action (Jeong *et al.* 2014; Lee *et al.* 2013; Ludewig *et al.* 2004; Lukasiewicz *et al.* 1999; Sahrmann 2002). Several authors suggest that these imbalances between the scapular muscles rather than global weakness of the scapulothoracic muscles are linked to altered scapular kin-ematics (Cools *et al.* 2005, 2007). To improve or restore shoulder function and stability, exer-cises and positions must be used that activate the lower trapezius, middle trapezius, and serratus anterior and minimally activate the upper trapezius (Andersen *et al.* 2012; Cools *et al.* 2005, 2007; Ludewig *et al.* 2004). It has been demonstrated that the push-up produces the strongest serratus anterior activation and the lowest upper trapezius/serratus anterior ratio from a range of exercises (Andersen *et al.* 2012; Ludewig *et al.* 2004). Increasing the intensity of the push-up by elevating the feet or applying external load will further augment serratus anterior activa-tion and reduce the upper trapezius/serratus anterior ratio (Andersen *et al.* 2012; Decker *et al.* 1999; Lear and Gross 1998; Ludewig *et al.* 2004). Next to exercise intensity, hand positioning during the push-up can also influence serratus anterior activation. Performing the push-up with the shoulder externally rotated (hands pointing lateral) further enhances serratus anterior activity (Lee *et al.* 2013; Yoon *et al.* 2010). A push-up training program has been shown to significantly increase serratus anterior activation and concomitantly reduce the neural activity of the upper trapezius in people with chronic shoulder pain (Choi 2008). This is in line with the recommendations of several other authors who stated that isolated movements are useful to strengthen weaker muscle groups, but to considerably enhance the strength and function of the entire rotator cuff, more compound and closed-kinetic chain exercises such as the push-up and pull-up are required (Beneka *et al.* 2002; Blievernicht 2000; Giannakopoulos *et al.* 2004; Malliou *et al.* 2004).

STARTING POSITION

Put your hands slightly wider than shoulder-width.

Keep the torso erect and the core tight. The knees and hips are extended and the spine is neutrally aligned.

EXECUTION

Lower your body by bending the arms until the chest touches the floor.

Return to the starting position by pushing the body up until the arms are fully extended.

COACHING KEYS

Make sure you perform the push-ups in the full range of motion with an erect torso and tight core. Avoid hip sagging.

To increase the intensity wear a weight vest or perform the push-up with a weight plate positioned on the back. Performing the push-up with the feet elevated onto a box or bench will also increase the exercise intensity.

9.4 Weight plate push-up

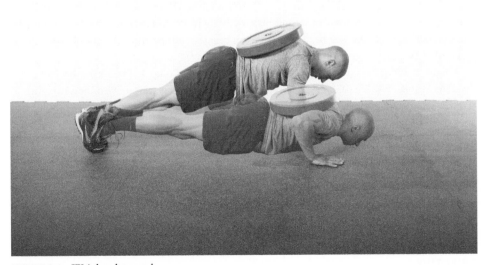

FIGURE 9.4 Weight plate push-up

TABLE 9.1 Example of weight calculation for the weight plate push-up

% of 1RM	Bodyweight + weight plate	Weight plate
60%	48.12 kg	0 kg – bodyweight push-up
70%	56.14 kg	7,5 kg
80%	64.16 kg	15 kg
90%	72.18 kg	(23.43 kg) 22.5–25 kg

OBJECTIVE

By adding resistance to the push-up, a high-intensity stimulus can be provided that produces maximal strength gains similar to the bench press exercise (Calatayud *et al.* 2014; Figure 9.4).

STARTING POSITION

Assume the push-up position. Let a lifting partner or trainer place one or more weight plates on your upper back.

EXECUTION

Perform the push-up through the full range of motion.

COACHING KEYS

Quantification of training load is important during resistance training. To accurately calculate training intensity it is necessary to determine the exact load that is lifted (Table 9.1). Verifying the exact percentage of the 1RM during the weight plate push-up is more complex because this exercise includes a portion of body weight. The approximate load on the upper body during a regular push-up is 65 percent of bodyweight (Ebben *et al.* 2011; Gouvali and Boudolos 2005). If a player of 75 kg can perform five push-ups with a weight plate of 20 kg placed on his upper back, according to Jim Wendler's formula he will be able to perform one repetition with a weight of 30–32.5 kg.

$1RM = (weight \times reps \times 0.0333) + weight$

Weight = 20 kg (weight plate) + 65% of bodyweight = 20 kg + 48.75 kg = 68.75 kg

$1RM = (68.75 \times 5 \times 0.0333) + 68.75 = 80.2$ kg (weight plate + 65% of bodyweight)

80.2 kg (weight plate + 65% of bodyweight) − 48.75 (65% of bodyweight) = 31.4 kg

9.5 Push-up progression

The push-up progression is comprised of variations of the push-up with a mounting level of difficulty. The activation of the prime movers, the anterior core muscles and/or scapular and rotator cuff muscles, progressively increases.

Medicine ball push-up on two balls

OBJECTIVE

Adding instability to movement challenges the abdominal muscles more to maintain good posture (Freeman *et al.* 2006; Figure 9.5).

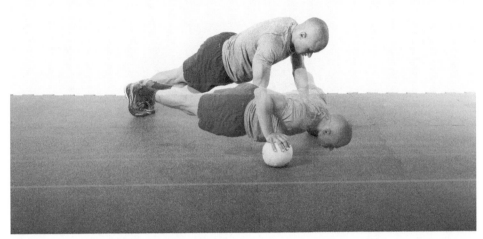

FIGURE 9.5 Medicine ball push-up on two balls

STARTING POSITION

Place each hand on a medicine ball.

EXECUTION

Lower your body until your chest reaches or is slightly below the level of the balls.

COACHING KEYS

Start with two medicine balls of the same size and move to two balls of a different size.

Medicine ball push-up on one ball

OBJECTIVE

The narrow base of support on one ball increases the activation of the pectoralis major and triceps brachii (Cogley *et al.* 2005; Gouvali and Boudolos 2005; Figure 9.6). Grasping the ball with the hands facing outward and shoulders placed in an externally rotated position also induces a stronger serratus anterior contraction (Lee *et al.* 2013; Yoon *et al.* 2010).

STARTING POSITION

Place both hands on a medicine ball.

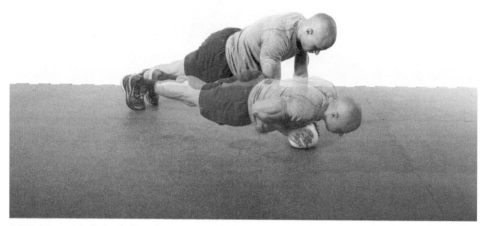

FIGURE 9.6 Medicine ball push-up on one ball

EXECUTION

Lower your body until the chest touches the ball.

COACHING KEYS

The smaller the ball, the less favorable the length–tension relationship at which the pectoralis major has to function and the greater its activation level will be.

Medicine ball crossover push-up

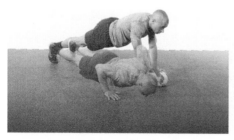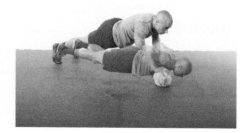

FIGURE 9.7 Medicine ball crossover push-up

OBJECTIVE

During this push-up variation (Figure 9.7) the lifter passes over the ball upon completing a push-up. By crossing over the lifter really has to balance on the ball, challenging the abdominal, scapular, and rotator cuff muscles more (Freeman *et al.* 2006). Pectoralis major and triceps brachii activity during this exercise is greater than during most other push-up variations (Freeman *et al.* 2006).

STARTING POSITION

Put your hands slightly wider than shoulder-width, with one hand on the floor and the other on a ball.

EXECUTION

Lower your body by bending the arms.
    Push your body up.
    Fully extend the arm of the hand that is balancing on the ball.
    Place both hands on the ball and cross over the ball to the other side.
    After every push-up cross over the ball to the opposite side until the prescribed number of repetitions is performed.

COACHING KEYS

Pass onto and over the ball in a fluid motion following the push-up.

Slide-board front lever push-up

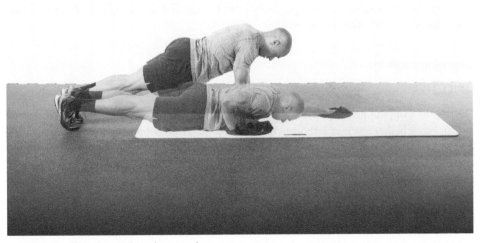

FIGURE 9.8   Slide-board front lever push-up

OBJECTIVE

This variation is practically a one-arm push-up. The slide-board front lever push-up (Figure 9.8) requires good rotational core stability. A high demand is placed on the obliques to stabilize the core and prevent twisting and lateral shifting of the spine throughout the exercise.

STARTING POSITION

Put both hands inside the slide-board booties.

Assume a push-up position, your hands placed on the slide-board, slightly wider than shoulder-width.

Keep the torso erect and the core tight. The knees and hips are extended and the spine is neutrally aligned.

EXECUTION

Lower your body, by flexing the right arm and sliding the left hand forward (the left arm remains extended), until your chest touches the floor.

Return to the starting position by extending the right arm and sliding your left hand back.

Perform the same movement on the opposite side.

Perform the prescribed number of repetitions.

COACHING KEYS

Start with a wide foot stance and progress to a narrow foot stance to augment rotational instability and the demand placed on the core muscles.

9.6 Plyometric push-ups

Plyometric push-ups are explosive push-ups to enhance upper body power (Crowder *et al.* 1993; Vossen *et al.* 2000). Plyometric push-ups elicit a strong activation of the upper body and core musculature (Freeman *et al.* 2006). Plyometric push-up programs have been shown to be more effective in improving upper body power compared to a regular push-up program (Crowder *et al.* 1993; Vossen *et al.* 2000).

Clapping push-up

OBJECTIVE

During the clapping push-up (Figure 9.9) the pectoralis major, anterior deltoid, and triceps brachii reach higher levels of activation compared to other push-up variations (Freeman *et al.* 2006; Garcia-Massó *et al.* 2011). While the force production is high, impact forces are lower compared to other plyometric upper body exercises (Garcia-Massó *et al.* 2011). This is important because the upper body is less efficient at absorbing impact forces.

STARTING POSITION

Put your hands slightly wider than shoulder-width.

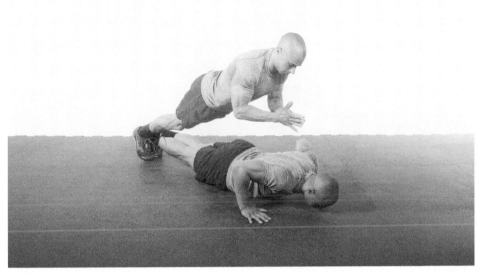

FIGURE 9.9 Clapping push-up

Keep the torso erect and the core tight. The knees and hips are extended and the spine is neutrally aligned.

EXECUTION

Lower your body by bending the arms until the chest touches the floor.

Perform an explosive push-up, pushing the upper body up off the ground, clapping the hands if possible.

COACHING KEYS

Maintain an erect torso and tight core throughout the entire exercise.

Depth-jump push-up

OBJECTIVE

Because the contact time during the depth-jump push-up is shorter compared to the clapping push-up, there is less time to absorb and produce force (Garcia-Massó et al. 2011). Rate of force development is therefore higher during the depth-jump push-up (Figure 9.10), which situates this exercise even more towards the speed-end of the force–velocity curve.

STARTING POSITION

Put your hands on one ball.

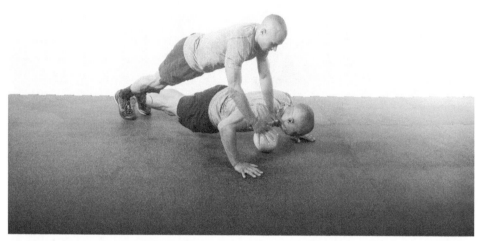

FIGURE 9.10   Depth-jump push-up

Keep the torso erect and the core tight. The knees and hips are extended and the spine is neutrally aligned.

EXECUTION

Release the ball with both hands.
　　On landing push up explosively off the floor.
　　Land with both hands on the ball.

COACHING KEYS

Minimize the time your hands are in contact with the ground.
　　As a progression use a bigger ball, so the height of the drop and ground reaction forces increase.

9.7 Staggered-stance, one-arm cable press

OBJECTIVE

Pressing from a standing position is a sport-specific, functional approach to develop pushing strength. The staggered-stance, one-arm cable press (Figure 9.11) is a total body exercise. Not only the activation of the prime movers, but also total-body stability and balance highly determine the amount of force that the lifter can produce (Santana *et al.* 2007).
　　The core muscles are highly challenged during standing pressing. This exercise strengthens the anterior oblique system (Santana *et al.* 2007). In the anterior oblique system the thigh

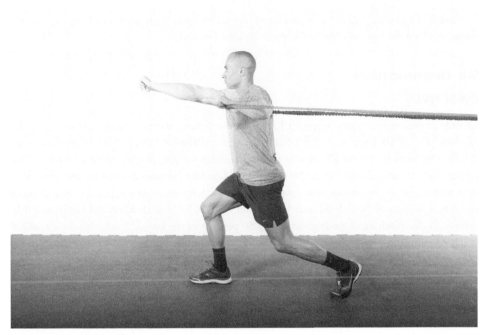

FIGURE 9.11 Staggered-stance, one-arm cable press

adductors are coupled with oblique abdominal muscles through the adductor-abdominal fascia. This system rotates the pelvis forward during the swing phase, playing an important role in locomotion and the soccer kick.

The staggered-stance, one-arm cable press can be considered as a ballistic exercise. The acceleration phase is critical for standing pressing performance (Santana *et al.* 2007). It is also during this phase that the highest muscle activation levels are observed (Santana *et al.* 2007). A powerful acceleration will enable the lifter to press a higher weight throughout the entire range of motion. The pulley machine allows the acceleration to be continued over the entire range of motion, enhancing motor unit recruitment.

STARTING POSITION

Position the handles at shoulder height.

Grasp one handle and step forward into a staggered stance with the handle to the lateral side of the chest.

Stand tall.

EXECUTION

Press the handle forward in front of your body until the arm is fully extended.

Return to the starting position by flexing the arm.

Perform the prescribed number of repetitions and then switch sides.

COACHING KEYS

In the staggered stance, make sure you stand hip-width apart with your toes pointing straight forward. Place the leg opposite to the pressing arm forward.

9.8 Overhead press

OBJECTIVE

Overhead pressing exercises (Figure 9.12) target the deltoid, triceps brachii, and core muscles (Kohler *et al.* 2010; Paoli *et al.* 2010; Saeterbakken and Fimland 2012, 2013; Willardson *et al.* 2009). The barbell version allows you to lift a heavier weight, placing more tension on the upper body muscles (Kohler *et al.* 2010; Saeterbakken and Fimland 2013). The dumbbell version requires more coordination and stabilization, which results in an enhanced coactivation of the different parts of the deltoid muscles (Kohler *et al.* 2010; Saeterbakken and Fimland 2013). Although dumbbell loads are approximately 80 percent of the barbell loads, deltoid activation levels are similar or even slightly higher during the dumbbell compared to barbell overhead press (Kohler *et al.* 2010; Saeterbakken and Fimland 2013).

STARTING POSITION

Position the barbell on the back of the shoulders. Place the hands just outside shoulder-width.
     Stand with the feet approximately shoulder-width apart.
     Keep the torso erect and the core tight. Look straight ahead.

EXECUTION

Press the barbell overhead.

COACHING KEYS

Push the barbell up as vertical as possible, while maintaining a straight body position. Avoid leaning back.
     The overhead press is an effective exercise to strengthen the serratus anterior and lower part of the trapezius (Andersen *et al.* 2012). Because the upper trapezius is activated to an even higher extent, the overhead press is not suited however to correct over-activation of the upper trapezius relative to the lower trapezius and serratus anterior (Andersen *et al.* 2012).
     Trapezius activity is higher when the bar is pressed behind the neck compared to in front of the neck, while serratus anterior activity is similar between both variants (Büll *et al.* 2001b). Grip width does not have an effect on the activity level of the trapezius and serratus anterior (Büll *et al.* 2001a).
     The highest muscle activation levels are obtained when the exercise is performed over the entire range of motion (Paoli *et al.* 2010). When moderate to heavy loads are used however, the activation level of the deltoid does not significantly reduce when the overhead press is performed over a partial range of motion (pressing from starting position to a 135° elbow angle, which is an incomplete elbow extension), while upper trapezius involvement is reduced (Paoli *et al.* 2010). The deltoid and upper trapezius muscles are synergists during shoulder abduction,

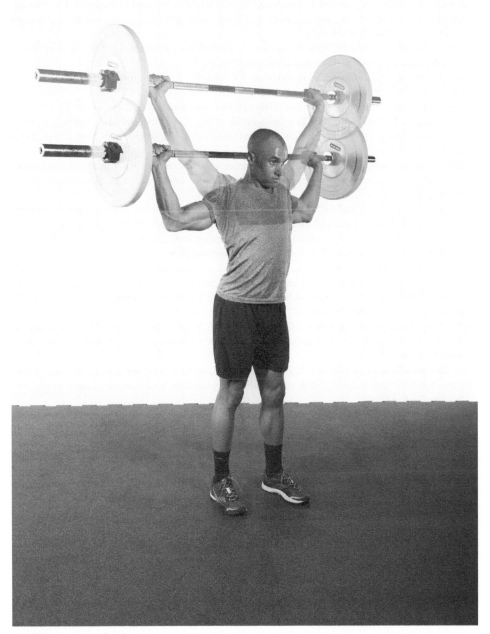

FIGURE 9.12 Overhead press

but pressing a moderate to high weight overhead in a partial range of motion might isolate the deltoid muscle to some extent (Paoli *et al.* 2010).

References

Andersen CH, Zebis MK, Saervoll C, Sundstrup E, Jakobsen MD, Sjøgaard G, Andersen LL. Scapular muscle activity from selected strengthening exercises performed at low and high intensities. *J Strength Cond Res.* 2012 Sep;26(9):2408–16.

Barnett C, Kippers V, Turner P. Effects of variations of the bench press exercise on EMG activity of five shoulder muscles. *J Strength Cond Res.* 1995 Nov;9(4):222–7.

Beneka A, Malliou P, Giannakopoulos K, Kyrialanis P, Godolias G. Different training modes for the rotator cuff muscle group. A comparative study. *Isokinet Exerc Sci.* 2002 Jan;10(2):73–9.

Blievernicht JA. Round shoulder syndrome. *IDEA health & fitness association;* 2000 Sep:44–53.

Büll ML, Vitti M, Freitas V, Rosa GJ. Electromyographic validation of the trapezius and serratus anterior muscles in military press exercises with open and middle grip. *Electromyogr Clin Neurophysiol.* 2001a Jun;41(4):203–7.

Büll ML, Vitti M, Freitas V, Rosa GJ. Electromyographic validation of the trapezius and serratus anterior muscles in military press exercises with middle grip. *Electromyogr Clin Neurophysiol.* 2001b Jul–Aug;41(5):263–8.

Calatayud J, Borreani S, Colado JC, Martin F, Rogers ME. Muscle activity levels in upper-body push exercises with different loads and stability conditions. *Phys Sportsmed.* 2014 Nov;42(4):106–19.

Choi JD. The effect of 7-week serratus anterior strengthening exercise on shoulder pain with serratus anterior weakness [dissertation]. [Seoul]: Yonsei University; 2008.

Chulvi-Medrano I, Martínez-Ballester E, Masiá-Tortosa L. Comparison of the effects of an eight-week push-up program using stable versus unstable surfaces. *Int J Sports Phys Ther.* 2012 Dec;7(6):586–94.

Clemons JM, Aaron C. Effect of grip width on myoelectric activity of the prime movers in the bench press. *J Strength Cond Res.* 1997 May;11(2):82–7.

Cogley RM, Archambault TA, Fibeger JF, Koverman MM, Youdas JW, Hollman JH. Comparison of muscle activation using various hand positions during the push-up exercise. *J Strength Cond Res.* 2005 Aug;19(3):628–33.

Cools AM, Witvrouw EE, Declercq GA, Danneels LA, Cambier DC. Scapular muscle recruitment patterns: trapezius muscle latency with and without impingement symptoms. *Am J Sports Med.* 2003 Jul–Aug;31(4):542–9.

Cools AM, Witvrouw EE, Mahieu NN, Danneels LA. Isokinetic scapular muscle performance in overhead athletes with and without impingement symptoms. *J Athl Train.* 2005 Jun;40(2):104–10.

Cools AM, Dewitte V, Lanszweert F, Notebaert D, Roets A, Soetens B, Cagnie B, Witvrouw EE. Rehabilitation of scapular muscle balance: which exercises to prescribe? *Am J Sports Med.* 2007 Oct;35(10):1744–51.

Crowder VS, Jolly SW, Collins B, Johnson J. The effect of plyometric push-ups on upper body power. *Track Field Q Rev.* 1993;93:58–9.

Decker MJ, Hintermeister RA, Faber KJ, Hawkins RJ. Serratus anterior muscle activity during selected rehabilitation exercises. *Am J Sports Med.* 1999 Nov–Dec;27(6):784–91.

Decker MJ, Tokish JM, Ellis HB, Torry MR, Hawkins RJ. Subscapularis muscle activity during selected rehabilitation exercises. *Am J Sports Med.* 2003 Jan–Feb;31(1):126–34.

Dillman CJ, Murray TA, Hintermeister RA, Faber KJ, Hawkins RJ. Biomechanical differences of open and closed chain exercises with respect to the shoulder. *J Sport Rehabil.* 1994 Aug;3(3):228–38.

Ebben WP, Wurm B, VanderZanden TL, Spadavecchia ML, Durocher JJ, Bickham CT, Petushek EJ. Kinetic analysis of several variations of push-ups. *J Strength Cond Res.* 2011 Oct;25(10):2891–4.

Escamilla RF, Yamashiro K, Paulos L, Andrews JR. Shoulder muscle activity and function in common shoulder rehabilitation exercises. *Sports Med.* 2009;39(8):663–85.

Fees M, Decker T, Snyder-Mackler L, Axe MJ. Upper extremity weight-training modifications for the injured athlete. A clinical perspective. *Am J Sports Med.* 1998 Sep–Oct;26(5):732–42.

Freeman S, Karpowicz A, Gray J, McGill S. Quantifying muscle patterns and spine load during various forms of the push-up. *Med Sci Sports Exerc.* 2006 Mar;38(3):570–7.

García-Massó X, Colado JC, González LM, Salvá P, Alves J, Tella V, Triplett NT. Myoelectric activation and kinetics of different plyometric push-up exercises. *J Strength Cond Res.* 2011 Jul;25(7):2040–7.

Giannakopoulos K, Beneka A, Malliou P, Godolias G. Isolated vs. complex exercise in strengthening the rotator cuff muscle group. *J Strength Cond Res.* 2004 Feb;18(1):144–8.

Glass SC, Armstrong T. Electromyographical activity of the pectoralis muscle during incline and decline bench presses. *J Strength Cond Res.* 1997 Aug;11(3):163–7.

Gouvali MK, Boudolos K. Dynamic and electromyographical analysis in variants of push-up exercise. *J Strength Cond Res.* 2005 Feb;19(1):146–51.

Green CM, Comfort P. The affect of grip width on bench press performance and risk of injury. *Strength Cond J.* 2007 Oct;29(5):10–14.

Haupt HA. Upper extremity injuries associated with strength training. *Clin Sports Med.* 2001 Jul;20(3):481–90.

Howarth SJ, Beach TA, Callaghan JP. Abdominal muscles dominate contributions to vertebral joint stiffness during the push-up. *J Appl Biomech.* 2008 May;24(2):130–9.

Jeong SY, Chung SH, Shim JH. Comparison of upper trapezius, anterior deltoid, and serratus anterior muscle activity during push-up plus exercise on slings and a stable surface. *J Phys Ther Sci.* 2014 Jun;26(6):937–9.

Kibler WB. Closed kinetic chain rehabilitation for sports injuries. *Phys Med Rehabil Clin N Am.* 2000 May;11(2):369–84.

Kohler JM, Flanagan SP, Whiting WC. Muscle activation patterns while lifting stable and unstable loads on stable and unstable surfaces. *J Strength Cond Res.* 2010 Feb;24(2):313–21.

Lander JE, Bates BT, Sawhill JA, Hamill J. A comparison between free-weight and isokinetic bench pressing. *Med Sci Sports Exerc.* 1985 Jun;17(3):344–53.

Lear LJ, Gross MT. An electromyographical analysis of the scapular stabilizing synergists during a push-up progression. *J Orthop Sports Phys Ther.* 1998 Sep;28(3):146–57.

Lee S, Lee D, Park J. The effect of hand position changes on electromyographic activity of shoulder stabilizers during push-up plus exercise on stable and unstable surfaces. *J Phys Ther Sci.* 2013 Aug;25(8):981–4.

Lehman GJ. The influence of grip width and forearm pronation/supination on upper-body myoelectric activity during the flat bench press. *J Strength Cond Res.* 2005 Aug;19(3):587–91.

Ludewig PM, Hoff MS, Osowski EE, Meschke SA, Rundquist PJ. Relative balance of serratus anterior and upper trapezius muscle activity during push-up exercises. *Am J Sports Med.* 2004 Mar;32(2):484–93.

Lukasiewicz AC, McClure P, Michiner L, Pratt N, Sennet B. Comparison of 3-dimensional scapular position and orientation between subjects with and without shoulder impingement. *J Orthop Sports Phys Ther.* 1999 Oct;29(10):574–86.

Madsen N, McLaughlin T. Kinematic factors influencing performance and injury risk in the bench press exercise. *Med Sci Sports Exerc.* 1984 Aug;16(4):376–81.

Malliou PC, Giannakopoulos K, Beneka AG, Gioftsidou A, Godolias G. Effective ways of restoring muscular imbalances of the rotator cuff muscle group: a comparative study of various training methods. *Br J Sports Med.* 2004 Dec;38(6):766–72.

Padulo J, Laffaye G, Chaouachi A, Chamari K. Bench Press exercise: the key points. *J Sports Med Phys Fitness.* 2014 May 13. [Epub ahead of print]

Page P. Shoulder muscle imbalance and subacromial impingement syndrome in overhead athletes. *Int J Sports Phys Ther.* 2011 Mar;6(1):51–8.

Paoli A, Marcolin G, Petrone N. Influence of different ranges of motion on selective recruitment of shoulder muscles in the sitting military press: an electromyographic study. *J Strength Cond Res.* 2010 Jun;24(6):1578–83.

Saeterbakken AH, Fimland MS. Muscle activity of the core during bilateral, unilateral, seated and standing resistance exercise. *Eur J Appl Physiol.* 2012 May;112(5):1671–8.

Saeterbakken AH, Fimland MS. Effects of body position and loading modality on muscle activity and strength in shoulder presses. *J Strength Cond Res.* 2013 Jul;27(7):1824–31.

Saeterbakken AH, van den Tillaar R, Fimland MS. A comparison of muscle activity and 1-RM strength of three chest-press exercises with different stability requirements. *J Sports Sci.* 2011 Mar;29(5):533–8.

Sahrmann S. *Diagnosis and treatment of movement impairment syndromes.* St Louis, MO: Mosby; 2002. Chapter 5, Movement impairment syndromes of the shoulder girdle; pp. 193–261.

Santana JC, Vera-Garcia FJ, McGill SM. A kinetic and electromyographic comparison of the standing cable press and bench press. *J Strength Cond Res.* 2007 Nov;21(4):1271–7.

Trebs AA, Brandenburg JP, Pitney WA. An electromyography analysis of 3 muscles surrounding the shoulder joint during the performance of a chest press exercise at several angles. *J Strength Cond Res.* 2010 Jul;24(7):1925–30.

Tucci HT, Ciol MA, de Araújo RC, de Andrade R, Martins J, McQuade KJ, Oliveira AS. Activation of selected shoulder muscles during unilateral wall and bench press tasks under submaximal isometric effort. *J Orthop Sports Phys Ther.* 2011 Jul;41(7):520–5.

Vossen JE, Kramer JE, Burke DG, Vossen DP. Comparison of dynamic push-up training and plyometric push-up training on upper-body power and strength. *J Strength Cond Res.* 2000 Aug;14(3):248–53.

Welsch EA, Bird M, Mayhew JL. Electromyographic activity of the pectoralis major and anterior deltoid muscles during three upper-body lifts. *J Strength Cond Res.* 2005 May;19(2):449–52.

Willardson JM, Fontana FE, Bressel E. Effect of surface stability on core muscle activity for dynamic resistance exercises. *Int J Sports Physiol Perform.* 2009 Mar;4(1):97–109.

Yoon JY, Kim TH, Oh JS. Effect of hand positions in electromyographic activity in scapulothoracic muscles during push-up plus. *J Phys Ther Korea.* 2010;17:8–15.

10

UPPER BODY PULL EXERCISES

Upper body pulling is the opposed movement pattern of upper body pressing. For a balanced upper body, opposing movements and muscle groups must be trained equally. An overemphasis of upper body pressing during training increases the likelihood of shoulder injuries (Durall et al. 2001).

Upper body pull exercises strengthen the muscles of the arms and upper back, while the muscles that stabilize the scapula and rotator cuff also display high levels of activity (Durall et al. 2001; Youdas et al. 2010).

More advanced pull exercises also strengthen the posterior core, the posterior oblique sling, and the deep longitudinal sling. The posterior oblique sling and the deep longitudinal sling dynamically stabilize the sacro-iliac joint and transfer forces from the ground to the upper body.

10.1 Pull-up

OBJECTIVE

The pull-up (Figure 10.1) is an excellent exercise to develop upper body strength because it requires the highest muscle activation of all upper body pull exercises (McGill et al. 2014). The pull-up will also help improve shoulder function and prevent shoulder complex injuries (Beneka et al. 2002; Giannakopoulos et al. 2004; Malliou et al. 2004). The movement is initiated with a strong contraction of the lower trapezius to pull the scapula down, followed by a strong contraction of the rotator cuff muscles (Youdas et al. 2010). The latissimus dorsi exhibits the highest level of activation during the pull-up. Next to the upper back and arm muscles, the sternocostal part of the pectoralis major, which extends the shoulder when the arm is positioned above the shoulder, also contributes during the early phase of the movement.

STARTING POSITION

Grasp an overhead bar about shoulder-width apart.

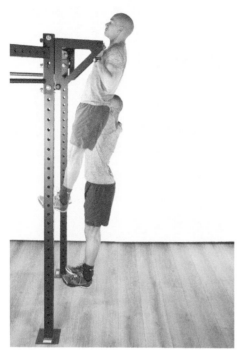

FIGURE 10.1 Pull-up

EXECUTION

Pull the body up until the chin is above the bar.

COACHING KEYS

Together with the parallel-grip pull-up, the chin-up (pull-up with underhand grip) is the easiest variant of the pull-up. The underhand grip enhances the involvement of the biceps brachii (Youdas *et al.* 2010).

When the lifter is not able to perform the prescribed number of repetitions during the pull-up, a form of assistance can be used to reduce the percentage of body weight that has to be lifted. An example of an assisted pull-up is the resistance band pull-up, in which one foot is placed into a resistance band that is looped over the pull-up bar. Through different bands of varying resistance the intensity of the pull-up can be further adjusted.

Extra weight can also be added to the pull-up by using a dip belt or by simply placing a dumbbell between the thighs.

10.2 Rowing

Rowing exercises are excellent exercises to develop strength in the upper back, the posterior shoulder region, and the arms. These exercises also strengthen the rotator cuff and scapula stabilizing muscles. During these exercises the lower and middle trapezius are predominantly activated over the upper trapezius (Andersen *et al.* 2012). The middle trapezius retracts the scapula together with the rhomboid muscles and shows high levels of activation (Andersen *et al.* 2012).

One-arm dumbbell row

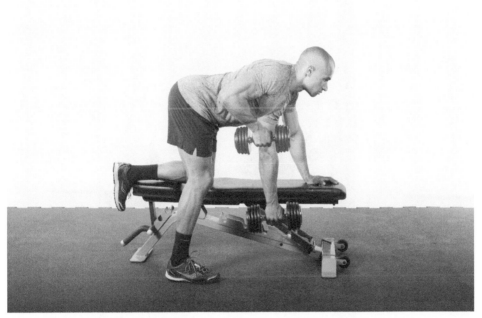

FIGURE 10.2 One-arm dumbbell row

OBJECTIVE

Due to the limited range of motion, the one-arm dumbbell row (Figure 10.2) is an appropri-ate exercise to integrate early in the rehabilitation process to restore shoulder function (Kibler *et al.* 2008).

This exercise is also well suited to overload the upper body for strengthening purposes. The one-arm dumbbell row requires less core strength to maintain good posture and can therefore be performed with a high load without the disruption of correct technique.

STARTING POSITION

Take a dumbbell in one hand.
Put the free hand at the upper end of the bench. Place the knee of the same side on the bench.
Keep your back neutrally aligned and your core tight.

EXECUTION

Pull the dumbbell up to your side.

COACHING KEYS

Do not rotate the torso to help raise the weight.

Inverse row

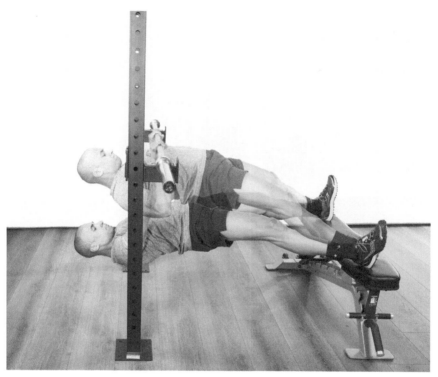

FIGURE 10.3   Inverse row

OBJECTIVE

Because the inverse row (Figure 10.3) combines a row and a bridge, it also strengthens the posterior muscles of the core.

Because an active scapular depression occurs during the inverse row, this row variation elicits higher levels of lower trapezius activity compared to other rowing exercises (De Mey *et al.* 2014).

STARTING POSITION

Place a bar in a rack in the bench press position. Place a bench parallel with the bar.
   Slide your body underneath the bar and grab it in the bench press position.
   Put your feet on a bench, with the toes pointing upward.
   Keep your body straight.

Stand with the feet hip–width apart.

Lower the bar to about kneecap level by bending forward at the hips. The hips are pushed back and the knees are flexed about 20°.

Keep the back straight and the torso tight. Look straight ahead.

EXECUTION

Retract the shoulder blades and row the bar up to the lower chest.

COACHING KEYS

Keep the back straight throughout the entire exercise.

Staggered-stance one-arm row

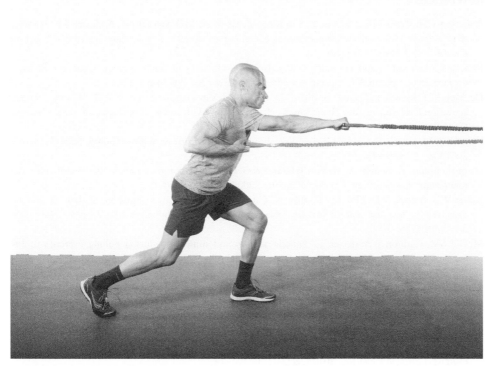

FIGURE 10.6   Staggered–stance one–arm row

OBJECTIVE

The staggered stance one-arm row (Figure 10.6) trains the posterior oblique sling.

STARTING POSITION

Position the handle at shoulder height.

Assume a staggered stance. Take a handle attached to a cable column in the hand opposite to the front leg.

Keep your back neutrally aligned and your core tight.

EXECUTION

Pull the handle back.

Perform the prescribed number of repetitions and then switch sides.

COACHING KEYS

The staggered-stance one-arm row can also be performed with the handle positioned at the bottom. Due to the low position of the handle, the trunk is inclined forward while performing the rowing motion. Therefore this exercise places a higher demand on the core to maintain proper form, compared to the staggered-stance one-arm row.

References

Andersen CH, Zebis MK, Saervoll C, Sundstrup E, Jakobsen MD, Sjøgaard G, Andersen LL. Scapular muscle activity from selected strengthening exercises performed at low and high intensities. *J Strength Cond Res.* 2012 Sep;26(9):2408–16.

Beneka A, Malliou P, Giannakopoulos K, Kyrialanis P, Godolias G. Different training modes for the rotator cuff muscle group. A comparative study. *Isokinet Exerc Sci.* 2002;Jan:10(2):73–9.

De Mey K, Danneels L, Cagnie B, Borms D, T'Jonck Z, Van Damme E, Cools AM. Shoulder muscle activation levels during four closed kinetic chain exercises with and without Redcord slings. *J Strength Cond Res.* 2014 Jun;28(6):1626–35.

Durall CJ, Manske RC, Davies GJ. Avoiding shoulder injury from resistance training. *Strength Cond J.* 2001 Oct;23(5):10–18.

Giannakopoulos K, Beneka A, Malliou P, Godolias G. Isolated vs. complex exercise in strengthening the rotator cuff muscle group. *J Strength Cond Res.* 2004 Feb;18(1):144–8.

Kibler WB, Sciascia AD, Uhl TL, Tambay N, Cunningham T. Electromyographic analysis of specific exercises for scapular control in early phases of shoulder rehabilitation. *Am J Sports Med.* 2008 Sep;36(9):1789–98.

McGill SM, Cannon J, Andersen JT. Muscle activity and spine load during pulling exercises: influence of stable and labile contact surfaces and technique coaching. *J Electromyogr Kinesiol.* 2014 Oct;24(5):652–65.

Malliou PC, Giannakopoulos K, Beneka AG, Gioftsidou A, Godolias G. Effective ways of restoring muscular imbalances of the rotator cuff muscle group: a comparative study of various training methods. *Br J Sports Med.* 2004 Dec;38(6):766–72.

Youdas JW, Amundson CL, Cicero KS, Hahn JJ, Harezlak DT, Hollman JH. Surface electromyographic activation patterns and elbow joint motion during a pull-up, chin-up, or perfect-pullup™ rotational exercise. *J Strength Cond Res.* 2010 Dec;24(12):3404–14.

11

HYBRID EXERCISES

Hybrid exercises consist of two or more exercises that are combined in one movement. These exercises are compound movements to develop total body strength and power. A high demand is placed on the core to stabilize the movement and transfer the power generated by the lower body to the upper body. These exercises also address and train the myofascial sling systems of the outer unit.

By combining two or more exercises, the training volume can be increased, workouts are more time efficient, and the monotony of training can be broken up. Hybrid exercises are also an excellent tool for metabolic training. Performing two or more exercises back-to-back increases the cardiovascular effect of your workout.

11.1 Battling ropes waves

OBJECTIVE

A great variety of exercises can be performed with the use of battling ropes (Figure 11.1). They are most used for wave training however. Battling rope exercises are total body movements. The legs, hips, and core generate and transfer power through the arms. Battling ropes can be used to increase strength and to trigger a potent metabolic response (Ratamess *et al.* 2015).

STARTING POSITION

Grasp both ends of the rope, which is anchored to a fixed point.
    Assume a stable position. The feet are shoulder-width apart and the knees slightly bend.

EXECUTION

Generate waves by forcefully moving the arms up and down.

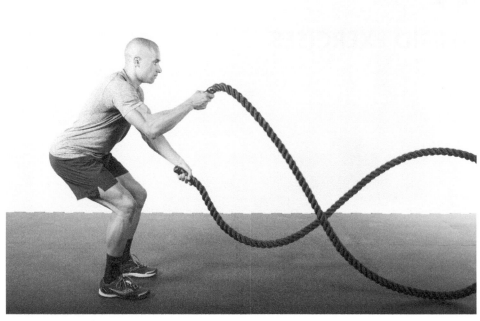

FIGURE 11.1   Battling ropes waves

COACHING KEYS

Maintain balance and a tight core throughout the entire exercise while generating explosive arm movements.

11.2 Single-leg squat and row

OBJECTIVE

This is a compound exercise that combines the single-leg squat with a one-arm row (Figure 11.2). It's a great exercise to develop upper back strength together with balance, stability, and single-leg strength. This exercise triggers a strong contraction from the gluteus maximus and trains the anti-rotation, anti-flexion, and anti-lateral flexion core functions.

STARTING POSITION

This exercise can be performed with elastic resistance, an adjustable cable column, or low pulley.
   Position the handle at shoulder height.
   Assume a single-leg stance.
   Reach forward with the opposite hand to grab the handle, and pull it to the side.

EXECUTION

Squat down and reach forward with the opposite hand.

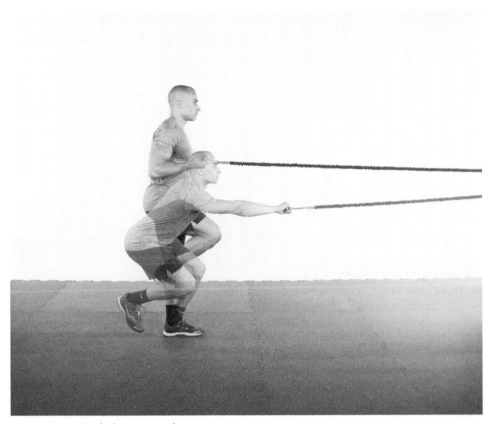

FIGURE 11.2   Single-leg squat and row

Return to the starting position by simultaneously squatting up and pulling the handle to the side.

COACHING KEYS

Avoid the knee of the supporting leg moving inward. Make sure it tracks over the second and third toe, staying well aligned between hip and ankle.

Make sure to perform the pull with the opposite arm of the stance leg.

11.3 Back lunge and one-arm press

OBJECTIVE

This total-body strengthening exercise combines the back lunge with a one-arm cable press (Figure 11.3). It places a high demand on balance and addresses the anterior oblique sling, which stores and releases energy to allow greater contraction velocities during rotational movements such as the soccer kick.

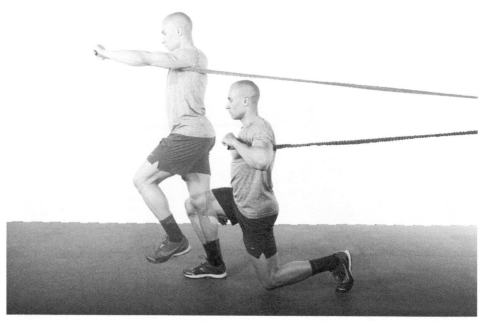

FIGURE 11.3   Back lunge and one-arm press

STARTING POSITION

Position the handles at shoulder height.

Grasp one handle.

Stand tall facing away from the pulley system and press the handle forward in front of your body.

EXECUTION

Step backwards as far as possible.

Descend onto the front leg while flexing the arm to move the handle to the lateral side of the chest.

Return to the starting position by performing a single-leg squat movement with the front leg while pressing the handle forward again.

COACHING KEYS

Keep the torso erect and the core tight during the whole exercise.

Make sure to perform the press with the opposite arm of the stance leg.

11.4 Single-leg Romanian deadlift and row

OBJECTIVE

The single-leg Romanian deadlift and row (Figure 11.4) is a compound exercise that targets the entire posterior chain: hamstrings, glutes, lower and upper back muscles.

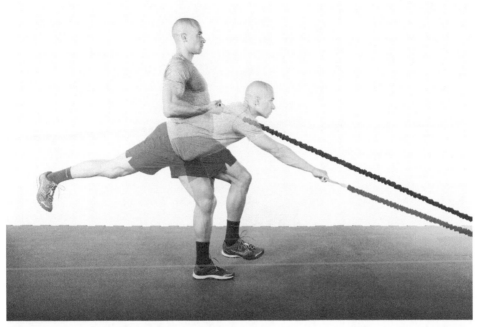

FIGURE 11.4   Single-leg Romanian deadlift and row

STARTING POSITION

This exercise can be performed with elastic resistance, an adjustable cable column, or low pulley.

Position the handle at the bottom.

Assume a single-leg stance. Take the handle in the hand opposite to the supporting leg.

Pull the handle up to your side.

EXECUTION

Lower the upper body by bending at the hip. Keep the back straight.

Push the hips back and slightly bend the knee during the descent.

Reach forward with the hand grasping the handle, by flexing the shoulder and extending the elbow.

Swing the free leg back so it stays in line with the torso.

Lower the upper body until a mild stretch is felt in the hamstrings.

Return to the starting position.

Perform the prescribed number of repetitions and switch sides.

COACHING KEYS

Focus on pushing the hips back and not on bending at the hips.

The movement occurs at hip level. Keep the spine neutrally aligned throughout the entire exercise.

11.5 Push–pull combination

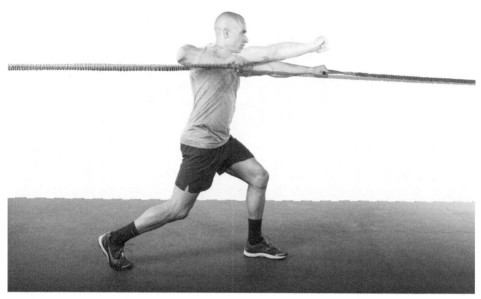

FIGURE 11.5   Push–pull combination

OBJECTIVE

This exercise combines a pressing and pulling movement, placing a high demand on the core to control and stabilize spinal rotation (Figure 11.5).

STARTING POSITION

This exercise can be performed with elastic resistance, a cable crossover, or functional trainer machine.

Position the handles at shoulder height.

Grasp both handles and assume a split stance with the left foot forward, perpendicular to the line of pull of the cables.

Hold the right handle at the lateral side of the chest. The left hand and handle are extended out in front of the left shoulder.

EXECUTION

Simultaneously pull the left handle back to the side while pressing the right handle out in front of the right shoulder.

Return to the starting position.

Perform the prescribed number of repetitions and switch sides.

COACHING KEYS

In the staggered stance, make sure you stand hip-width apart with your toes pointing straight forward.

Keep your back neutrally aligned and your core tight throughout the entire exercise.

11.6 Squat and press

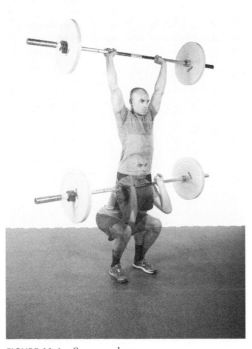

FIGURE 11.6   Squat and press

OBJECTIVE

The squat and press (Figure 11.6) hits 90 percent of the muscles in the body. It is a great hybrid exercise to develop total body strength and power. A high demand is placed on the core to stabilize the movement and transfer the power generated by the lower body to the upper body.

STARTING POSITION

Grab the bar slightly wider than shoulder-width. Rotate the elbows around the bar and lift the elbows up and forward to position the bar on front of the shoulders.

Choose between a jump stance and an athletic stance.

EXECUTION

Descend with control until the top of the thighs is at least parallel to the floor.

Squat back up explosively by extending the knees and hips, using this momentum to lift the barbell overhead.

COACHING KEYS

Use the impulse generated by the lower body to push the barbell overhead.

Push the barbell up as vertically as possible, while maintaining a straight body position. Avoid leaning back.

Reference

Ratamess NA, Rosenberg JG, Klei S, Dougherty BM, Kang J, Smith C, Ross RE, Faigenbaum AD. Comparison of the acute metabolic responses to traditional resistance, body-weight, and battling rope exercises. *J Strength Cond Res*. 2015 Jan;29(1):47–57.

12
MUSCLE ANATOMY AND FUNCTION

Lower extremity and lower back injuries can change the neuromuscular activity patterns of some of the core, hip, and thigh muscles (Brindle *et al.* 2003; Bullock-Saxton *et al.* 1994; Nelson-Wong *et al.* 2012). These altered muscle activation patterns may be the result of compensation patterns and can persist after recovery (Brindle *et al.* 2003; Gamble 2013). The altered muscle function or inhibition affects both strength and function, compromising performance and increasing the risk of (re-)injury (Ingersoll *et al.* 2008). Injury is therefore considered as an important risk factor for future injury (Mendiguchia *et al.* 2012). Rehabilitation and training need to focus on restoring correct muscle function and intermuscular coordination. When training for injury prevention the player's previous injuries should be taken into account, because they might still be associated with persisting altered muscle function (Gamble 2013).

The main purpose of this chapter is to explore the anatomy and function of some muscle groups, including the gluteal muscles, hamstrings, hip adductors, and vastus medialis obliquus. These muscles play a crucial role in providing neuromuscular control of the lower extremity, and altered activation patterns of these muscles are a contributing factor for various lower extremity injuries (Hewett and Myer 2011; Mendiguchia *et al.* 2011).

There is evidence to support that these altered activation patterns are also implicated in the mechanism of hamstring and adductor strain injuries and re-injuries (Crosier *et al.* 2008; Crow *et al.* 2010; Prior *et al.* 2014; Sahrmann 2002; Sole *et al.* 2011). Muscle strains are the most prevalent type of injury in soccer, with the majority affecting the hamstring and adductor muscles (Arnason *et al.* 2004; Carling *et al.* 2011; Ekstrand *et al.* 2011b, 2013; Mallo *et al.* 2011; Mohib *et al.* 2014; Schmikli *et al.* 2011; Stubbe *et al.* 2014). There is also a high incidence of recurring strains, which are more serious than the original injury and require a longer absence from training and competition (Carling *et al.* 2011; Dick *et al.* 2007; Ekstrand *et al.* 2011b.

In spite of the belief in sports medicine that especially muscle injuries are preventable, muscle strain injury and re-injury rates have not improved over the last 30 years (Mendiguchia *et al.* 2012). In this chapter the injury mechanisms and risk factors associated with hamstring and groin strain injury are identified. This chapter also focuses on the training interventions to address the risk factors and exercises that may help to restore proper activation patterns and intermuscular coordination.

12.1 The gluteal muscles

Introduction

The gluteus maximus is the strongest and biggest muscle of the body. It is not only a powerful hip extensor but also plays an important role in pelvic and spinal stabilization (Lafond et al. 1998; Noe et al. 1992; Snijders et al. 1993; Vakos et al. 1994; Vleeming et al. 1989). The gluteal muscles (gluteus maximus, gluteus medius, and gluteus minimus) stabilize the hip by counteracting gravity's hip adduction torque and maintain proper leg alignment by eccentrically controlling adduction and internal rotation of the thigh (Distefano et al. 2009; Moore and Dalley 1999).

The gluteus maximus may also function as a knee stabilizer in addition to the hamstring muscles (Alkjaer et al. 2012). Through the connection with the iliotibial tract, which inserts on the tibia, a contraction of the gluteus maximus can control the anterior tibial translation to reduce the anterior cruciate ligament strain (Alkjaer et al. 2012; Standring 2008).

The gluteus maximus allows us to maintain an upright position needed for bipedalism (Jenkins 2008; Marzke et al. 1988). Through evolution the gluteus maximus enlarged in humans as a means to stabilize the trunk while standing and counteracts the high impact forces that tend to flex the trunk anteriorly during running and sprinting (Jenkins 2008; Marzke et al. 1988).

The terms "gluteal amnesia" and "sleeping giant" probably sound familiar. These terms refer to inhibition and delayed activation of the gluteal muscles, which in time leads to weakness of these muscles. Low back pain and lower body injuries result in delayed and reduced gluteal activation with concurrent hamstring and low back compensation (Bullock-Saxton et al. 1994; Burger et al. 1996; Freeman et al. 1965; Leinonen et al. 2000; Vogt et al. 2003). Gluteal inhibition negatively affects performance and lower body strength and is a root cause for many injuries and chronic pain (Fredericson et al. 2000; Friel et al. 2006; Hewett et al. 2005, 2006; Ireland 2002, 2003; Lewis et al. 2007; Powers and Flynn 2003; Sahrmann 2002; Tyler et al. 2006).

Implementing exercises into the workout, warm-up, or activation session that targets the gluteal muscles and re-establish correct muscle recruitment patterns can positively affect lower body strength and function, improve your core stability, prevent lower body injuries, and enhance athletic performance.

The gluteus maximus and lower back stability

Activating and strengthening the glutes needs to form an important part of your core routine.

Co-contraction of the gluteus maximus with the psoas major (part of the iliopsoas muscle) contributes to lumbosacral stabilization (Gibbons 2005; Gibbons and Comerford 2001). The gluteus maximus provides stability to the sacroiliac joint by bracing and compression (Snijders et al. 1993; Vleeming et al. 1989). Excess movement at the sacroiliac joint would compromise the L5–S1 intervertebral joints and disc and could lead to sacroiliac joint dysfunction and low back pain.

The gluteus maximus also provides lower back stability through its connection with the erector spinae and thoracolumbar fascia (Snijders et al. 1997; Vleeming et al. 1995). Some of its fibers are continuous with the fibers of the erector spinae. A contraction of the gluteus maximus will generate tension in the erector spinae muscle on the same side, providing stiffness to the spinal column (Snijders et al. 1997; Vleeming et al. 1995).

Gluteus maximus contraction also exerts a pull on the lower end of the thoracolumbar fascia, which is a thick layer of ligamentous connective tissue. Tightening of this fascia stabilizes the vertebras. People with low back pain often have weak and deconditioned glutes (Kankaanpää et al. 1998).

Inhibition of the gluteal muscles

Low back pain has been associated with inhibition of the gluteus maximus (Leinonen et al. 2000; Nelson-Wong et al. 2012; Vogt et al. 2003). The activation of the gluteus maximus during hip extension is delayed in people with a history of low back pain compared to people with no back pain. In people with low back pain, hip extension is initiated by the hamstrings and erector spinae instead of the gluteus maximus (Janda 1985; Leinonen et al. 2000; Nelson-Wong et al. 2012). Even after the episode of low back pain has resolved, the altered firing patterns in the gluteus maximus remain (Ferreira et al. 2004).

A similar pattern of delayed activation of the gluteus medius during hip abduction has been described in patients with low back pain and also in people with anterior knee pain (Brindle et al. 2003; Janda 1985).

People suffering from ankle sprain injuries also have been shown to have reduced activation levels of the gluteus maximus (Bullock-Saxton et al. 1994).

Inhibition and delayed activation of the gluteus maximus compromises pelvic stability (Wilson et al. 2005). This can result in compensation by the lower back and more altered muscular firing patterns and function. In the case of low back pain, ankle and probably all lower body injuries, rehabilitation needs to focus on reactivating the gluteal muscles.

Weak or inhibited gluteal muscles contribute to injury

Weak or delayed activation of the gluteus maximus and gluteus medius is a root cause for many injuries and chronic pain.

- Hamstring strains: Due to delayed gluteus maximus activity, the hamstring muscles become dominant during hip extension, which can cause hamstring strains (Sahrmann 2002). A lot of athletes that pulled a hamstring keep suffering re-injuries despite their focus and efforts to strengthen the hamstrings. They are reinforcing a compensation pattern instead of reactivating their inhibited glutes. Shirley Sahrmann says that any time you see an injured muscle, you need to look for a weak synergist.
- Low back pain: Gluteus maximus activation plays an important role in stabilizing the pelvis during the task of lifting (Noe et al. 1992; Vakos et al. 1994). Delayed gluteus maximus activation also causes excessive compensation of the back extensors (Nelson-Wong et al. 2012).
- Anterior knee pain: The excessive internal rotation of the femur as a result of gluteal weakness increases the pressure on the patellar cartilage (Ireland et al. 2003; Powers et al. 2003; Tyler et al. 2006).
- Anterior hip pain: Decreased force production from the gluteus maximus during hip extension is associated with increased anterior translation of the femur in the acetabulum. The increased femoral anterior glide could lead to increased force and wear and tear on the anterior hip joint structures (Lewis et al. 2007; Sahrmann 2002).

- Lower body malalignment: Weak glutes result in increased internal rotation of the femur, knee valgus, and foot pronation (Lephart *et al.* 2002).
- Gluteal weakness also has been associated with anterior cruciate ligament (ACL) sprains (Hewett *et al.* 2005, 2006; Ireland 2002), chronic ankle instability (Friel *et al.* 2006), and iliotibial friction syndrome (Fredericson *et al.* 2000).

Exercises to reactivate the gluteal muscles

Reactivating the gluteal muscles can re-establish correct muscle recruitment patterns and enhance strength and performance.

The gluteus maximus is the strongest muscle of the body and has a multitasking function (Comerford 2004). This muscle is able to combine a local stabilizer, global stabilizer, and global mobilizer role (Table 12.1).

The gluteus maximus is especially active during stair climbing, running, and activities that involve stabilizing the trunk against flexion (McLay *et al.* 1990; Marzke *et al.* 1988; Stern *et al.* 1980; Zimmermann *et al.* 1994). An exercise that combines these movements would trigger a strong contraction of the gluteus maximus and addresses both the stabilizing and movement role. Single-leg stance exercises require the gluteus medius and upper part of the gluteus maximus to resist gravity's hip adduction torque.

In the resisted slide-board back lunge (Figure 12.1) the pull of the cable creates a hip flexion force against which the gluteus maximus has to stabilize. The movement also mimics the

TABLE 12.1 The multitasking function of the gluteus maximus

Local stabilizer	*Global stabilizer*	*Global mobilizer*
Segmental stabilization	Eccentric lengthening or isometric holding to control range of motion	Produce high force or power
- Force closure of the sacroiliac joint - Control and centralize the femur in the hip socket (acetabulum) - Co-contraction with psoas major provides pelvic stability - Segmental stabilization of the vertebras: 1. directly by tensing the thoracolumbar fascia; 2. indirectly by triggering the deep lumbar multifidus	- Sagittal plane stabilization of the trunk during walking, running, and standing - Control of trunk rotation during gait through the connection with contralateral latissimus dorsi (posterior oblique system) - Frontal plane stabilization of the pelvis during single-leg stance (resisting gravity's hip adduction torque) - Control of the stance leg in the frontal (preventing adduction of the thigh) and transverse plane (preventing internal rotation of the thigh)	- Hip extension - External rotation - Superior fibers: hip abduction - Lower fibers: hip adduction

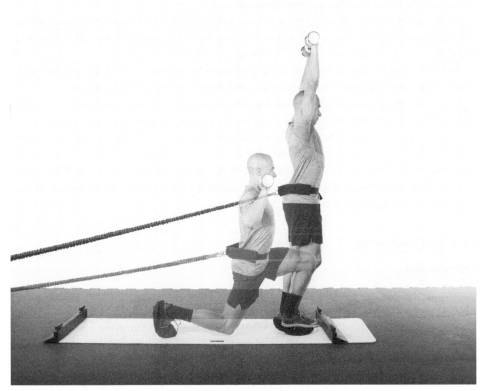

FIGURE 12.1   Resisted slide-board back lunge with overhead press

hip action of running and stair climbing. Like in running, the body has to be pulled over the foot by a powerful hip extension.

As an advanced progression the exercise can be combined with a shoulder press. This compound exercise emphasizes the stabilizing role of the gluteus maximus even more. Pressing dumbbells overhead requires anti-flexion stability from the core. The co-contraction of the gluteus maximus and deeper trunk muscles stabilize the spine, so forces can be effectively transferred from the lower to the upper body.

Other exercises that elicit a high gluteus maximus and medius activity are the single-leg squat and the single-leg Romanian deadlift (Ayotte *et al.* 2007; Distefano *et al.* 2009; Zeller *et al.* 2003). These single-leg exercises require concentric or eccentric hip extension throughout a large range of motion. The need to stabilize the hip in the frontal (resisting gravity's hip adduction torque) and transverse plane (preventing internal rotation of the thigh) while generating movement in the frontal plane (concentric/eccentric hip extension) results in a high neural drive of the gluteus maximus, medius, and minimus.

In the single-leg squat and pull and the single-leg Romanian deadlift and pull the hand opposite to the stance leg is loaded. The added rotary force stimulates the external rotator capability of the gluteus maximus and medius and gives these exercises a multi-planar character. These exercises also train the cross-body connection (posterior oblique system), which transmits forces from the ground through the leg and hip, across the sacroiliac joint via the thoracolumbar fascia, into the opposite latissimus dorsi.

High activation levels of the gluteus medius, upper part of the gluteus maximus, and lateral system muscles have also been observed during the side bridge and the side bridge with abduction exercises (Ekstrom *et al.* 2007; Selkowitz *et al.* 2013).

The slide-board lateral slide combines a powerful hip extension and abduction and really activates the gluteal muscles. Skating develops and shapes the hips and glutes best.

Due to low back pain, an ankle sprain, or other injuries the gluteal muscles may be inhibited and do not fire when they are supposed to. Because of compensatory patterns it may be difficult to target and strengthen the glutes. Exercises that require single-leg balance, stability of the lumbo-pelvic region, hip extension, or eccentric control of hip flexion, which are all major functions of the gluteus maximus, result in the greatest level of activation. These exercises can help to reactivate the gluteal muscles and re-establish correct intermuscular coordination and movement patterns.

12.2 The hamstrings

Introduction

Hamstring injuries are a major problem in sports. There is especially a high prevalence in athletes who participate in sports that require sprinting and kicking such as soccer and rugby (Kujala *et al.* 1997; Orchard and Seward 2002; Woods *et al.* 2004). Hamstring injuries also have a high propensity for re-injury. One-third of the injuries will recur with the greatest risk during the initial two weeks following return to sport (Orchard and Seward 2002). The risk for re-injury remains elevated for at least a year and the subsequent injury is often more severe than the original strain (Gabbe *et al.* 2006a; Hagglund *et al.* 2006; Warren *et al.* 2010). In some cases a strained hamstring can cause long-term problems and have a severe impact on a player's career.

The majority of hamstring injuries occur during the late swing phase of running and 80 percent of the hamstring strains affect the long head of the biceps femoris (Chumanov *et al.* 2007; Koulouris and Connell 2003). Architectural and functional differences between the hamstring muscles contribute to the tendency of the biceps femoris to be more often injured than the other muscles.

The very high risk to recur in the early phase after returning to sport suggests that most rehabilitation plans are inadequate. To design effective rehabilitation programs several questions need to be posed and answered. What are the risk factors that increase the hamstring injury rate and how can the training or rehab plan have an impact on these risk factors? A previous hamstring strain is probably the most important risk factor for future injury. Which muscle properties are altered following a hamstring strain and why do they put the athlete at a higher risk for recurrence when he/she returns to play? Which exercise selection and training parameters can help prevent injury or are important in the rehabilitation in order to avoid re-injury?

Architectural characteristics, activation patterns, and function

The hamstrings consist of four muscles. The semitendinosus, the semimembranosus, and the long head of the biceps femoris are bi-articular and cross the hip and knee joint. The short head of the biceps femoris only spans the knee joint (Table 12.2).

TABLE 12.2 Function of the hamstring muscles

	Local stabilizer	*Global stabilizer*	*Global mobilizer*
	Segmental stabilization	Eccentric lengthening or isometric holding to control range of motion	Produce high force or power
Semitendinosus		- Provide stability to valgus stress at the knee	- Hip extension - Hip internal rotation when the hip is extended - Knee flexion - Internal knee rotation when the knee is flexed
Semimembranosus		- Provide dynamic support to the posterior capsule - Resist excessive hip abduction - Resist external knee rotation	- Hip extension - Hip internal rotation when the hip is extended - Knee flexion - Internal knee rotation when the knee is flexed
Biceps femoris (long and short heads)	- Force-closure of the sacroiliac joint through its origin at the sacrotuberous ligament (deep longitudinal system)	- Resist internal knee rotation - Resist anterioposterior knee stress - Provide stability to varus stress at the knee	- Hip extension - Knee flexion - External knee rotation when the knee is flexed

Before, the hamstring muscles were considered as one muscle group of which the muscles had similar activation patterns during knee flexion or hip extension. The anatomical characteristics of a muscle are the primary determinants of its function (Lieber *et al.* 1993, 2000). Architectural differences between the hamstring muscles indicate that each muscle has its inherent function.

The semitendinosus and the short head of the biceps femoris are thin muscles with a lower cross-sectional area and long, parallel-arranged fibers. This makes them more suited to contract over larger distances with high speed and lower force. The long head of the biceps femoris and the semimembranosus on the other hand are bulky muscles with shorter pennate fibers, more suited for high force production (Kellis *et al.* 2012; Lieber *et al.* 1993, 2000; Makihara *et al.* 2006).

Function of the hamstring muscles during sprinting

The prolonged activity of the hamstrings shows the importance of these muscles for running. EMG recordings have shown that the hamstring muscles are active from mid-swing until the

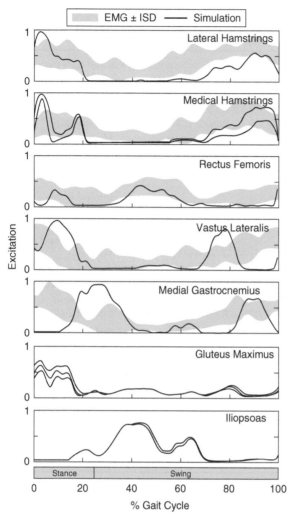

FIGURE 12.2 Muscle activity during maximal sprinting speed (Chumanov et al. 2011)

terminal stance phase of running (Chumanov *et al.* 2011; Higashihara *et al.* 2010; Jonhagen *et al.* 1996; Kyrolainen *et al.* 1999, 2005; Simonsen *et al.* 1985; Yu *et al.* 2008; Figure 12.2). Most of the hamstring injuries occur during the terminal swing phase (Chumanov *et al.* 2012; Petersen *et al.* 2005). During this phase the knee extends while the hip is in flexion, lengthening the bi-articular hamstrings over both joints they cross. The hamstring muscles lengthen and contract eccentrically to brake the knee extension of the swing leg (Chumanov *et al.* 2012).

Just before foot-strike the hamstrings reach peak force and peak lengths (Schache *et al.* 2009; Simonsen *et al.* 1985; Thelen *et al.* 2005a, 2005b; Wood 1987; Yamaguchi and Zajak 1989). At high speeds the EMG activity of the hamstring muscles during the terminal swing phase has been shown to exceed the activity of a maximal voluntary contraction (Kyrolainen *et al.* 1999).

The peak lengths during terminal swing are approximately 10 percent greater than the hamstring lengths during an upright stance (Schache *et al.* 2009; Simonsen *et al.* 1985). Because of the differences in hip extension (origin on the pelvis) and knee flexion moment arms (insertion on the tibia), peak lengths are significantly larger in the long head of the biceps femoris than the semitendinosus and semimembranosus (Thelen *et al.* 2005a). The greater incurred musculo-tendon stretch by the biceps femoris may contribute to its tendency to be more often injured than the other two hamstring muscles (Thelen *et al.* 2005a).

Peak lengths do not increase significantly with faster sprinting speeds, while hamstring muscle force and power steadily increase with speed (Chumanov *et al.* 2007, 2011; Schache *et al.* 2010; Thelen *et al.* 2005a).

Just before foot-strike the hamstrings undergo a stretch–shortening cycle to begin the concentric hip extension contraction that is continuous throughout the stance phase. Before, there was hesitation to consider the hamstrings as prime movers during sprinting (Mero and Komi 1987). The reason for this hesitation is that the hamstrings beside hip extension also flex the knee, while during the stance phase of sprinting knee extension is required (Bober and Mularczyk 1990; McClay *et al.* 1990; Wood 1986). The Lombard paradox shows however that the hamstrings simultaneously perform a hip and knee extension during running (Andrews 1985; Molbech 1965; Wiemann and Tidow 1995). The lower leg is guided during running by foot contact with the ground and the force output of the quads. The hamstrings shorten over the hip joint during hip extension and contract eccentrically around the knee joint to pull the knee backwards into extension.

The hamstrings are active until the end of the stance phase. They are silent from the early swing phase until mid-swing (Chumanov *et al.* 2011; Mero and Komi 1987).

The way the hamstring muscles function during running explains the high propensity for injury during high-speed running.

The role of the hamstrings as a knee stabilizer

The hamstring muscles provide additional valgus and varus stability to the knee and help protect the ligamentous structures of the knee.

Explosive stopping, cutting, and turning actions require a high amount of strength and neuromuscular control from the hamstrings to stabilize the knee and decrease ACL loading (Besier *et al.* 2003; Fujii *et al.* 2012; Lloyd *et al.* 2005). Reduced hamstring strength significantly increases the ACL loading during cutting actions (Weinhandl *et al.* 2014).

Peak ACL tensile force occurs around 20° of knee flexion (Biscarini 2008; Escamilla *et al.* 2012; Kulas *et al.* 2012; Nagura *et al.* 2006; Shelburne and Pandy 2002; Shelburne *et al.* 2005; Shin *et al.* 2007). Around this knee angle a contraction of the semitendinosus and biceps femoris (long and short heads) provides the greatest decrease of ACL loading (Biscarini *et al.* 2013).

The biceps femoris is an important dynamic stabilizer of the knee (Fujii *et al.* 2012). Its tendon consists of three layers that insert on the crural fascia, the knee capsule, and the head of the fibula (Ellenbecker *et al.* 2009; Terry and LaPrade 1996). The middle part of the tendon also surrounds the lateral collateral ligament (Ellenbecker *et al.* 2009; Terry and LaPrade 1996). The short head of the biceps femoris is mono-articular with a deep tendon insertion, which makes it perfectly suitable to stabilize the knee. Because the tendon inserts into the posterolateral capsule, rotary and anterioposterior stress on the knee joint will trigger a contraction of the biceps femoris (Ellenbecker *et al.* 2009).

At the medial side of the knee, the conjoined tendon of the sartorius, gracilis, and semitendinosus lies superficial to the medial collateral ligament and fuses with the crural fascia. These

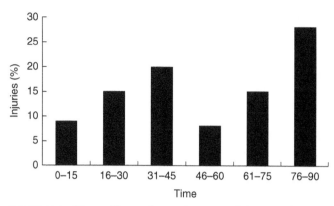

FIGURE 12.3 Time of hamstring strain sustained during a football match (Woods et al. 2004)

muscles, tendons, and membranes stabilize the medial side of the knee joint to prevent knee valgus (Mochizuki *et al.* 2004).

Risk factors

Strength imbalances, bilateral asymmetries, and fatigue: A large prospective study of professional football players indicates that quadriceps-to-hamstring strength imbalances or bilateral asymmetries can identify players at higher risk of hamstring strain and that the normalization of these imbalances significantly reduces hamstring injury rates (Croisier *et al.* 2008). A strength imbalance between the hamstrings and quadriceps is the injury risk factor that has been most supported by research (Arnason *et al.* 2008; Croisier *et al.* 2008; Yeung *et al.* 2009).

During sprinting and kicking the hamstrings have to brake the knee extension generated by the quadriceps muscles (Chumanov *et al.* 2012). Because the quads are stronger than the hamstrings, the hamstrings will become fatigued faster. Strength imbalances between both muscle groups will result in a faster decrease of the eccentric knee flexor torque and increase the risk for hamstring strain (Croisier *et al.* 2008).

Fatigue: Hamstring injuries are more likely to occur at the latter stages of a game (Ekstrand *et al.* 2011a; Greig and Siegler 2009; Woods *et al.* 2004; Figure 12.3). Eccentric hamstring strength decreases with playing time. The fatigue effect is also speed dependent. Faster running speeds result in a greater decrease of the peak eccentric hamstring torque (Greig and Siegler 2009). The decreased ability of the hamstring muscles to generate force reduces the energy absorption capacity and predisposes them to strain-type injuries (Garrett 1990). The activity of the biceps femoris, the muscle in which the vast majority of hamstring strains occur, also progressively increases during each half and markedly the second half (Greig *et al.* 2006).

Core instability: The force and stretch of the iliopsoas during the late stance phase and early swing phase induces an increased anterior tilt of the pelvis. This anterior pelvic tilt results in a greater hamstring stretch of the opposite limb, which is simultaneously in the late swing phase. Increased pelvic tilting when sprinting, due to core instability and compromised pelvic control, results in greater musculo-tendon stretch and strain of the hamstring muscles during the terminal swing phase (Chumanov *et al.* 2007).

Weak or inhibited gluteal muscles: Due to delayed gluteus maximus activity, the hamstring muscles become dominant during hip extension, which can cause hamstring strains (Sahrmann 2002).

The gluteus maximus and long head of the biceps femoris play an important role in stabilizing the pelvis. Pelvic instability can alter the muscle activation timing and the load transfer through the sacro-iliacal joint (Janda 1985; Leinonen et al. 2000; Nelson-Wong et al. 2012).

Lack of proper warm-up: beneficial effects of warm-up, temperature, and stretching on the mechanical properties of muscle. These benefits potentially reduce the risks of strain injury to the muscle (Garrett 1996).

How does a hamstring strain-type injury alter the muscles' properties and why do these altered properties put the athlete at a higher risk for recurrence?

Previous hamstring injury has been associated with a shifted length–tension curve towards shorter muscle lengths and reduced eccentric hamstring strength towards full knee extension (Brockett et al. 2004). This indicates that after a hamstring strain the hamstring muscles can produce their greatest force at shorter muscle lengths compared to the pre-injury state. This also means that the end-range strength of the hamstrings is reduced. The presence of scar tissue at the site of the injury might be responsible for the shift of peak torque towards shorter muscle lengths (Kaariainen et al. 2000). Scar tissue is less compliant than contractile tissue and can therefore alter the mechanical properties of the muscle (Butler et al. 2004).

Because the peak force during sprinting occurs at longer muscle lengths, a shifted peak torque towards shorter lengths and reduced end-range strength place the muscle at a higher risk for re-injury (Brockett et al. 2004). This is probably a major cause of the very high recurrence rate during the first month after returning to play.

Another reason for the reduced end-range eccentric hamstring strength is a decreased activation of the biceps femoris towards full knee extension (Sole et al. 2011). A lot of athletes return to sport with inhibition and selective atrophy of the long head of the biceps (Croisier et al. 2002; Silder et al. 2008).

Scar tissue appears as early as six weeks after the muscle strain and persists a minimum of five months at the site of the injury (Silder et al. 2008). Because the scar tissue is less compliant than muscle tissue, extensive scarring requires the muscle fibers in proximity of the scar tissue to lengthen a greater amount to reach the same overall muscle length (Butler et al. 2004). Because the muscle region near the scar tissue is subjected to higher strain, re-injuries mostly occur near the site of prior injury. The neuromuscular inhibition is probably a protective mechanism to reduce the risk of re-injury. As a result of the inhibition the majority of athletes return to sport with atrophy, strength deficits, and a shifted peak torque towards shorter muscle lengths, which places them at a higher risk for re-injury (Sanfilippo et al. 2013). The atrophy is not limited to the injured muscle but can also affect the agonist muscles (Sanfilippo et al. 2013). Sanfilippo et al. showed that the healing and remodeling process continues after return to sport and that the atrophy and strength deficits of the injured leg returned to normal after six months (Sanfilippo et al. 2013). Other studies demonstrate however that the strength abnormalities and scar tissue remodeling and hence an elevated risk of re-injury can persist a lot longer than six months after the initial muscle strain (Croisier et al. 2002; Silder et al. 2008). This emphasizes the importance of functional loading and progressive rehabilitation programs.

And of course if the initial risk factors that were associated with the first injury are not addressed in the rehabilitation, they will remain to put the athlete at a higher risk of recurrence.

Rehabilitation

The high early re-injury rate following return to sport after hamstring injury indicates that the players return prematurely or that most rehabilitation programs are inadequate. Studies have shown that on return to sport the player has developed maladaptations that increase the risk of re-injury. These maladaptations include:

- reduced eccentric hamstring strength especially towards leg extension (Brockett *et al.* 2004; Brughelli *et al.* 2009; Sanfilippo *et al.* 2013);
- inhibition and atrophy of the long head of biceps femoris (Croisier *et al.* 2002; Sanfilippo *et al.* 2013; Silder *et al.* 2008; Sole *et al.* 2011);
- a shift of the length–tension curve towards shorter muscle lengths (Brockett *et al.* 2004; Brughelli *et al.* 2009; Sanfilippo *et al.* 2013).

These factors together with the initial risk factors that were associated with the original hamstring injury have to be addressed in the rehabilitation program.

The Nordic hamstring exercise and eccentric hamstring exercises

Most of the hamstring strains occur in the terminal swing phase, when the hamstrings are contracting eccentrically at peak length (Chumanov *et al.* 2012; Petersen and Hölmich 2005). The ratio of eccentric hamstring strength to concentric quadriceps strength has also been shown to be a more accurate way to identify players with an increased risk for hamstring injury (Arnason *et al.* 2008; Croisier *et al.* 2008; Yeung *et al.* 2009). Strengthening the hamstring muscles eccentrically in an elongated range of motion should therefore form an important part of rehab or training (Arnason *et al.* 2008; Askling *et al.* 2003; Brockett *et al.* 2004; Gabbe *et al.* 2006b; Petersen and Hölmich 2011). Eccentric training has been shown to shift the force–length curve to longer muscle lengths (Brockett *et al.* 2001; Brughelli *et al.* 2009, 2010; Kilgallon *et al.* 2007; Schmitt *et al.* 2012). Sarcomerogenesis, which is the process of adding the number of sarcomeres in series, gradually adapts the optimal muscle length to the zone in which it is operating. Not only eccentric training, but also regular strength training using exercises that are more challenging at lengthened ranges of motion can shift peak torque towards greater muscle lengths (Goldspink 1999; Seynnes *et al.* 2007).

The Nordic hamstring exercise is an eccentric hamstring strengthening exercise that is also more challenging towards a more extended knee position (Iga *et al.* 2012). A Nordic hamstring exercise program has been shown to substantially reduce the incidence of new (60 percent) and recurrent (85 percent) hamstring injuries of soccer players (Thorborg 2012). After only ten days of eccentric hamstring training a shift of the peak torque towards greater muscle lengths has been detected (Brockett *et al.* 2001, 2004; Brughelli *et al.* 2009, 2010; Seynnes *et al.* 2007).

The hamstrings function at long lengths during sprinting (Chumanov *et al.* 2012; Petersen and Hölmich 2005). Shifting the length–tension curve and increasing the end-range strength of the hamstrings counteract the maladaptations following hamstring injury and prevent fibers from reaching a length where they are susceptible to tearing (Brughelli *et al.* 2010).

Static flexibility programs have been shown to be unable to influence the length–tension relationship and are therefore ineffective in preventing hamstring strains (Arnason *et al.* 2008). Because static stretching does not require muscle contraction it is likely unable to positively affect the length–tension curve of the hamstrings in the same way as eccentric strength training.

A number of studies provide evidence that a Nordic exercise program is effective in reducing the risk of hamstring injury and recurrence, as well as improving eccentric hamstring muscle strength and sprint ability (Arnason *et al.* 2008; Häkkinen and Komi 1985; Mjølsnes *et al.* 2004; Petersen *et al.* 2011; Thorborg 2012).

For these reasons mentioned the Nordic hamstring exercise is imperative for soccer players.

Re-activating the long head of the biceps femoris

Rehabilitation programs also need to focus on the re-activation of the long head of the biceps femoris muscle to counter the inhibition and atrophy associated with hamstring injury. Because research started to focus only recently on the inherent function of each of the hamstring muscles, there is limited evidence about the activation pattern of the different muscles. The anatomical characteristics of a muscle are the primary determinants of its function, so based on the architecture of the long head of the biceps femoris its function during movement can be derived (Lieber *et al.* 1993, 2000). It is a thick muscle with a large cross-sectional area and short, pennate fibers, especially suited for high force contractions over a shorter distance (Kellis *et al.* 2012; Lieber *et al.* 1993; Makihara *et al.* 2006). During the stance phase of running the hamstring muscles have to contract forcefully while there is less change in muscle length because of the simultaneous hip and knee extension. This is in accordance with research that revealed the forward lunge, which involves simultaneous knee and hip extension, especially loads the long head of the biceps femoris (Mendiguchia *et al.* 2013). Exercises where leg action is similar to the stance phase of running, like a resisted slide-board back lunge, a step-up, or a walking lunge can counter the inhibition and atrophy associated with hamstring injury. These exercises also require horizontal force production and contribute to enhanced sprinting performance. On return to sport after hamstring injury, athletes are slower and demonstrate substantially lower horizontal force and power outputs during sprinting (Mendiguchia *et al.* 2014). This inability to produce a high level of horizontal force is probably related to the inhibition of the long head of the biceps femoris and stresses the importance of hamstring exercises that mimic the muscle actions during a sprint.

Enhancing hamstring strength and endurance

Strength and endurance of the hamstring muscles play an important role in the prevention of hamstring strain and recurrence. Therefore rehabilitation and training need to emphasize these bio-motor abilities.

Rehabilitation needs to focus on re-establishing adequate strength ratios between the quadriceps and hamstrings. An eccentric hamstring/concentric quadriceps strength ratio superior to 1.0, a concentric hamstring/concentric quadriceps ratio superior to 0.6, and right–left hamstring strength deficit of less than 5 percent have been associated with a lower risk for hamstring injury (Croisier *et al.* 2008). Athletes with strength imbalances have been found to be four to five times more prone to sustain a hamstring injury compared to athletes with proper strength ratios (Croisier *et al.* 2008). Especially the eccentric hamstring to concentric quadriceps ratio gives a good indication of the energy absorption capacity of the hamstring muscles during sprinting. Implementing hamstring strengthening, particularly in the eccentric mode will help normalize strength imbalances and reduce the risk of re-injury.

Because the hamstrings consist of a higher percentage of fast-twitch muscle fibers and co-contract with the stronger quadriceps muscles, they are prone to fatigue. To enhance the capacity of hamstrings to cope with fatigue the volume of hamstring work needs to be increased progressively during rehabilitation. Another possibility to enhance the strength endurance of the hamstring muscles is to perform some regular or eccentric strengthening exercises at the end of the rehabilitation session or soccer practice.

Core stability

Rehab also needs to integrate exercises to promote core stability and develop neuromuscular control. Sherry *et al.* demonstrated a significant reduction in injury recurrence when the rehabilitation program for acute hamstring strain included core stability exercises (Sherry and Best 2004). The powerful contraction of the iliopsoas in the stance leg greatly increases the stretch that the hamstrings of the opposite side incur during the terminal swing phase (Chumanov *et al.* 2007). Enhanced lumbo-pelvic control will better counteract the forces of the iliopsoas and hence reduce the anterior pelvic tilt and stretch of the hamstrings of the swing leg (Sherry and Best 2004).

Reactivating the gluteus maximus and enhancing intermuscular coordination

The gluteus maximus is a very powerful hip extensor and also plays an important role in the stabilization of the lumbo-pelvic region. Pelvic instability, back pain, or other lower body injuries can alter the muscle activation timing (Janda 1985; Leinonen *et al.* 2000; Nelson-Wong *et al.* 2012). The hamstring muscles then become dominant during hip extension as a result of gluteal inhibition or weakness (Sahrmann 2002). Hip extension is initiated by the hamstrings and erector spinae while the activation of the gluteus maximus is delayed (Janda 1985; Leinonen *et al.* 2000; Nelson-Wong *et al.* 2012). The gluteus maximus should be the primary hip extensor. Diminished gluteal function will place a higher load on the hamstrings and increases the risk of hamstring injury. Rehabilitation programs for hamstring injury should focus on restoring proper coordination patterns, consist of exercises that (re)activate the glutes, and enhance the intermuscular coordination between the glutes and hamstrings.

Ballistic exercises

An adequate rehab program for hamstring injury progressively integrates exercises that are more ballistic in nature (Schmitt *et al.* 2012). Several studies show that training adaptations are velocity-specific and that training adaptations are greatest near the training velocity (Häkkinen and Komi 1985; McBride *et al.* 2002; Mero and Komi 1986). The strength and eccentric exercises develop the high-force/low-speed end of the force–velocity curve, but they do not work the hamstrings near the contraction speeds of sprinting (Häkkinen and Komi 1985; McBride *et al.* 2002; Mero and Komi 1986). An acute hamstring strain is a high-velocity injury (Chumanov *et al.* 2007). Exercises that develop the low-force/high-speed end of the spectrum will progressively prepare the hamstrings to handle high eccentric loads during the terminal swing phase (Häkkinen and Komi 1985; McBride *et al.* 2002; Mero and Komi 1986). Stair bounds, hops, alternate leg bounds will all reinforce hamstring stiffness without placing an excessive eccentric load on the hamstrings during terminal swing (Cormie *et al.* 2010, 2011). Stiffer hamstring muscles can store more elastic energy during active lengthening, thereby reducing peak muscle stretch and reducing the susceptibility to injury (Thelen *et al.* 2005b). Ballistic exercises provide a functional eccentric loading and are a good progression towards higher-intensity running.

Progressive sprint loading

An increase in running speed from 80 percent to 100 percent effort is associated with a 1.4-fold increase of peak hamstring force and a 1.9-fold increase of energy absorption during the terminal swing phase (Chumanov *et al.* 2007). This means hamstring load significantly increases during the swing, but not the stance phase (Chumanov *et al.* 2007).

During rehabilitation the volume and intensity of sprinting progressively have to be augmented to prepare the player to return to playing soccer. Uphill and resisted sprinting can help to make the transition from 80 percent to maximal speed. While the effort during uphill and resisted sprinting is maximal, the top speed is lower. The hamstring forces during the stance phase will be equal or slightly elevated compared to regular sprinting, but the amount of energy that has to be absorbed during terminal swing is significantly less. Because the hamstring muscles are especially vulnerable to strain-type injury during the late swing phase, the change of re-injury is less during resisted and uphill maximal sprinting.

12.3 The hip adductors

The group of hip adductor muscles consists of the pectineus, gracilis, adductor brevis, adductor longus, and adductor magnus (Williams and Warwick 1980). This muscle group's main function is adducting the thigh (Williams and Warwick 1980). In addition to generating movement they also stabilize the hip and lower extremity to perturbations in the three planes of motion during closed kinetic chain movements (Sedaghati *et al.* 2013; Tyler *et al.* 2014). Depending on the position of the thigh, each hip adductor muscle separately can also contribute to hip flexion and hip rotation (Delp *et al.* 1999; Leighton 2006). The adductor magnus is a powerful hip extensor as well.

The hip adductor muscles have long muscle fiber lengths, which makes them perfectly suited to move the thigh through a large range of motion (Lieber and Ward 2011; Takizawa *et al.* 2014; Ward *et al.* 2009). The adductor minimus on the other hand (the upper part of the adductor magnus) has shorter muscle fiber lengths and appears to primarily function as a stabilizer of the hip (Retchford *et al.* 2013; Takizawa *et al.* 2014). The adductor minimus forms part of what is described as the rotator cuff of the hip (Retchford *et al.* 2013).

Groin injuries are frequently encountered in soccer. They account for 10–18 percent of all injuries in soccer and are the most common type of injury for goalkeepers (Eirale *et al.* 2014; Ekstrand and Gillquist 1983; Hölmich 2007; Nielsen and Yde 1989; Sedaghati *et al.* 2013). There are multiple causes of groin pain, but a strain of the adductor muscles is the major cause in soccer players (Ibrahim *et al.* 2007; Renström and Peterson 1980). The adductor longus is the most frequently injured muscle (Tyler *et al.* 2014).

Groin strains typically occur during movements that require a strong eccentric contraction of the hip adductors to decelerate the lower extremity during rapid abduction (Hrysomallis 2009). The adductor muscle group is exposed to high eccentric forces at longer muscle lengths during sudden changes of direction and kicking the ball (Charnock et al. 2009; Hureibi and McLatchie 2010). The multiple abrupt changes of direction, kicking, and body contact during competition and practice explain why soccer players are at a high risk of sustaining groin injury (Macintyre et al. 2006; Sedaghati et al. 2013). Goalkeepers are even more prone to adductor injuries than field players due to the many explosive lateral movements and jumps (Eirale et al. 2014).

An association between adductor strength and groin injuries has been reported in soccer players (Engebretsen et al. 2010; Malliaras et al. 2009; Thorborg et al. 2014). An adductor/abductor strength ratio of less than 80 percent considerably increases the risk of developing an adductor strain injury (Tyler et al. 2001). Functional exercises to strengthen the adductor muscles can therefore help protect the player against groin injury (Nicholas and Tyler 2002). In line with this, Tyler reported that a pre-season strengthening program that mainly emphasized to restore the hip adductor-to-abductor strength imbalance drastically reduced the risk of sustaining a groin strain injury during the following season (Tyler et al. 2002).

Restoring the strength of the adductor muscle group is also key during rehabilitation and for players that have a history of groin injuries (Sedaghati et al. 2013; Tyler et al. 2002). A previous groin strain increases the possibility for a reoccurring adductor injury. Recurrence rates for groin strains of 32–44 percent have been reported in a variety of sports (Seward et al. 1993; Tyler et al. 2002). Large eccentric hip adduction strength deficits have been observed in soccer players with adductor-related groin pain (Thorborg et al. 2014). Reduced eccentric muscle strength can impair the energy-absorbing capacity and increase the susceptibility to strain injury (Garrett 1990). A program to improve the eccentric strength of the hip adductors has been proven very effective for athletes with long-standing adductor-related groin pain to return to full sport participation without pain (Hölmich et al. 1999).

Other identified risk factors for groin strain injury include core muscle weakness and poor flexibility of the hip adductors (Arnason et al. 2004; Ekstrand and Gillquist 1983; Ibrahim et al. 2007; Maffey and Emery 2007). The association between a reduced range of motion for hip abduction and an increased risk of groin strain injury has only been observed in soccer players (Arnason et al. 2004; Ekstrand and Gillquist 1983; Ibrahim et al. 2007). Studies conducted with ice hockey and rugby players did not find an association (Emery and Meeuwisse 2001; O'Connor 2004; Tyler et al. 2001). Why poor adductor flexibility is more likely to increase the risk of groin injury in soccer may depend upon sport-specific factors such as movement patterns and velocity (Hrysomallis 2009).

Due to the high prevalence of groin strains in soccer it is important to address the risk factors associated with a greater injury incidence in training and rehabilitation. Correcting hip adductor weakness, which is considered the main risk factor, should not be limited to exercises that isolate the inner thigh muscles. A better way to strengthen the hip adductors however is to include a few movements that emphasize the various functions of the adductor muscle group. During soccer these muscles are engaged in both open and closed kinetic chain movements. The progressive hip adductor strengthening should therefore also include closed kinetic chain exercises. Closed kinetic chain movements such as the lateral lunge and the slide-board lateral lunge place a high eccentric emphasis on the adductor muscles. These exercises also challenge the adductor muscles at long lengths, which can induce an increased active and passive range of motion. The slide-board lateral slide is another effective exercise to eccentrically strengthen the hip adductors (Chang *et al.* 2009; Tyler *et al.* 2014). Exercises to enhance the neuromuscular control and strength of the core should also be incorporated into the rehabilitation or preventive program (Maffey and Emery 2007). Single-leg and some multiple-joint exercises, including the back lunge and one-arm press, the staggered-stance one-arm press, the split stance core press, and the barbell torque, enhance core stability and train the hip stabilization function of the adductors simultaneously. It is also recommended to progressively incorporate some plyometric exercises. Plyometrics will help improve the neuromuscular control, the musculo-tendinous stiffness, and energy-absorbing capacity of the adductor muscles, reducing the susceptibility to strain injuries (Chimera *et al.* 2004; Fouré *et al.* 2011; Wilson and Flanagan 2008).

12.4 The vastus medialis obliquus

The quadriceps femoris is a powerful extensor of the knee among four muscles: the biarticular rectus femoris and the monoarticular vastus medialis, vastus intermedius, and vastus lateralis (VL). Based on the different fiber orientation, a further division of vastus medialis into an oblique (vastus medialis obliquus, VMO) and long part (vastus medialis longus) was introduced (Bose *et al.* 1980; Smith *et al.* 2009a; Travnik *et al.* 1995). The vastus medialis obliquus is the distal part of the vastus medialis and is positioned at the inside and just above the kneecap. While the fibers of the vastus medialis longus are directed vertically, the vastus medialis obliquus fibers run medially in a 50–55° angle with the long axis of the femur and attach to the upper medial border of the patella (Bose *et al.* 1980; Travnik *et al.* 1995). Some fibers of the vastus medialis obliquus do not attach to the medial margin of the patella but have direct continuity with the patellar tendon (Toumi *et al.* 2007).

There is controversy whether the vastus medialis longus and obliquus have a shared or separate innervation, but both parts have a different fiber type composition and function (Dhaher and Khan 2002; Nozic *et al.* 1997; Smith *et al.* 2009b; Tanino and Suzuki 2014). The vastus medialis longus consists of a higher proportion of type I (slow-twitch) fibers and a lower proportion of type IIb (fast-twitch) fibers compared to the vastus medialis obliquus (Travnik *et al.* 1995). While the vastus medialis longus is mainly a knee extensor, it also stabilizes the patella similar to the vastus medialis obliquus (Dhaher and Khan 2002; Nozic *et al.* 1997; Tanino and Suzuki 2014). The vastus medialis obliquus is a weak knee extensor, but plays an important role to counteract the laterally directed forces of the vastus lateralis to control the tracking of the patella in the patellar groove (Basmajian and De Luca 1985). The vastus medialis obliquus also prevents external rotation of the tibia via the insertion of the patellar tendon on the top of the tibial shinbone and can therefore resist knee valgus (Cerny 1995; Hanten and Schulthies 1990; Müller 1983; Toumi *et al.* 2007; van Kampen and Huiskes 1990). Weakness or inhibition of the vastus medialis obliquus can lead to abnormal patellar tracking and subsequent elevated patellofemoral contact pressures (Smith *et al.* 2009a; Travnik *et al.* 1995). Knee injuries are associated with altered activation and possible atrophy of the vastus medialis obliquus (Giles *et al.* 2013; Pattyn *et al.* 2011).

It has been suggested that concurrent hip adductor co-contraction or performing the exercise with the tibia externally rotated may enhance the activity of the vastus medialis obliquus (Hodges and Richardson 1993; Willis *et al.* 2005). There is however also an extensive body of evidence to suggest that altering the lower limb position or simultaneous hip adductor

TABLE 12.3 VMO/VL ratios across different exercises

Study	Exercise	Mean VMO/VL ratio
Cerny 1995	Step-down	1.3
	Squat (1/4)	1.2
	Leg extension	1.1
	Isometric leg extension	1.2
Earl et al. 2001	Squat	Left leg: 1.02
		Right leg: 1.28
Hertel et al. 2004	Squat (1/2)	3.00
Hodges and Richardson 1993	Squat	1.29
	Leg extension	0.93
Hung and Gross 1999	Squat	1.31
	Isometric leg extension	1.02
Irish et al. 2010	Squat (with isometric hip adduction)	1.14
	Lunge	1.18
	Leg extension	0.72
Miller et al. 1997	Squat (1/2)	2.08
	Step-up–step-down	2.18

contraction does not result in preferential vastus medialis obliquus activation (Smith *et al.* 2009a).

To improve the medial stabilization of the patella it has been proposed that the vastus medialis obliquus should be preferentially strengthened to correct the strength imbalance between the vastus medialis obliquus and vastus lateralis. It is suggested that exercises with a VMO/VL activity ratio greater than 1 can address this imbalance (Table 12.3). That the lower body is a closed kinetic chain during most of its functions also has to be taken into consideration (Houglum 2010). Malalignment at the hip or foot can cause knee valgus and result in abnormal patellar tracking and increased patellofemoral compressive forces (Houglum 2010). Knee valgus is the result of hip adduction, hip internal rotation, and external rotation of the tibia. The gluteal muscles (hip abductors and external rotators), medial hamstrings, gracilis, sartorius, and vastus medialis (internal rotation of tibia) all work in concert to resist knee valgus. Exercises such as the lunge, step-up, step-down, single-leg squat, and the double-leg squat have VMO/VL activity ratios greater than 1 and address the entire kinetic chain (Hertel *et al.* 2004; Hodges and Richardson 1993; Hung and Gross 1999; Irish *et al.* 2010; Miller *et al.* 1997). Squat strength is also the best predictor of knee valgus during movement (McCurdy *et al.* 2014). People with patellofemoral pain syndrome have been shown to have hip and knee strength deficits (Baldon *et al.* 2009; Cowan and Crossley 2009; Nakagawa *et al.* 2011; Souza and Powers 2009). Training programs that focus on the whole kinetic chain report superior outcomes compared to exercise programs that only address the knee extensor strength deficit and quadriceps muscle imbalance (Harvie *et al.* 2011; Mascal *et al.* 2003; Nakagawa *et al.* 2008).

The vastus medialis obliquus activity and VMO/VL ratios are more pronounced during weight-bearing activities compared to open-chain kinetic exercises (exercises in which the foot is free to move) (Cerny 1995; Hodges and Richardson 1993; Hung and Gross 1999; Irish *et al.* 2010; Toumi *et al.* 2007). This may come as no surprise regarding the double role the vastus medialis obliquus fulfills in closed kinetic chain movements (movements in which the force is applied to the ground). The vastus medialis obliquus does not only stabilize the patella, but also contracts to resist knee valgus of the stance leg. Single-leg weight-bearing exercises, which challenge the stability of the knee joint more compared to bilateral movements, may also elicit greater vastus medialis obliquus activation (Toumi *et al.* 2007).

References

Alkjaer T, Wieland MR, Andersen MS, Simonsen EB, Rasmussen J. Computational modeling of a forward lunge: towards a better understanding of the function of the cruciate ligaments. *J Anat.* 2012 Dec;221(6):590–7.

Andrews JG. A general method for determining the functional role of a muscle. *J Biomech Eng.* 1985 Nov;107(4):348–53.

Arnason A, Sigurdsson SB, Gudmundsson A, Holme I, Engebretsen L, Bahr R. Risk factors for injuries in football. *Am J Sports Med.* 2004 Jan–Feb;32(1 Suppl):5S–16S.

Arnason A, Andersen TE, Holme I, Engebretsen L, Bahr R. Prevention of hamstring strains in elite soccer: an intervention study. *Scand J Med Sci Sports.* 2008 Feb;18(1):40–8.

Askling C, Karlsson J, Thorstensson A. A hamstring injury occurrence in elite soccer players after preseason training with eccentric overload. *Scand J Med Sci.* 2003 Aug;13(4):244–50.

Ayotte N, Stetts D, Keenan G, Greensway E. Electromyographical analysis of selected lower extremity muscles during 5 unilateral weight-bearing exercises. *J Orthop Sports Phys Ther.* 2007 Feb;37(2):48–55.

Baldon Rde M, Nakagawa TH, Muniz TB, Amorim CF, Maciel CD, Serrão FV. Eccentric hip muscle function in females with and without patellofemoral pain syndrome. *J Athl Train.* 2009 Sep–Oct;44(5):490–6.

Basmajian JV, De Luca CJ. *Muscles alive: their functions revealed by electromyography.* 5th ed. Baltimore, MD: Lippincott Williams & Wilkins; 1985. 561 pp.

Besier TF, Lloyd DG, Ackland TR. Muscle activation strategies at the knee during running and cutting maneuvers. *Med Sci Sports Exerc.* 2003 Jan;35(1):119–27.

Biscarini A. Minimization of the knee shear joint load in leg-extension equipment. *Med Eng Phys.* 2008 Oct;30(8):1032–41.

Biscarini A, Botti FM, Pettorossi VE. Selective contribution of each hamstring muscle to anterior cruciate ligament protection and tibiofemoral joint stability in leg-extension exercise: a simulation study. *Eur J Appl Physiol.* 2013 Sep;113(9):2263–73.

Bober T, Mularczyk W. The mechanics of the leg swing in running. In: Brüggemann GP, Rühl JK, editors. *Proceedings of the first international conference on techniques in athletics;* 1990 Jun 7–9; Cologne. Cologne: Deutsche Sporthochschule Köln; 1990. pp. 507–10.

Bose K, Kanagasuntheram R, Osman MB. Vastus medialis oblique: an anatomic and physiologic study. *Orthopedics.* 1980 Sep;3(9):880–3.

Brindle TJ, Mattacola C, McCrory J. Electromyographic changes in the gluteus medius during stair ascent and descent in subjects with anterior knee pain. *Knee Surg Sports Traumatol Arthrosc.* 2003 Jul;11(4):244–51.

Brockett CL, Morgan DL, Proske U. Human hamstring muscles adapt to eccentric exercise by changing optimum length. *Med Sci Sports Exerc.* 2001 May;33(5):783–90.

Brockett CL, Morgan DL, Porske U. Predicting hamstring strain injury in elite athletes. *Med Sci Sports Exerc.* 2004 Mar;36(3):379–87.

Brughelli M, Nosaka K, Cronin J. Application of eccentric exercise on an Australian rules football player with recurrent hamstring injuries. *Phys Ther Sport.* 2009 May;10(2):75–80.

Brughelli M, Cronin J, Mendiguchia J, Kinsella D, Nosaka K. Contralateral leg deficits in kinetic and kinematic variables during running in Australian rules football players with previous hamstring injuries. *J Strength Cond Res.* 2010 Sep;24(9):2539–44.

Bullock-Saxton JE, Janda V, Bullock MI. The influence of ankle sprain injury on muscle activation during hip extension. *Int J Sports Med.* 1994 Aug;15(6):330–4.

Burger H, Valencic V, Marincek C, Kogovsek N. Properties of musculus gluteus maximus in above-knee amputees. *Clin Biomech (Bristol, Avon).* 1996 Jan;11(1):35–38.

Butler DL, Juncosa N, Dressler MR. Functional efficacy of tendon repair processes. *Annu Rev Biomed Eng.* 2004;6:303–29.

Carling C, Le Gall F, Orhant E. A four-season prospective study of muscle strain reoccurrences in a professional football club. *Res Sports Med.* 2011 Apr;19(2):92–102.

Cerny K. Vastus medialis oblique/vastus lateralis muscle activity ratios for selected exercises in persons with and without patellofemoral pain syndrome. *Phys Ther.* 1995 Aug;75(8):672–83.

Chang R, Turcotte R, Pearsall D. Hip adductor muscle function in forward skating. *Sports Biomech.* 2009 Sep;8(3):212–22.

Charnock BL, Lewis CL, Garrett WE Jr, Queen RM. Adductor longus mechanics during the maximal effort soccer kick. *Sports Biomech.* 2009 Sep;8(3):223–34.

Chimera NJ, Swanik KA, Swanik CB, Straub SJ. Effects of plyometric training on muscle-activation strategies and performance in female athletes. *J Athl Train.* 2004 Mar;39(1):24–31.

Chumanov ES, Heiderscheit BC, Thelen DG. The effect of speed and influence of individual muscles on hamstring mechanics during the swing phase of sprinting. *J Biomech.* 2007;40(16):3555–62.

Chumanov ES, Heiderscheit BC, Thelen DG. Hamstring musculotendon dynamics during stance and swing phases of high-speed running. *Med Sci Sports Exerc.* 2011 Mar;43(3):525–32.

Chumanov ES, Schache AG, Heiderscheit BC, Thelen DG. Hamstrings are most susceptible to injury during the late swing phase of sprinting. *Br J Sports Med.* 2012 Feb;46(2):90.

Comerford MJ. Core stability: priorities in rehab of the athlete. *Sport Ex Medicine.* 2004;22:15–22.

Cormie P, McGuigan MR, Newton RU. Changes in the eccentric phase contribute to improved stretch-shorten cycle performance after training. *Med Sci Sports Exerc.* 2010 Sep;42(9):1731–44.

Cormie P, McGuigan MR, Newton RU. Developing maximal neuromuscular power: Part 1–biological basis of maximal power production. *Sports Med.* 2011 Jan;41(1):17–38.

Cowan SM, Crossley KM. Does gender influence neuromotor control of the knee and hip? *J Electromyogr Kinesiol.* 2009 Apr;19(2):276–82.

Croisier J, Forthomme B, Namurois M, Vanderthommen M, Crielaard J. Hamstring muscle strain recurrence and strength performance disorders. *Am J Sports Med.* 2002 Mar–Apr;30(2):199–203.

Croisier JL, Ganteaume S, Binet J, Genty M, Ferret JM. Strength imbalances and prevention of hamstring injury in professional soccer players: a prospective study. *Am J Sports Med.* 2008 Aug;36(8):1469–75.

Crow JF, Pearce AJ, Veale JP, Vander Westhuizen D, Coburn PT, Pizzari T. Hip adductor muscle strength is reduced preceding and during the onset of groin pain in elite junior Australian football players. *J Sci Med Sport.* 2010 Mar;13(2):202–4.

Delp SL, Hess WE, Hungerford DS, Jones LC. Variation of rotation moment arms with hip flexion. *J Biomech.* 1999 May;32(5):493–501.

Dhaher YY, Kahn LE. The effect of vastus medialis forces on patello-femoral contact: a model-based study. *J Biomech Eng.* 2002 Dec;124(6):758–67.

Dick R, Putukian M, Agel J, Evans TA, Marshall SW. Descriptive epidemiology of collegiate women's soccer injuries: National Collegiate Athletic Association Injury Surveillance System, 1988–1989 through 2002–2003. *J Athl Train.* 2007 Apr–Jun;42(2):278–85.

Distefano LJ, Blackburn JT, Marshall SW, Padua DA. Gluteal muscle activation during common therapeutic exercises. *J Orthop Sports Phys Ther.* 2009 Jul;39(7):532–40.

Earl JE, Schmitz RJ, Arnold BL. Activation of the VMO and VL during dynamic mini-squat exercises with and without isometric hip adduction. *J Electromyogr Kinesiol.* 2001 Dec;11(6):381–6.

Eirale C, Tol JL, Whiteley R, Chalabi H, Hölmich P. Different injury pattern in goalkeepers compared to field players: a three-year epidemiological study of professional football. *J Sci Med Sport.* 2014 Jan;17(1):34–8.

Ekstrand J, Gillquist J. The avoidability of soccer injuries. *Int J Sports Med.* 1983 May;4(2):124–8.

Ekstrand J, Hagglund M, Walden M. Injury incidence and injury patterns in professional football: the UEFA injury study. *Br J Sports Med.* 2011a;45:553–8.

Ekstrand J, Hägglund M, Waldén M. Epidemiology of muscle injuries in professional football (soccer). *Am J Sports Med.* 2011b Jun;39(6):1226–32.

Ekstrand J, Hägglund M, Kristenson K, Magnusson H, Waldén M. Fewer ligament injuries but no preventive effect on muscle injuries and severe injuries: an 11-year follow-up of the UEFA Champions League injury study. *Br J Sports Med*. 2013 Aug;47(12):732–7.

Ekstrom R, Donatelli R, Carp K. Electromyographical analysis of core trunk, hip, and thigh muscles during 9 rehabilitation exercises. *J Orthop Sports Phys Ther*. 2007 Dec;37(12):754–62.

Ellenbecker T, De Carlo M, DeRosa C. *Effective functional progressions in sport rehabilitation*. Champaign, IL: Human Kinetics; 2009. 248 pp.

Emery CA, Meeuwisse WH. Risk factors for groin injuries in hockey. *Med Sci Sports Exerc*. 2001 Sep;33(9):1423–33.

Engebretsen AH, Myklebust G, Holme I, Engebretsen L, Bahr R. Intrinsic risk factors for groin injuries among male soccer players: a prospective cohort study. *Am J Sports Med*. 2010 Oct;38(10):2051–7.

Escamilla RF, Macleod TD, Wilk KE, Paulos L, Andrews JR. Anterior cruciate ligament strain and tensile forces for weight-bearing and non-weight-bearing exercises: a guide to exercise selection. *J Orthop Sports Phys Ther*. 2012 Mar;42(3):208–20.

Ferreira PH, Ferreira ML, Hodges PW. Changes in recruitment of the abdominal muscles in people with low back pain: ultrasound measurement of muscle activity. *Spine (Phila Pa 1976)*. 2004 Nov;29(22):2560–6.

Fouré A, Nordez A, McNair P, Cornu C. Effects of plyometric training on both active and passive parts of the plantarflexors series elastic component stiffness of muscle-tendon complex. *Eur J Appl Physiol*. 2011 Mar;111(3):539–48.

Fredericson M, Cookingham CL, Chaudhari AM, Dowdell BC, Oestreicher N, Sahrmann SA. Hip abductor weakness in distance runners with iliotibial band syndrome. *Clin J Sport Med*. 2000 Jul;10(3):169–75.

Freeman MA, Dean MR, Hanham IW. The etiology and prevention of functional instability of the foot. *J Bone Joint Surg Br*. 1965 Nov;47(4):678–85.

Friel K, McLean N, Myers C, Caceres M. Ipsilateral hip abductor weakness after inversion ankle sprain. *J Athl Train*. 2006 Jan–Mar;41(1):74–8.

Fujii M, Sato H, Takahira N. Muscle activity response to external moment during single-leg drop landing in young basketball players: the importance of biceps femoris in reducing internal rotation of knee during landing. *J Sports Sci Med*. 2012 Jun;11(2):255–9.

Gabbe BJ, Bennell KL, Finch CF, Wajswelner H, Orchard JW. Predictors of hamstring injury at the elite level of Australian football. *Scand J Med Sci Sports*. 2006a Feb;16(1):7–13.

Gabbe BL, Branson R, Bennel KL. A pilot randomised controlled trial of eccentric exercise to prevent hamstring injuries in community-level Australian football. *J Sci Med Sport*. 2006b May;9(1–2):103–9.

Gamble P. *Strength and conditioning for team sports: sport-specific physical preparation for high performance*. 2nd ed. New York: Routledge; 2013. 304 pp.

Garrett WE Jr. Muscle strain injuries: clinical and basic aspects. *Med Sci Sports Exerc*. 1990 Aug;22(4):436–43.

Garrett WE Jr. Muscle strain injuries. *Am J Sports Med*. 1996;24(6 Suppl):S2–8.

Gibbons SGT. Integrating the psoas major and deep sacral guteus maximus muscles into the lumbar cylinder model. Presented at The Spine – World Congress on Manual Therapy; Oct 7–9, 2005; Rome, Italy.

Gibbons SGT, Comerford MJ. Strength versus stability: Part 1: Concept and terms. *Orthopaedic Division Review*. 2001 Mar–Apr:21–7.

Giles LS, Webster KE, McClelland JA, Cook J. Does quadriceps atrophy exist in individuals with patellofemoral pain? A systematic literature review with meta-analysis. *J Orthop Sports Phys Ther*. 2013 Nov;43(11):766–76.

Goldspink G. Changes in muscle mass and phenotype and the expression of autocrine and systemic growth factors by muscle in response to stretch and overload. *J Anat*. 1999 Apr;194(Pt 3):323–34.

Greig M, Siegler JC. Soccer-specific fatigue and eccentric hamstrings muscle strength. *J Athl Train*. 2009;44:180–4.

Greig MP, McNaughton LR, Lovell RJ. Physiological and mechanical response to soccer-specific intermittent activity and steady-state activity. *Res Sports Med*. 2006 Jan–Mar;14(1):29–52.

Hagglund M, Walden M, Ekstrand J. Previous injury as a risk factor for injury in elite football: a prospective study over two consecutive seasons. *Br J Sports Med*. 2006 Sep;40(9):767–72.

Häkkinen K, Komi PV. Effect of explosive-type strength training on electromyographic and force production characteristics of leg extensor muscles during concentric and various stretch-shortening cycle exercises. *Scand J Sports Sci*. 1985;7:65–76.

Hanten WP, Schulthies SS. Exercise effect on electromyographic activity of the vastus medialis oblique and vastus lateralis muscles. *Phys Ther*. 1990 Sep;70(9):561–5.

Harvie D, O'Leary T, Kumar S. A systematic review of randomized controlled trials on exercise parameters in the treatment of patellofemoral pain: what works? *J Multidiscip Healthc*. 2011;4:383–92.

Hertel J, Earl JE, Tsang KK, Miller SJ. Combining isometric knee extension exercises with hip adduction or abduction does not increase quadriceps EMG activity. *Br J Sports Med*. 2004 Apr;38(2):210–13.

Hewett TE, Myer GD. The mechanistic connection between the trunk, hip, knee, and anterior cruciate ligament injury. *Exerc Sport Sci Rev*. 2011 Oct;39(4):161–6.

Hewett TE, Myer GD, Ford KR, Heidt RS Jr, Colosimo AJ, McLean SG, van den Bogert AJ, Paterno MV, Succop P. Biomechanical measures of neuromuscular control and valgus loading of the knee predict anterior cruciate ligament injury risk in female athletes: a prospective study. *Am J Sports Med*. 2005 Apr;33(4):492–501.

Hewett TE, Myer GD, Ford KR. Anterior cruciate ligament injuries in female athletes: Part 1, mechanisms and risk factors. *Am J Sports Med*. 2006 Feb;34(2):299–311.

Higashihara A, Ono T, Kubota J, Okuwaki T, Fukubayashi T. Functional differences in the activity of the hamstring muscles with increasing running speed. *J Sports Sci*. 2010 Aug;28(10):1085–92.

Hodges PW, Richardson CA. The influence of isometric hip adduction on quadriceps femoris activity. *Scand J Rehabil Med*. 1993 Jun;25(2):57–62.

Hölmich P. Long-standing groin pain in sportspeople falls into three primary patterns, a "clinical entity" approach: a prospective study of 207 patients. *Br J Sports Med*. 2007 Apr;41(4):247–52.

Hölmich P, Uhrskou P, Ulnits L, Kanstrup IL, Nielsen MB, Bjerg AM, Krogsgaard K. Effectiveness of active physical training as treatment for long-standing adductor-related groin pain in athletes: randomised trial. *Lancet*. 1999 Feb 6;353(9151):439–43.

Houglum PA. *Therapeutic exercise for musculoskeletal injuries (athletic training education series)*. Champaign, IL: Human Kinetics; 2010. Chapter 23, Knee and thigh; pp. 847–915.

Hrysomallis C. Hip adductors' strength, flexibility, and injury risk. *J Strength Cond Res*. 2009 Aug;23(5):1514–17.

Hung YJ, Gross MT. Effect of foot position on electromyographic activity of the vastus medialis oblique and vastus lateralis during lower-extremity weight-bearing activities. *J Orthop Sports Phys Ther*. 1999 Feb;29(2):93–102; discussion 103–5.

Hureibi KA, McLatchie GR. Groin pain in athletes. *Scott Med J*. 2010 May;55(2):8–11.

Ibrahim A, Murrell GA, Knapman P. Adductor strain and hip range of movement in male professional soccer players. *J Orthop Surg (Hong Kong)*. 2007 Apr;15(1):46–9.

Iga J, Fruer CS, Deighan M, Croix MD, James DV. 'Nordic' hamstrings exercise – engagement characteristics and training responses. *Int J Sports Med*. 2012 Dec;33(12).1000–4.

Ingersoll CD, Grindstaff TL, Pietrosimone BG, Hart JM. Neuromuscular consequences of anterior cruciate ligament injury. *Clin Sports Med*. 2008 Jul;27(3):383–404.

Ireland ML. The female ACL: why is it more prone to injury? *Orthop Clin North Am*. 2002 Oct;33(4):637–51.

Ireland ML, Willson JD, Ballantyne BT, Davis IM. Hip strength in females with and without patellofemoral pain. *J Orthop Sports Phys Ther*. 2003 Nov;33(11):671–6.

Irish SE, Millward AJ, Wride J, Haas BM, Shum GL. The effect of closed-kinetic chain exercises and open-kinetic chain exercise on the muscle activity of vastus medialis oblique and vastus lateralis. *J Strength Cond Res*. 2010 May;24(5):1256–62.

Janda V. Pain in the locomotor system – a broad approach. In: Glasgow EF, Twomey LT, Scull ER, Kleynhans AM, Idczak RM, editors. *Aspects of manipulative therapy*. Edinburgh: Churchill Livingstone; 1985. pp. 148–51.

Jenkins D. *Hollinshead's functional anatomy of the limbs and back*. 9th ed. Philadelphia: Saunders; 2008. 480 pp.

Jonhagen S, Ericson MO, Nemeth G, Eriksson E. Amplitude and timing of electromyographic activity during sprinting. *Scand J Med Sci Sports*. 1996 Feb;6(1):15–21.

Kaariainen M, Jarvinen T, Jarvinen M, Rantanen J, Kalimo H. Relation between myofibers and connective tissue during muscle injury repair. *Scand J Med Sci Sports*. 2000 Dec;10(6):332–7.

Kankaanpää M, Taimela S, Laaksonen D, Hänninen O, Airaksinen O. Back and hip extensor fatigability in chronic low back pain patients and controls. *Arch Phys Med Rehabil*. 1998 Apr;79(4):412–17.

Kellis E, Galanis N, Kapetanos G, Natsis K. Architectural differences between the hamstring muscles. *J Electromyogr Kinesiol*. 2012 Aug;22(4):520–6.

Kilgallon M, Donnelly AE, Shafat A. Progressive resistance training temporarily alters hamstring torque-angle relationship. *Scand J Med Sci Sports*. 2007 Feb;17(1):18–24.

Koulouris G, Connell D. Evaluation of the hamstring muscle complex following acute injury. *Skeletal Radiol*. 2003 Oct;32(10):582–9.

Kujala UM, Orava S, Järvinen M. Hamstring injuries. Current trends in treatment and prevention. *Sports Med*. 1997 Jun;23(6):397–404.

Kulas AS, Hortobagyi T, DeVita P. Trunk position modulates anterior cruciate ligament forces and strains during a single-leg squat. *Clin Biomech (Bristol, Avon)*. 2012 Jan;27(1):16–21.

Kyrolainen H, Komi PV, Belli A. Changes in muscle activity patterns and kinetics with increasing running speed. *J Strength Cond Res*. 1999 Nov;13(4):400–6.

Kyrolainen H, Avela J, Komi PV. Changes in muscle activity with increasing running speed. *J Sports Sci*. 2005 Oct;23(10):1101–9.

Lafond D, Normand MC, Gosselin G. Rapport force. *J Can Chiropr Assoc*. 1998;42(2):90–100.

Leighton RD. A functional model to describe the action of the adductor muscles at the hip in the transverse plane. *Physiother Theory Pract*. 2006 Nov;22(5):251–62.

Leinonen V, Kankaanpää M, Airaksinen O, Hänninen O. Back and hip extensor activities during trunk flexion/extension: effects of low back pain and rehabilitation. *Arch Phys Med Rehabil*. 2000 Jan;81(1):32–7.

Lephart SM, Ferris CM, Riemann BL, Myers JB, Fu FH. Gender differences in strength and lower extremity kinematics during landing. *Clin Orthop Relat Res*. 2002 Aug;(401):162–9.

Lewis CL, Sahrmann SA, Moran DW. Anterior hip joint force increases with hip extension, decreased gluteal force, or decreased iliopsoas force. *J Biomech*. 2007;40(16):3725–31.

Lieber RL, Bodine-Fowler SC. Skeletal muscle mechanics: implications for rehabilitation. *Phys Ther*. 1993 Dec;73(12):844–56.

Lieber RL, Friden J. Functional and clinical significance of skeletal muscle architecture. *Muscle Nerve*. 2000 Nov;23(11):1647–66.

Lieber RL, Ward SR. Skeletal muscle design to meet functional demands. *Phil Trans R Soc B*. 2011 Apr;366:1466–1476.

Lloyd DG, Buchanan TS, Besier TF. Neuromuscular biomechanical modeling to understand knee ligament loading. *Med Sci Sports Exerc*. 2005 Nov;37(11):1939–47.

McBride JM, Triplett-McBride T, Davie A, Newton RU. The effect of heavy- vs. light-load jump squats on the development of strength, power, and speed. *J Strength Cond Res*. 2002 Feb;16(1):75–82.

McCurdy K, Walker J, Armstrong R, Langford G. The relationship between selected measures of strength and hip and knee excursion during unilateral and bilateral landings in females. *J Strength Cond Res*. 2014 Sep;28(9):2429–36.

Macintyre J, Johnson C, Schroeder EL. Groin pain in athletes. *Curr Sports Med Rep*. 2006 Dec;5(6):293–9.

McLay IS, Lake MJ, Cavanagh PR. Muscle activity in running. In: Cavanagh PR, editor. *Biomechanics of distance running*. Champaign, IL: Human Kinetics Books; 1990. pp. 165–86.

Maffey L, Emery C. What are the risk factors for groin strain injury in sport? A systematic review of the literature. *Sports Med*. 2007;37(10):881–94.

Makihara Y, Nishino A, Fukubayashi T, Kanamori A. Decrease of knee flexion torque in patients with ACL reconstruction: combined analysis of the architecture and function of the knee flexor muscles. *Knee Surg Sports Traumatol Arthrosc*. 2006 Apr;14(4):310–17.

Malliaras P, Hogan A, Nawrocki A, Crossley K, Schache A. Hip flexibility and strength measures: reliability and association with athletic groin pain. *Br J Sports Med*. 2009 Oct;43(10):739–44.

Mallo J, González P, Veiga S, Navarro E. Injury incidence in a Spanish sub-elite professional football team: a prospective study during four consecutive seasons. *J Sports Sci Med*. 2011 Dec 1;10(4):731–6.

Marzke MW, Longhill JM, Rasmussen SA. Gluteus maximus muscle function and the origin of hominid bipedality. *Am J Phys Anthropol*. 1988 Dec;77(4):519–28.

Mascal CL, Landel R, Powers C. Management of patellofemoral pain targeting hip, pelvis, and trunk muscle function: 2 case reports. *J Orthop Sports Phys Ther*. 2003 Nov;33(11):647–60.

Mendiguchia J, Ford KR, Quatman CE, Alentorn-Geli E, Hewett TE. Sex differences in proximal control of the knee joint. *Sports Med*. 2011 Jul 1;41(7):541–57.

Mendiguchia J, Alentorn-Geli E, Brughelli M. Hamstring strain injuries: are we heading in the right direction? *Br J Sports Med*. 2012 Feb;46(2):81–5.

Mendiguchia J, Garrues MA, Cronin JB, Contreras B, Los Arcos A, Malliaropoulos N, Maffulli N, Idoate F. Nonuniform changes in MRI measurements of the thigh muscles after two hamstring strengthening exercises. *J Strength Cond Res*. 2013 Mar;27(3):574–81.

Mendiguchia J, Samozino P, Martinez-Ruiz E, Brughelli M, Schmikli S, Morin JB, Mendez-Villanueva A. Progression of mechanical properties during on-field sprint running after returning to sports from a hamstring muscle injury in soccer players. *Int J Sports Med*. 2014 Jul;35(8):690–5.

Mero A, Komi PV. Force-, EMG-, and elasticity-velocity relationships at submaximal, maximal and supramaximal running speeds in sprinters. *Eur J Appl Physiol*. 1986;55(5):553–61.

Mero A, Komi PV. Electromyographic activity in sprinting at speeds ranging from sub-maximal to supra-maximal. *Med Sci Sports Exerc*. 1987 Jun;19(3):266–74.

Miller JP, Sedory D, Croce RV. Leg rotation and vastus medialis oblique/vastus lateralis electromyogram activity ratio during closed chain kinetic exercises prescribed for patellofemoral pain. *J Athl Train*. 1997 Jul;32(3):216–20.

Mjølsnes R, Arnason A, Østhagen T, Raastad T, Bahr R. A 10-week randomized trial comparing eccentric vs. concentric hamstring strength training in well-trained soccer players. *Scand J Med Sci Sports*. 2004 Oct;14(5):311–17.

Mochizuki T, Akita K, Muneta T, Sato T. Pes anserinus: layered supportive structure on the medial side of the knee. *Clin Anat*. 2004 Jan;17(1):50–4.

Mohib M, Moser N, Kim R, Thillai M, Gringmuth R. A four year prospective study of injuries in elite Ontario youth provincial and national soccer players during training and matchplay. *J Can Chiropr Assoc*. 2014 Dec;58(4):369–76.

Molbech S. On the paradoxical effect of some two-joint muscles. *Acta Morphologica Neerlando-Scandinavica*. 1965;6:171–8.

Moore KL, Dalley AF. *Clinically oriented anatomy*. 4th ed. Baltimore, MD: Lippincott Williams & Wilkins; 1999. 1163 pp.

Müller W. *The knee: form, function, and ligament reconstruction*. 3rd ed. Berlin: Springer-Verlag; 1983. Chapter 3, Rotation; pp. 76–115.

Nagura T, Matsumoto H, Kiriyama Y, Chaudhari A, Andriacchi TP. Tibiofemoral joint contact force in deep knee flexion and its consideration in knee osteoarthritis and joint replacement. *J Appl Biomech*. 2006 Nov;22(4):305–13.

Nakagawa TH, Muniz TB, Baldon Rde M, Dias Maciel C, de Menezes Reiff RB, Serrão FV. The effect of additional strengthening of hip abductor and lateral rotator muscles in patellofemoral pain syndrome: a randomized controlled pilot study. *Clin Rehabil*. 2008 Dec;22(12):1051–60.

Nakagawa TH, Baldon Rde M, Muniz TB, Serrão FV. Relationship among eccentric hip and knee torques, symptom severity and functional capacity in females with patellofemoral pain syndrome. *Phys Ther Sport*. 2011 Aug;12(3):133–9.

Nelson-Wong E, Alex B, Csepe D, Lancaster D, Callaghan JP. Altered muscle recruitment during extension from trunk flexion in low back pain developers. *Clin Biomech*. 2012 Dec;27(10):994–8.

Nicholas SJ, Tyler TF. Adductor muscle strains in sport. *Sports Med*. 2002;32(5):339–44.

Nielsen AB, Yde J. Epidemiology and traumatology of injuries in soccer. *Am J Sports Med*. 1989 Nov–Dec;17(6):803–7.

Noe DA, Mostardi RA, Jackson ME, Porterfield JA, Askew MJ. Myoelectric activity and sequencing of selected trunk muscles during isokinetic lifting. *Spine (Phila Pa 1976)*. 1992 Feb;17(2):225–9.

Nozic M, Mitchell J, de Klerk D. A comparison of the proximal and distal parts of the vastus medialis muscle. *Aust J Physiother.* 1997;43(4):277–81.

O'Connor D. Groin injuries in professional rugby league players: a prospective study. *J Sports Sci.* 2004 Jul;22(7):629–36.

Orchard J, Seward H. Epidemiology of injuries in the Australian Football League, seasons 1997–2000. *Br J Sports Med.* 2002 Feb;36(1):39–44.

Pattyn E, Verdonk P, Steyaert A, Vanden Bossche L, Van den Broecke W, Thijs Y, Witvrouw E. Vastus medialis obliquus atrophy: does it exist in patellofemoral pain syndrome? *Am J Sports Med.* 2011 Jul;39(7):1450–5.

Petersen J, Hölmich P. Evidence based prevention of hamstring injuries in sport. *Br J Sports Med.* 2005 Jun;39(6):319–23.

Petersen J, Thorborg K, Nielsen MB, Budtz-Jørgensen E, Hölmich P. Preventive effect of eccentric training on acute hamstring injuries in men's soccer: a cluster-randomized controlled trial. *Am J Sports Med.* 2011 Nov;39(11):2296–303.

Powers CM, Flynn T. Research forum. Presented at the Combined Sections Meeting of the American Physical Therapy Association; 2003 Feb; Tampa, FL.

Prior S, Mitchell T, Whiteley R, O'Sullivan P, Williams BK, Racinais S, Farooq A. The influence of changes in trunk and pelvic posture during single leg standing on hip and thigh muscle activation in a pain free population. *BMC Sports Sci Med Rehabil.* 2014 Mar 27;6(1):13.

Renström P, Peterson L. Groin injuries in athletes. *Br J Sports Med.* 1980 Mar;14(1):30–6.

Retchford TH, Crossley KM, Grimaldi A, Kemp JL, Cowan SM. Can local muscles augment stability in the hip? A narrative literature review. *J Musculoskelet Neuronal Interact.* 2013 Mar;13(1):1–12.

Sahrmann S. *Diagnosis and treatment of movement impairment syndromes.* St Louis, MO: Mosby; 2002. 384 pp.

Sanfilippo JL, Silder A, Sherry MA, Tuite MJ, Heiderscheit BC. Hamstring strength and morphology progression after return to sport from injury. *Med Sci Sports Exerc.* 2013 Mar;45(3):448–54.

Schache AG, Wrigley TV, Baker R, Pandy MG. Biomechanical response to hamstring muscle strain injury. *Gait Posture.* 2009 Feb;29(2):332–8.

Schache AG, Kim HJ, Morgan DL, Pandy MG. Hamstring muscle forces prior to and immediately following an acute sprinting-related muscle strain injury. *Gait Posture* 2010 May;32(1):136–40.

Schmikli SL, de Vries WR, Inklaar H, Backx FJ. Injury prevention target groups in soccer: injury characteristics and incidence rates in male junior and senior players. *J Sci Med Sport.* 2011 May;14(3):199–203.

Schmitt B, Tim T, McHugh M. Hamstring injury rehabilitation and prevention of reinjury using lengthened state eccentric training: a new concept. *Int J Sports Phys Ther.* 2012 Jun;7(3):333–41.

Sedaghati P, Alizadeh MH, Shirzad E, Ardjmand A. Review of sport-induced groin injuries. *Trauma Mon.* 2013 Dec;18(3):107–12.

Selkowitz DM, Beneck GJ, Powers CM. Which exercises target the gluteal muscles while minimizing activation of the tensor fascia lata? Electromyographic assessment using fine-wire electrodes. *J Orthop Sports Phys Ther.* 2013 Feb;43(2):54–64.

Seward H, Orchard J, Hazard H, Collinson D. Football injuries in Australia at the élite level. *Med J Aust.* 1993 Sep 6;159(5):298–301.

Seynnes OR, de Boer M, Narici MV. Early skeletal muscle hypertrophy and architectural changes in response to high-intensity resistance training. *J Appl Physiol.* 2007 Jan;102(1):368–73.

Shelburne KB, Pandy MG. A dynamic model of the knee and lower limb for simulating rising movements. *Comput Methods Biomech Biomed Engin.* 2002 Apr;5(2):149–59.

Shelburne KB, Torry MR, Pandy MG. Muscle, ligament, and joint-contact forces at the knee during walking. *Med Sci Sports Exerc.* 2005 Nov;37(11):1948–56.

Sherry MA, Best TM. A comparison of 2 rehabilitation programs in the treatment of acute hamstring strains. *J Orthop Sports Phys Ther.* 2004 Mar;34(3):116–25.

Shin CS, Chaudhari AM, Andriacchi TP. The influence of deceleration forces on ACL strain during single-leg landing: a simulation study. *J Biomech.* 2007;40(5):1145–52.

Silder A, Heiderscheit BC, Thelen DG, Enright T, Tuite MJ. MR observations of long-term musculoten-don remodeling following a hamstring strain injury. *Skeletal Radiol.* 2008 Dec;37(12):1101–9.

Simonsen EB, Thomsen L, Klausen K. Activity of mono- and biarticular leg muscles during sprint running. *Eur J Appl Physiol Occup Physiol.* 1985;54(5):524–32.

Smith TO, Bowyer D, Dixon J, Stephenson R, Chester R, Donell ST. Can vastus medialis oblique be preferentially activated? A systematic review of electromyographic studies. *Physiother Theory Pract.* 2009a Feb;25(2):69–98.

Smith TO, Nichols R, Harle D, Donell ST. Do the vastus medialis obliquus and vastus medialis longus really exist? A systematic review. *Clin Anat.* 2009b Mar;22(2):183–99.

Snijders CJ, Vleeming A, Stoeckart R. Transfer of lumbosacral load to iliac bones and legs Part 1: bio-mechanics of self-bracing of the sacroiliac joints and its significance for treatment and exercise. *Clin Biomech (Bristol, Avon).* 1993 Nov;8(6):285–94.

Snijders CJ, Vleeming A, Stoeckart R, Mens JM, Kleinrensink GJ. Biomechanics of the inter-face between the spine and pelvis in different postures. In: Vleeming A, Mooney V, Snijders CJ, Dorman TA, Stoeckart A, editors. *Movement, stability and low back pain: the essential role of the pelvis.* Edinburgh: Churchill Livingstone; 1997. pp. 103–13.

Sole G, Milosavljevic S, Nicholson HD, Sullivan SJ. Selective strength loss and decreased muscle activity in hamstring injury. *J Orthop Sports Phys Ther.* 2011 May;41(5):354–63.

Souza RB, Powers CM. Differences in hip kinematics, muscle strength, and muscle activation between subjects with and without patellofemoral pain. *J Orthop Sports Phys Ther.* 2009 Jan;39(1):12–19.

Standring S. *Gray's anatomy: the anatomical basis of clinical practice.* 40th ed. Edinburgh: Churchill & Livingstone; 2008. 1576 pp.

Stern JT Jr, Paré EB, Schwartz JM. New perspectives on muscle use during locomotion: electromyo-graphic studies of rapid and complex behaviors. *J Am Osteopath Assoc.* 1980 Dec;80(4):287–91.

Stubbe J, van Beijsterveldt AM, van der Knaap S, Stege J, Verhagen E, van Mechelen W, Backx FJ. Injuries in professional male soccer players in the Netherlands: a prospective cohort study. *J Athl Train.* 2014 Dec 22. [Epub ahead of print]

Takizawa M, Suzuki D, Ito H, Fujimiya M, Uchiyama E. Why adductor magnus muscle is large: the function based on muscle morphology in cadavers. *Scand J Med Sci Sports.* 2014 Feb;24(1):197–203.

Tanino Y, Suzuki T. Spinal reflex arc excitability corresponding to the vastus medialis obliquus and vastus medialis longus muscles. *J Phys Ther Sci.* 2014 Jan;26(1):101–4.

Terry GC, LaPrade RF. The posterolateral aspect of the knee. Anatomy and surgical approach. *Am J Sports Med.* 1996 Nov–Dec;24(6):732–9.

Thelen DG, Chumanov ES, Hoerth DM, Best TM, Swanson SC, Li L, Young M, Heiderscheit BC. Hamstring muscle kinematics during treadmill sprinting. *Med Sci Sports Exerc.* 2005a Jan;37(1):108–14.

Thelen DG, Chumanov ES, Best TM, Swanson SC, Heiderscheit BC. Simulation of biceps femoris musculotendon mechanics during the swing phase of sprinting. *Med Sci Sports Exerc.* 2005b; 37(11):1911–18.

Thorborg K. Why hamstring eccentrics are hamstring essentials. *Br J Sports Med.* 2012;46:463–5.

Thorborg K, Branci S, Nielsen MP, Tang L, Nielsen MB, Hölmich P. Eccentric and isometric hip adduc-tion strength in male soccer players with and without adductor-related groin pain. An assessor-blinded comparison. *Orthopaedic Journal of Sports Medicine.* 2014 Feb;2(2):1–7.

Toumi H, Poumarat G, Benjamin M, Best TM, F'Guyer S, Fairclough J. New insights into the function of the vastus medialis with clinical implications. *Med Sci Sports Exerc.* 2007 Jul;39(7):1153–9.

Travnik L, Pernus F, Erzen I. Histochemical and morphometric characteristics of the normal human vastus medialis longus and vastus medialis obliquus muscles. *J Anat.* 1995 Oct;187 (Pt 2):403–11.

Tyler TF, Nicholas SJ, Campbell RJ, McHugh MP. The association of hip strength and flexibility with the incidence of adductor muscle strains in professional ice hockey players. *Am J Sports Med.* 2001 Mar–Apr;29(2):124–8.

Tyler TF, Nicholas SJ, Campbell RJ, Donellan S, McHugh MP. The effectiveness of a preseason exercise program to prevent adductor muscle strains in professional ice hockey players. *Am J Sports Med.* 2002 Sep–Oct;30(5):680–3.

Tyler TF, Nicholas SJ, Mullaney MJ, McHugh MP. The role of hip muscle function in the treatment of patellofemoral pain syndrome. *Am J Sports Med.* 2006 Apr;34(4):630–6.

Tyler TF, Fukunaga T, Gellert J. Rehabilitation of soft tissue injuries of the hip and pelvis. *Int J Sports Phys Ther.* 2014 Nov;9(6):785–97.

Vakos JP, Nitz AJ, Threlkeld AJ, Shapiro R, Horn T. Electromyographic activity of selected trunk and hip muscles during a squat lift. Effect of varying the lumbar posture. *Spine (Phila Pa 1976).* 1994 Mar;19(6):687–95.

van Kampen A, Huiskes R. The three-dimensional tracking pattern of the human patella. *J Orthop Res.* 1990 May;8(3):372–82.

Vleeming A, Van Wingerden JP, Snijders CJ, Stoeckart R, Stijnen T. Load application to the sacrotuberous ligament; influences on sacroiliac joint mechanics. *Clin Biomech (Bristol, Avon).* 1989;4(4):204–9.

Vleeming A, Pool-Goudzwaard AL, Stoeckart R, van Wingerden JP, Snijders CJ. The posterior layer of the thoracolumbar fascia. Its function in load transfer from spine to legs. *Spine (Phila Pa 1976).* 1995 Apr;20(7):753–8.

Vogt L, Pfeifer K, Banzer W. Neuromuscular control of walking with chronic low-back pain. *Man Ther.* 2003 Feb;8(1):21–8.

Ward SR, Eng CM, Smallwood LH, Lieber RL. Are current measurements of lower extremity muscle architecture accurate? *Clin Orthop Relat Res.* 2009 Apr;467(4):1074–82.

Warren P, Gabbe BJ, Schneider-Kolsky M, Bennell KL. Clinical predictors of time to return to competition and of recurrence following hamstring strain in elite Australian footballers. *Br J Sports Med.* 2010 May;44(6):415–19.

Weinhandl JT, Earl-Boehm JE, Ebersole KT, Huddleston WE, Armstrong BS, O'Connor KM. Reduced hamstring strength increases anterior cruciate ligament loading during anticipated sidestep cutting. *Clin Biomech (Bristol, Avon).* 2014 Aug;29(7):752–9.

Wiemann K, Tidow G. Relative activity of hip and knee extensors in sprinting – implications for training. *New Studies in Athletics.* 1995;10(1):29–49.

Williams PL, Warwick R. *Gray's anatomy.* 36th ed. Edinburgh: Churchill Livingstone; 1980. 1578 pp.

Willis FB, Burkhardt EJ, Walker JE, Johnson MA, Spears TD. Preferential vastus medialis oblique activation achieved as a treatment for knee disorders. *J Strength Cond Res.* 2005 May;19(2):286–91.

Wilson J, Ferris E, Heckler A, Maitland L, Taylor C. A structured review of the role of gluteus maximus in rehabilitation. *New Zeal J Physioth.* 2005;33(3):95–100.

Wilson JM, Flanagan EP. The role of elastic energy in activities with high force and power requirements: a brief review. *J Strength Cond Res.* 2008 Sep;22(5):1705–15.

Wood GA. Optimal performance criteria and limiting factors in sprint running. *New Stud Athlet.* 1986;2:SS–63.

Wood GA. Biomechanical limitations to sprint running. In: Van Gheluwe B, Atha J, editors. *Current research in sports biomechanics (medicine and sport science).* Basel, Switzerland: S Karger Pub; 1987. pp. 58–71.

Woods C, Hawkins RD, Maltby S, Hulse M, Thomas A, Hodson A; Football Association Medical Research Programme. The Football Association Medical Research Programme: an audit of injuries in professional football – analysis of hamstring injuries. *Br J Sports Med.* 2004 Feb;38(1):36–41.

Yamaguchi GT, Zajac FE. A planar model of the knee joint to characterise the knee extensor mechanism. *J Biomech.* 1989;22(1):1–10.

Yeung SS, Suen AM, Yeung EW. A prospective cohort study of hamstring injuries in competitive sprinters: preseason muscle imbalance as a possible risk factor. *Br J Sports Med.* 2009 Aug;43(8):589–94.

Yu B, Queen RM, Abbey AN, Liu Y, Moorman CT, Garrett WE. Hamstring muscle kinematics and activation during overground sprinting. *J Biomech.* 2008 Nov;41(15):3121–6.

Zeller BL, McCrory J, Kibler B, Uhl TL. Differences in kinematics and electromyographic activity between men and women during the single-legged squat. *Am J Sports Med.* 2003 May–Jun;31(3):449–56.

Zimmermann CL, Cook TM, Bravard MS, Hansen MM, Honomichl RT, Karns ST, Lammers MA, Steele SA, Yunker LK, Zebrowski RM. Effects of stair-stepping exercise direction and cadence on EMG activity of selected lower extremity muscle groups. *J Orthop Sports Phys Ther.* 1994 Mar;19(3):173–80.

PART IV
Speed-strength training

13

TRAINING PRINCIPLES TO DEVELOP POWER

Success in soccer depends highly on the level of power and speed the player can exert (Cormie et al. 2011; Haugen et al. 2014).

With beginners, strength training will enhance both strength and power as a result of hypertrophy and neural adaptations (Cormie et al. 2010a, 2010b; Häkkinen and Komi 1985a). An improvement in strength results in an increase of power and athletic performance (Cormie et al. 2010a, 2010b; Häkkinen and Komi 1985a). With players that have developed a solid strength base however, heavy resistance strength training does not necessarily result in simultaneous improvements in power and athletic performance (Cormie et al. 2011; Häkkinen 1989). Trained athletes require more specific training interventions to further enhance power output (Cormie et al. 2011; Wilson et al. 1993).

High-intensity strength training is only half of the equation (Power = force × velocity). Zatsiorsky states that it takes 0.4 seconds to achieve maximal muscle force (Zatsiorsky 1995). During soccer actions time is limited however. The player has to exert as much force as possible in a short period of time. Compare the 0.4 seconds necessary to achieve peak force to the ground contact times of 0.08–0.1 seconds while sprinting and you will understand that strength gains do not necessarily transfer to faster sprinting (Taylor and Beneke 2012; Table 13.1).

High-force/low-speed strength training will only raise one end of the strength–velocity curve and is not enough to improve explosiveness and speed of movement. To phrase L.S. Dvorkin: "There is no connection between the ability to generate great force and the ability to realize it at maximum speed" (Dvorkin 2005).

The SAID principle (specific adaptations to imposed demands) also applies to speed. Training with a specific load and thus velocity results in velocity-specific increases in muscle activation (Häkkinen and Komi 1985b; McBride et al. 2002; Mero and Komi 1986). The adaptations to the nervous system in response to power training differ from the changes seen with training to increase muscle strength (Häkkinen and Komi 1985b). Power training results in high-frequency motor unit activation and the selective recruitment and synchronization of the high-threshold motor units (Behm and Sale 1993; Desmedt and Godaux 1978; Hannerz and Grimby 1979). The increased neural activation of the muscles, the improved interaction

TABLE 13.1 Duration of force production in various athletic movements (Čoh et al. 2011; Dintiman and Ward 2003; Lockie et al. 2012; Marshall et al. 2014; Taube et al. 2012; Zatsiorsky 2003; Zatsiorsky and Kraemer 2006)

Movement	Ground contact time (in seconds)
Sprint running	0.08–0.10
Accelerating (0–5 m)	0.15
Accelerating (5–10 m)	0.125
Cut 20–60°	0.25
Cut 75–90°	0.3–0.4
Running vertical jump	0.17–0.18
Vertical jump	0.39
Depth jump (25 cm)	0.17
Depth jump (75 cm)	0.22
Kicking (stance foot)	0.285

between synergists, and decreased co-contraction of antagonists contribute to athletic performance enhancement (Behm 1995; Carroll et al. 2001).

To maximally increase power and performance different resistances that span the force–velocity curve have to be incorporated into a combined strength and ballistic training, so players present their neuromuscular systems with a variety of different stimuli.

13.1 Maximum strength is a contributing factor to explosive power

The use of heavy resistance strength training is theoretically based on the size principle, which states that motor units are recruited in an orderly manner from the smaller (lower threshold) to the larger (higher threshold) motor units (Fleck and Kraemer 1987; Sale 1992). The low-threshold motor units are predominantly composed of slow-twitch fibers, which are well suited for low-intensity, long-duration activities. The high-threshold motor units consist of a large number of fast-twitch fibers, which produce more power output than slow-twitch motor units and are responsible for athletic performance (Faulkner et al. 1986; Harris et al. 2000). The high-threshold fast-twitch motor units will be recruited as the force required increases (Harris et al. 2000; McBride et al. 2002; Schmidtbleicher 1992; Wilson et al. 1993).

There also exists a high and positive correlation between peak power and maximum strength (r=0.77–0.94) in both the upper body (Baker 2001a, 2001b; Baker et al. 2001a; Moss et al. 1997) and lower body (Baker 2001a; Baker and Newton 2008; Baker et al. 2001b; McLellan et al. 2011; Nuzzo et al. 2008; Peterson et al. 2006).

Maximum strength (high-force/low-speed) is a contributing factor to explosive power. All explosive movements start from zero or slow velocities, and it is at this acceleration phase of the movement that slow-velocity strength can contribute to power development. At the higher-velocity component of the movement, however, slow-velocity strength capacity has a reduced impact on the ability to produce high force (Duchateau et al. 1984; Kanehisa and Miyashita 1983; Kaneko et al. 1983). Training to enhance leg strength has excellent transference to agility and vertical jump performance, but considerably less to sprinting performance (Kawamori and Haff 2004; Wilson et al. 1996).

The longer the contact time, the longer the time that force can be exerted and the higher the performance benefit that can be expected from enhanced strength. The time to apply force during most athletic movements is around 0.1–0.2 seconds however. The rate of force development – the ability of the neuromuscular system to produce the greatest possible force in the shortest possible time – determines success in soccer and should be a major focus of training.

13.2 Force–velocity curve and peak power output

Research shows that the force output during heavy lifting increases when the load is increased (Cormie *et al.* 2007). Second, as the load increases, the velocity of the lift decreases with a greater factor than the force increases (Cormie *et al.* 2007). Third, since power equals force times speed, the loads that lead to the highest power output are 30–40 percent of 1RM (Kaneko *et al.* 1983; Swinton *et al.* 2011; Wilson *et al.* 1993). The peak power output is typically seen with lifting loads of 30 percent of 1RM, but might vary between upper and lower body and also depends on the exercise and experience of the trainee (Baker *et al.* 2001a, 2001b; Kaneko *et al.* 1983; Swinton *et al.* 2011; Wilson *et al.* 1993). The study of Cormie *et al.* clearly indicates that the load of peak power output occurs at various percentages of 1RM in different exercises (Cormie *et al.* 2007). Loads of 0 percent maximize power in the jump squat, while peak power in the squat and power clean were produced at 56 percent and 80 percent of 1RM respectively (Cormie *et al.* 2007).

13.3 Rate of force development and ballistic training

During the vast majority of soccer actions time is limited and the player does not have the time to produce maximal force. Not the strongest players, but those that can produce the greatest force in the shortest amount of time have an advantage. To reach higher forces and velocities during fast movement, training should focus on improving rate of force development. While heavy resistance training increases the highest point of the force–velocity curve, rate of force development training improves the slope of the curve (Jones *et al.* 2001; Kaneko *et al.* 1983; Kawamori and Haff 2004; McBride *et al.* 2002; Moss *et al.* 1997; Figure 13.1). An increase in rate of force development allows reaching a higher level of muscle force in the early phase of muscle contraction.

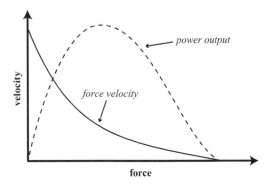

FIGURE 13.1   Force–velocity curve and peak power output

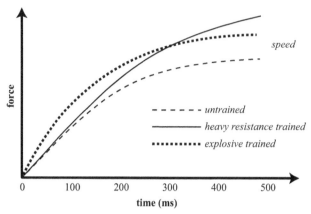

FIGURE 13.2 Effects of explosive and heavy resistance training on maximal strength and rate of force development

Several studies have shown that to enhance maximal power, athletes should train with the velocity and resistance that maximizes mechanical power output (McBride *et al.* 2002; Newton and Kraemer 1994; Wilson *et al.* 1993). In single-joint movements maximal power is produced at 30 percent of 1RM. Speed repetitions performed with 30 percent of 1RM will not improve the rate of force development however (Newton *et al.* 1996). Newton and co-workers demonstrated that when 45 percent of 1RM was lifted as explosively as possible, power decreased significantly during the final half of the range of motion (Newton *et al.* 1996). The reduction in power is due to activation of the antagonist muscles and lack of agonist neural activation, in order to decelerate the bar and reach zero velocity at the end of the movement (Newton and Kraemer 1994; Newton *et al.* 1996). Deceleration accounts for 24 percent of the movement with a heavy weight and 52 percent of the movement with a light weight (Elliott *et al.* 1989).

With the use of ballistic movements, movements in which the weight can be released, power and acceleration are enhanced throughout the entire range of motion (Newton *et al.* 1996). Jump squat and bench throws are therefore far superior to speed reps for power development (Clark *et al.* 2008). Speed reps merely train the neuromuscular system to decelerate the movement towards the end of the range of motion and are therefore counterproductive. Ballistic exercises, Olympic lifts, and plyometrics allow the athlete to accelerate throughout the entire range of motion.

Explosive movements do not adhere to the size principle (Figure 13.2). During high-velocity movements the high-threshold motor units, which are composed of a large number of fast-twitch fibers, are preferentially recruited (Sale 1992). The low-threshold motor units, which mainly consist of the smaller slow-twitch fibers, are skipped over to facilitate power production. Part of the training effect from ballistic training is the enhanced ability to activate the highest-threshold motor units (Sale 1992).

13.4 Load specificity to enhance power performance

In analogy of a car, high-load strength training will enhance the engine capacity while rate of force development training maximizes the engine power. To improve the rate of force development, ballistic exercises in which the weight can be accelerated over the entire range of motion are superior over speed reps without propelling the bar into the air. What remains to be determined is the training load of these ballistic exercises to optimally enhance power output. Some authors recommend training with the load that produces maximal power output, because this results in the greatest increase in power and force over the entire velocity range of the curve (Baker *et al.* 2001b; Kaneko *et al.* 1983; Wilson *et al.* 1993). Monotonous power training however, in which one load is prescribed, is not recommended. Training monotony does not optimally enhance performance and increases the likelihood of neuromuscular fatigue (Stone *et al.* 1991).

Several studies also demonstrate that training adaptations are velocity-specific. Training adaptations are greatest at or near the training velocity (Häkkinen and Komi 1985b; Kaneko *et al.* 1983; McBride *et al.* 2002; Mero and Komi 1986). Training with heavy resistance results in the greatest increase in power at high-force/low-speed movements, while ballistic training with low loads produces the greatest increase in unloaded movement velocity (Kaneko *et al.* 1983; McBride *et al.* 2002; Mero and Komi 1986). To maximally increase power performance different loads that span the entire force–velocity curve have to be incorporated into the training. Soccer also involves motor skills that cover the entire force–velocity curve.

Verkhoshansky made a distinction between speed-strength and strength-speed (Verkhoshansky 1966). These are separate training modalities that pertain to defined areas of the force–velocity curve and both need to be addressed to maximize power.

13.5 Different modalities of force–velocity curve

To improve each modality and each part of the speed-strength spectrum, there is an appropriate choice of exercises and selection of the training load (Figure 13.3).

To maximize strength gains, loads that require a high peak force output should be used (Kirby *et al.* 2010). Peak force outputs increase with the percentage of 1RM (Cormie *et al.* 2007; Swinton *et al.* 2011, 2012). Lifting heavy loads above 90 percent of your 1RM, however, leads to very slow bar speeds and low power outputs (Cormie *et al.* 2007; Zatsiorsky 1995). The peak power output during the squat occurs at 56 percent of 1RM, while the peak force output is still high (Cormie *et al.* 2007). Explosively lifting loads in the range of 50–70 percent

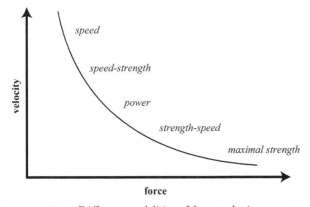

FIGURE 13.3 Different modalities of force–velocity curve

of 1RM will serve to develop power in the high-force range of the spectrum and can simultaneously help maintain strength levels (Haff and Nimphius 2012; Kirby *et al.* 2010).

Plyometrics and sprints are performed with high movement speeds and the total force production is lower because there is no additional external load. This places plyometrics and sprints more towards the speed end of the spectrum.

Maximal peak power outputs for the jump squat are seen with loads between 10 percent and 45 percent of 1RM (Kaneko *et al.* 1983; Stone *et al.* 2003; Wilson *et al.* 1993; Zatsiorsky 1995). Performing jump squats with these loads will therefore result in the greatest increase in speed-strength. The optimal load to maximize power outputs in Olympic lifts are higher compared with the jump squat (Cormie *et al.* 2007). Maximum power outputs in Olympic lifts occur between 60 percent and 80 percent of 1RM and are therefore perfect to develop strength-speed (Cormie *et al.* 2007; Garhammer 1993; Haff *et al.* 1997; Kawamori and Haff 2004). Jump squats are far from ideal to develop the strength-speed modality, for two reasons. First, jump squats with a load above 60 percent of 1RM pose safety concerns because of the high impact forces on landing. Second, the optimal loads to maximize power outputs in the jump squat appear to be lower (Kaneko *et al.* 1983; Wilson *et al.* 1993). Some authors see jump squats as the perfect replacement for the technically more complex Olympic lifts. This is a misconception however, because jump squats and Olympic lifts perfectly complement each other to maximize power and speed.

13.6 Combined training

Because strength is a prerequisite of power, the athlete should progress from strength training to power training in a logical sequence. Bompa and Carrera note that power is developed in two stages (Bompa and Carrera 2005). The first stage involves the recruitment of fast-twitch fibers through heavy resistance training based on the size principle. The second stage involves an increased firing rate and synchronization of these high-threshold, fast-twitch motor units through ballistics (Bompa and Carrera 2005). Periodization to maximize power performance suggests a training emphasis for either strength or power and does not suggest either should be trained in isolation. The increases in power and motor performance with combined strength and plyometric training are greater than with either training method alone (Adams *et al.* 1992; Lyttle *et al.* 1996). Research also supports the superiority of concurrent heavy resistance training/ballistics (Harris *et al.* 2000; McBride *et al.* 2002), heavy-resistance training/sports-specific task (Cronin *et al.* 2001; Mayhew *et al.* 1997), and ballistics/sports-specific task (Cronin *et al.* 2001). By integrating strength, power, and speed modalities into the same workout, the different areas of the force–velocity curve can be targeted. The Russian complex and the Bulgarian method vertically integrate different modalities of the speed-strength spectrum to maximize power output and overall performance.

The optimal development of power and speed also requires a sequencing of the training focus in a periodized manner in which different phases or workouts emphasize hypertrophy, strength, strength-speed, or speed-strength (Bompa and Carrera 2005; Haff and Nimphius 2012).

Russian complex and post-activation potentiation

Verkhoshansky states that resistance training programs which incorporate plyometrics are superior to those that do not include plyometrics (Verkhoshanski 1966; Verkhoshansky and Tatyan 1983; Tables 13.2 and 13.3).

TABLE 13.2 Example of Russian complex: perform this combination for three to four sets

Exercise	Intensity	Reps	Rest interval
Front squat	80% of 1RM	4 reps	2'
Hurdle jump (multiple response)	Body weight	2 x 5 reps	30"

TABLE 13.3 Example of Bulgarian method: Start with heavy-resistance strength exercise and progressively work down to plyometric exercise. Repeat three to four times

Exercise	Intensity	Reps	Rest interval
Front squat	85% of 1RM	3 reps	2'
Power clean	75% of 1RM	4 reps	2'
Jump squat	30% of 1RM	5 reps	2'
Hurdle jump (multiple response)	Body weight	2 x 5 reps	30"

In the Russian complex, a set of heavy-strength training is followed by a set of a bio-mechanically similar plyometric exercise. Lifting a heavy load will enhance the power output in the subsequent set of plyometrics (Docherty *et al.* 2004; Hilfiker *et al.* 2007). The enhanced explosiveness has been attributed to the post-activation potentiation phenomenon. Performing a near-maximal contraction before the unresisted drill stimulates the central nervous system, which results in enhanced high-threshold motor unit recruitment (Docherty *et al.* 2004; Hilfiker *et al.* 2007). The increased amount of recruited fast-twitch muscle fibers as a result of lifting the heavy load will carry over to the subsequent unresisted explosive exercise. This enables the player to move faster, more explosively (Sale 2002).

Bulgarian method

The Bulgarian method starts with a high-intensity exercise, followed by progressively working down to a plyometric exercise. In one workout all the modalities of the force–velocity curve are addressed (maximum strength, strength-speed, speed-strength, and speed) to increase the power output across the entire loading spectrum.

References

Adams K, O'Shea JP, O'Shea KL, Climstein M. The effect of six weeks of squat, plyometric and squat-plyometric training on power production. *J Strength Cond Res.* 1992 Feb;6(1):36–41.

Baker D. A series of studies on the training of high intensity muscle power in rugby league football players. *J Strength Cond Res.* 2001a May;15(2):198–209.

Baker D. The effects of an in-season of concurrent training on the maintenance of maximal strength and power in professional and college-aged rugby league football players. *J Strength Cond Res.* 2001b May;15(2):172–7.

Baker D, Newton RU. Observation of 4-year adaptations in lower body maximal strength and power output in professional rugby league players. *J Aust Strength Cond.* 2008;16(1):3–10.

Baker D, Nance S, Moore M. The load that maximizes the average mechanical power output during explosive bench press throws in highly trained athletes. *J Strength Cond Res.* 2001a Feb;15(1):20–4.

Baker D, Nance S, Moore M. The load that maximizes the average mechanical power output during jump squats in power-trained athletes. *J Strength Cond Res.* 2001b Feb;15(1):92–7.

Behm DG, Sale DG. Velocity specificity of resistance training. *Sports Med*. 1993;15(6):374–88.

Behm DG. Neuromuscular implications and applications of resistance training. *J Strength Cond Res*. 1995 Nov;9(4):264–74.

Bompa TO, Carrera MC. *Periodization training for sports*. 2nd ed. Champaign, IL: Human Kinetics; 2005. Chapter 11, Phase 4: Conversion; pp. 187–222.

Carroll TJ, Riek S, Carson RG. Neural adaptations to resistance training. Implications for movement control. *Sports Med*. 2001;31(12):829–40.

Clark RA, Bryant AL, Humphries B. A comparison of force curve profiles between the bench press and ballistic bench throws. *J Strength Cond Res*. 2008 Nov;22(6):1755–9.

Čoh M, Bračič M, Peharec S, Bačić P, Bratić M, Aleksandrović M. Biodynamic characteristics of vertical and drop jumps. *Acta Kinesiologiae Universitatis Tartuensis*. 2011;17:24–36.

Cormie P, McCaulley GO, Triplett NT, McBride JM. Optimal loading for maximal power output during lower-body resistance exercises. *Med Sci Sports Exerc*. 2007 Feb;39(2):340–9.

Cormie P, McGuigan MR, Newton RU. Influence of strength on magnitude and mechanisms of adaptation to power training. *Med Sci Sports Exerc*. 2010a Aug;42(8):1566–81.

Cormie P, McGuigan MR, Newton RU. Adaptations in athletic performance after ballistic power versus strength training. *Med Sci Sports Exerc*. 2010b Aug;42(8):1582–98.

Cormie P, McGuigan MR, Newton RU. Developing maximal neuromuscular power: part 2 – training considerations for improving maximal power production. *Sports Med*. 2011 Feb 1;41(2):125–46.

Cronin J, McNair PJ, Marshall RN. Velocity specificity, combination training and sport specific tasks. *J Sci Med Sport*. 2001 Jun;4(2):168–78.

Desmedt JE, Godaux E. Ballistic contractions in fast or slow human muscles: discharge patterns of single motor units. *J Physiol*. 1978 Dec;285:185–96.

Dintiman G, Ward B. *Sports speed*. 3rd ed. Champaign, IL: Human Kinetics; 2003. Chapter 11, Cutting and accelerating; pp. 218–30.

Docherty D, Robbins D, Hodgson M. Complex training revisited: a review of its current status as a viable training approach. *Strength Cond J*. 2004 Dec;26(6):52–7.

Duchateau J, Hainaut K. Isometric or dynamic training: differential effects on mechanical properties of a human muscle. *J Appl Physiol Respir Environ Exerc Physiol*. 1984 Feb;56(2):296–301.

Dvorkin LS. *Tiiazhelaya atletika. Uchebnik dlja vuzov*. Moscow: Sovyetsky sport publishers; 2005. 600 pp.

Elliott BC, Wilson GJ, Kerr GK. A biomechanical analysis of the sticking region in the bench press. *Med Sci Sports Exerc*. 1989 Aug;21(4):450–62.

Faulkner JA, Claflin DR, McCully KK. Power output of fast and slow fibers from human skeletal muscles. In: Jones NL, McCartney NM, McComas AJ, editors. *Human muscle power*. Champaign, IL: Human Kinetics; 1986. pp. 81–94.

Fleck SJ, Kraemer WJ. *Designing resistance training programs*. 2nd ed. Champaign, IL: Human Kinetics; 1987. 275 pp.

Garhammer, J. A review of power output studies of Olympic and powerlifting: methodology, performance prediction, and evaluation tests. *J Strength Cond Res*. 1993 May;7(2):76–89.

Haff GG, Nimphius S. Training principles for power. *Strength Cond J*. 2012 Oct;34(5):2–12.

Haff GG, Stone M, O'Bryant HS, Harman E, Dinan C, Johnson R, Han KH, Force-time dependent characteristics of dynamic and isometric muscle actions. *J Strength Cond Res*. 1997 Nov;11(4):269–72.

Häkkinen K. Neuromuscular and hormonal adaptations during strength and power training. *J Sports Med Phys Fitness*. 1989;29:9–26.

Häkkinen K, Komi PV. Changes in electrical and mechanical behavior of leg extensor muscles during heavy resistance strength training. *Scand J Sports Sci*. 1985a;7:55–64.

Häkkinen K, Komi PV. Effect of explosive-type strength training on electromyographic and force production characteristics of leg extensor muscles during concentric and various stretch-shortening cycle exercises. *Scand J Sports Sci*. 1985b;7:65–76.

Hannerz J, Grimby L. The afferent influence on the voluntary firing range of individual motor units in man. *Muscle Nerve*. 1979 Nov–Dec;2(6):414–22.

Harris GR, Stone MH, O'Bryant HS, Proulx CM, Johnson RL. Short-term performance effects of high power, high force, or combined weight-training methods. *J Strength Cond Res.* 2000 Feb;14(1):14–20.

Haugen T, Tønnessen E, Hisdal J, Seiler S. The role and development of sprinting speed in soccer. *Int J Sports Physiol Perform.* 2014 May;9(3):432–41.

Hilfiker R, Hubner K, Lorenz T, Marti B. Effects of drop jumps to the warm-up of elite sports athletes with a high capacity for explosive force development. *J Strength Cond Res.* 2007 May;21(2):550–5.

Jones K, Bishop P, Hunter G, Fleisig G. The effects of varying resistance-training loads on intermediate-and high-velocity-specific adaptations. *J Strength Cond Res.* 2001 Aug;15(3):349–56.

Kanehisa H, Miyashita M. Effect of isometric and isokinetic muscle training on static strength and dynamic power. *Eur J Appl Physiol Occup Physiol.* 1983;50(3):365–71.

Kaneko M, Fuchimoto T, Toji H, Suei K. Training effect of different loads on the force-velocity relationship and mechanical power output in human muscle. *Scand J Med Sci Sports.* 1983;5:50–5.

Kawamori N, Haff GG. The optimal training load for the development of muscular power. *J Strength Cond Res.* 2004 Aug;18(3):675–84.

Kirby TJ, Erickson T, McBride JM. Model for progression of strength, power, and speed training. *Strength Cond J.* 2010 Oct;32(5):86–90.

Lockie RG, Murphy AJ, Schultz AB, Knight TJ, Janse de Jonge XA. The effects of different speed training protocols on sprint acceleration kinematics and muscle strength and power in field sport athletes. *J Strength Cond Res.* 2012 Jun;26(6):1539–50.

Lyttle AD, Wilson GJ, Ostrowski KJ. Enhancing performance: maximal power versus combined weights and plyometrics training. *J Strength Cond Res.* 1996;10(3):173–9.

McBride JM, Triplett-McBride T, Davie A, Newton RU. The effect of heavy- vs. light-load jump squats on the development of strength, power, and speed. *J Strength Cond Res.* 2002 Feb;16(1):75–82.

McLellan CP, Lovell DI, Gass GC. The role of rate of force development on vertical jump performance. *J Strength Cond Res.* 2011 Feb;25(2):379–85.

Marshall BM, Franklyn-Miller AD, King EA, Moran KA, Strike SC, Falvey ÉC. Biomechanical factors associated with time to complete a change of direction cutting maneuver. *J Strength Cond Res.* 2014 Oct;28(10):2845–51.

Mayhew JL, Ware JS, Johns RA, Bemben MG. Changes in upper body power following heavy-resistance strength training in college men. *Int J Sports Med.* 1997 Oct;18(7):516–20.

Mero A, Komi PV. Force-, EMG-, and elasticity-velocity relationships at submaximal, maximal and supramaximal running speeds in sprinters. *Eur J Appl Physiol Occup Physiol.* 1986;55(5):553–61.

Moss BM, Refsnes PE, Abildgaard A, Nicolaysen K, Jensen J. Effects of maximal effort strength training with different loads on dynamic strength, cross-sectional area, load-power and load-velocity relationships. *Eur J Appl Physiol Occup Physiol.* 1997;75(3):193–9.

Newton RU, Kraemer WJ. Developing explosive muscular power: implications for a mixed methods training strategy. *Strength Cond J.* 1994 Oct;16(5):20–31.

Newton RU, Kraemer WJ, Hakkinen K, Humphries BJ, Murphy AJ. Kinematics, kinetics, muscle activation during explosive upper body movements: implications for power development. *J Appl Biomech.* 1996 Feb;12(1):31–43.

Nuzzo JL, McBride JM, Cormie P, McCaulley GO. Relationship between countermovement jump performance and multijoint isometric and dynamic tests of strength. *J Strength Cond Res.* 2008 May;22(3):699–707.

Peterson MD, Alvar BA, Rhea MR. The contribution of maximal force production to explosive movement among young collegiate athletes. *J Strength Cond Res.* 2006 Nov;20(4):867–73.

Sale D. Postactivation potentiation: role in performance. *Br J Sports Med.* 2004 Aug;38(4):386–7.

Sale DG. Neural adaptations to strength training. In: Komi PV, editor. *Strength and power in sport.* Oxford, UK: Blackwell Scientific; 1992. pp. 249–65.

Sale DG. Postactivation potentiation: role in human performance. *Exerc Sport Sci Rev.* 2002 Jul; 30(3):138–43.

Schmidtbleicher D. Training for power events. In: Komi PV, editor. *Strength and power in sport.* Oxford, UK: Blackwell Scientific; 1992. pp. 381–95.

Stone MH, Keith RE, Kearney JT, Fleck SJ, Wilson GD, Triplett NT. Overtraining: a review of the signs, symptoms and possible causes. *J Appl Sport Sci Res*. 1991;5:35–50.

Stone MH, O'Bryant HS, McCoy L, Coglianese R, Lehmkuhl M, Schilling B. Power and maximum strength relationships during performance of dynamic and static weighted jumps. *J Strength Cond Res*. 2003 Feb;17(1):140–7.

Swinton PA, Stewart A, Agouris I, Keogh JW, Lloyd R. A biomechanical analysis of straight and hexagonal barbell deadlifts using submaximal loads. *J Strength Cond Res*. 2011 Jul;25(7):2000–9.

Swinton PA, Lloyd R, Keogh JW, Agouris I, Stewart AD. A biomechanical comparison of the traditional squat, powerlifting squat, and box squat. *J Strength Cond Res*. 2012 Jul;26(7):1805–16.

Taube W, Leukel C, Lauber B, Gollhofer A. The drop height determines neuromuscular adaptations and changes in jump performance in stretch-shortening cycle training. *Scand J Med Sci Sports*. 2012 Oct;22(5):671–83.

Taylor MJ, Beneke R. Spring mass characteristics of the fastest men on earth. *Int J Sports Med*. 2012 Aug;33(8):667–70.

Verkhoshansky Y. Perspectives in the improvement of speed-strength preparation of jumpers. *Legkaya Atletika*. 1966; 9:11–12.

Verkhoshanski Y, Tatyan V. Speed-strength preparation of future champions. *Sov Sports Rev*. 1983; 18(4):166–70.

Wilson GJ, Newton RU, Murphy AJ, Humphries BJ. The optimal training load for the development of dynamic athletic performance. *Med Sci Sports Exerc*. 1993 Nov;25(11):1279–86.

Wilson GJ, Murphy AJ, Walshe A. The specificity of strength training: the effect of posture. *Eur J Appl Physiol Occup Physiol*. 1996;73(3–4):346–52.

Zatsiorsky VM. *Science and practice of strength training*. Champaign, IL: Human Kinetics; 1995. 243 pp.

Zatsiorsky VM. Biomechanics of strength and strength training. In: Komi PV, editor. *Strength and power in sport*. 2nd ed. Oxford, UK: Blackwell Science; 2003. pp. 114–33.

Zatsiorsky VM, Kraemer WJ. *Science and practice of strength training*. 2nd ed. Champaign, IL: Human Kinetics; 2006. Chapter 8, Goal-specific strength training; pp. 155–70.

14

PLYOMETRICS

Yuri Verkhoshanski, a Russian sports scientist, introduced the concept of plyometrics in 1968 (Verkhoshanski 1968, 1969). He stated that progressive jumping exercises could significantly improve jumping and sprinting ability. Plyometrics are defined as exercises that involve a stretch-shortening cycle in which a rapid lengthening of a muscle is followed by an immediate shortening (Macaluso *et al.* 2012; Sáez-Sáez de Villarreal *et al.* 2009). During the deceleration or lengthening the muscle is stretched and elastic energy is stored, which is released again during the subsequent shortening of the muscle (Adams *et al.* 1992; Verkhoshanski 1968). The pre-stretch enables the muscles to contract more powerfully as a result of the combined effect of the storage of elastic energy and the reflex activation of the muscle (Chu and Plummer 1984). Plyometrics, also named stretch-shortening cycle training, enable the muscles to reach maximum force in the shortest possible time and are therefore widely used by athletes in various sports to improve power performance (Baechle and Earle 2000).

14.1 Physiology of plyometrics

Plyometric training enhances the effect of the stretch-shortening cycle by inducing neural and morphological changes.

The neuromuscular changes induced by plyometric training include:

- Improved intermuscular coordination (Markovic and Mikulic 2010).
- Desensitization of the Golgi tendon organ: The Golgi tendon organ, which is located at the junction between the tendon and the muscle, protects the muscle from excessive tension. On activation the Golgi tendon organ has an inhibitory effect on the muscle, reducing the force output. Plyometric training results in a desensitization of the Golgi tendon organ, allowing the elastic components of the muscle to be stretched further and store more energy (Wilk *et al.* 1993).
- Stretch reflex potentiation: The stretch reflex (myotatic reflex) is generated by the muscle spindles. These spindles run parallel with the muscle fibers and are stretched when the muscle is lengthened. The stretch reflex functions to prevent overstretching and injury of

the muscle. Plyometric training upregulates the stretch reflex, which results in enhanced motor unit recruitment and force production during the ensuing concentric contraction (Macaluso et al. 2012; Vissing et al. 2008).

The morphological changes induced by plyometric training consist of:

• Changes in elastic properties of the muscle and connective tissue that increase the ability of the muscle–tendon complex to store and release more elastic energy (Fouré et al. 2010, 2011; Kubo et al. 2007; Markovic and Mikulic 2010; Vissing et al. 2008).
• Increases in muscle cross-sectional area (Markovic et al. 2010; Vissing et al. 2008).

14.2 Efficient movement mechanics and performance

The neuromuscular adaptations and increased ability to store elastic energy following plyometric training result in a reduced loss of energy during the stretch-shortening cycle and a more powerful concentric muscle contraction (Wilk et al. 1993). Plyometrics play an important role in efficient movement mechanics and performance enhancement (Sáez-Sáez de Villarreal et al. 2009). Plyometric training will improve the player's strength, power, coordination, and overall athletic performance (Adams et al. 1992; Sáez-Sáez de Villarreal et al. 2009, 2010; Michailidis et al. 2013; Rimmer and Sleivert 2000; Siegler et al. 2003; Thomas et al. 2009).

All movements in soccer involve repeated bouts of stretch-shortening cycles and require a high rate of force development (Michailidis et al. 2013; Ramírez-Campillo et al. 2014).

Plyometrics will therefore besides improving a wide range of overall athletic abilities such as sprinting and jumping also enhance soccer-related activities such as endurance performance, kicking velocity and distance (Markovic et al. 2010; Michailidis et al. 2013; Wong et al. 2010). The better use of elastic energy and ability to develop explosiveness is considered the key mechanism behind the performance improvement (Adams et al. 1992).

14.3 Increased joint stability and injury prevention

Plyometrics also play an important role in increased joint stability and injury prevention (Hewett et al. 1996). Plyometrics are believed to enhance joint stability through an improved preparatory and reactive neuromuscular control (Chimera et al. 2004; Hewett et al. 1996). In time-critical movements, the central nervous system uses feedback information from previous movement experiences to update feedforward muscle activation patterns (see perception–action coupling). Plyometric training has been shown to improve the feedforward neuromuscular control of the lower extremity (Chimera et al. 2004, Hewett et al. 1996). The beneficial neuromuscular adaptations following plyometric training include earlier and greater muscle pre-activation before landing, increased reactive muscle activation upon landing, and a more symmetric agonist and antagonist cocontraction (Chimera et al. 2004; Hewett et al. 1996).

Greater medially and laterally directed torques at the knee during landing can increase the knee varus or valgus alignment during landing (Chimera et al. 2004; Cuoco and Tyler 2012). A more symmetric preparatory adductor–abductor co-activation will decrease the force and torque that act on the knee, resulting in a better lower limb alignment and more stable knee position at landing (Chimera et al. 2004; Cuoco and Tyler 2012). Plyometric training can also help correct hamstring-to-quadriceps torque imbalances, which reduces the strain on the anterior cruciate ligament and can decrease the incidence of knee injury (Hewett *et al.* 1996).

The enhanced muscle activation and stiffness of the muscle–tendon complex following plyometric training will also increase the load absorbed by the muscles and tendons and diminishes the load transmitted through the joint and ligaments (Chimera et al. 2004; Fouré et al. 2010, 2011).

14.4 Plyometric training parameters (Table 14.1)

Organization: Plyometrics replicate the ballistic movement patterns involved in sports, and various authors describe plyometrics as the link between speed and strength (Adams et al. 1992; Chu et al. 1984; Vissing et al. 2008). Plyometrics are high-velocity movements that mainly target the fast-twitch fibers and enable to train the velocity component of power (Macaluso et al. 2012; Morrissey et al. 1995). Verkhoshanski believed that plyometrics had to be included into the strength training to enhance explosiveness (Adams et al. 1992). Strength training combined with plyometrics has been shown to increase leg extension power more compared to either training program in isolation (Adams et al. 1992; Ebben 2002; Sáez-Sáez de Villarreal et al. 2010). This holds various benefits to develop and maintain explosiveness during the in-season when the time to develop physical qualities is limited due to the emphasis on technical and tactical training. Plyometrics can also easily be integrated into the warm-up to facilitate subsequent strength and athletic performance through post-activation potentiation (Brandenburg and Czajka 2010; Tobin and Delahunt 2014).

Rest interval: To maintain explosiveness and movement quality throughout the entire workout, a complete recovery between sets is required. The use of cluster sets, which involve a nontraditional training organization characterized by built-in intra-set rest periods, has been shown to improve the overall quality and efficiency of the plyometric routine (Moreno et al. 2014). Cluster sets of 2–5 jumps with a 30–45 second recovery time between sets allow for maximal recovery and result in greater conservation of power output, compared to a traditional set configuration (Moreno et al. 2014).

Exercise selection: Combining slow stretch-shortening cycle movements such as a countermovement or squat jump and fast stretch-shortening cycle movements such as hurdle or

TABLE 14.1 Plyometrics training parameters

Training parameter	Work
Intensity	Higher intensity maximizes performance improvements
Exercise selection	Combination of slow (>250 ms) and fast (<250 ms) stretch-shortening cycle movements
Organization	Complex training in combination with strength training
	Warm-up to induce post-activation potentiation effect
Rest interval	Cluster sets with intra-set rest intervals
	E.g., 4 x 5 with 30" RI or 10 x 2 with 10" RI
Speed of execution	Dynamic/explosive
Volume	>40 jumps/session is recommended for maximal performance improvements

box jumps into the same workout may be the best strategy to improve performance in a wide range of athletic abilities (Sáez-Sáez de Villarreal et al. 2009). The different athletic movements during soccer make different use of the stretch-shortening characteristics and require different strength properties. Sprinting is characterized by short contact times and a very rapid switch from a lengthening to a shortening of the muscle–tendon complex. On the other hand the movement amplitude is greater and contact time is longer during a change of direction or countermovement jump when heading. Both stretch-shortening cycle variations are mutually exclusive and require specific training (Schmidtbleicher 1990; Young et al. 1995). Soccer players therefore benefit from combining both slow (>250 ms contact time) and fast (<250 ms contact time) stretch-shortening movements into their plyometric workout.

Intensity: Intensity of the plyometric exercises is a very important training parameter (Ebben et al. 2011). Using higher-intensity exercise, with the premise that the player can perform these with correct technique, has been shown to maximize performance improvements (Sáez-Sáez de Villarreal et al. 2009). It has been shown that high-intensity plyometric exercises can be safely and effectively incorporated into the training of soccer players (Ramírez-Campillo et al. 2014; Thomas et al. 2009).

Several studies quantified the intensity of varies plyometric exercises based on the ground reaction forces during landing and take-off (Bobbert et al. 1987; Ebben et al. 2011; Fowler and Lees 1998; Jensen and Ebben 2007; Van Soest et al. 1985). The ground reaction force is highly related to jump height (Bobbert et al. 1987; Ebben et al. 2011). Exercises with lower jump heights such as cone hops can therefore be considered as submaximal or moderately intense (Ebben et al. 2011). Unilateral plyometric drills, in which the trainee intends to jump as high or as far as possible, are of the highest intensity because the ground reaction forces amount to 75 percent of those experienced during bilateral plyometrics (Ebben et al. 2011; Jensen and Ebben 2007; Van Soest et al. 1985). Box jumps or depth jumps are not more intense than regular jumps as long as the height of the box does not exceed jump height (Ebben et al. 2011; Jensen and Ebben 2007).

Volume: Because higher intensities require lower training volumes, plyometric programs consisting of only 20 contacts per session have been shown successful in improving athletic and soccer-specific performance of soccer players (Ramírez-Campillo et al. 2014). To maximize performance gains an amount of 40 high-intensity jumps or more, integrated into the strength workout, is recommended (Sáez-Sáez de Villarreal et al. 2009, 2010). Based on the literature there seems to be a threshold for the maximal number of jumps per session (Sáez-Sáez de Villarreal et al. 2009). Increasing the total number of jumps past this volume threshold does not seem to further enhance performance and can even be counterproductive (Luebbers et al. 2003; Sáez-Sáez de Villarreal et al. 2009). The study of Luebbers et al. shows that a high-intensity, high-volume plyometric program (4x/week 272 jumps/session) can decrease performance due to fatigue (Luebbers et al. 2003). The exercise intensity, competition period, and the available post-training recovery time should be considered to determine the total amount of jumps per session. Studies carried out with soccer players demonstrate that a range of 20–120 jumps per session can induce remarkable improvements in athletic and soccer-specific performance (Chelly et al. 2010; Maio Alves et al. 2010; Meylan and Malatesta 2009; Michailidis et al. 2013; Ramírez-Campillo et al. 2014; Sedano Campo et al. 2009; Thomas et al. 2009; Váczi et al. 2013). A low-intensity, high-volume plyometric training (90–220 jumps/session) performed once a week can also significantly enhance sprint and jump performance in soccer players (Ozbar et al. 2014).

14.5 Exercises

Box jumps

Two variations of the box jumps (Figure 14.1) can be performed: the single-response versus the multiple-response box jump. During the single-response box jump the trainee performs a countermovement jump to land on top of a box. The multiple-response box jump on the other hand is a more reactive plyometric drill. Muscle activation is higher during the single-response compared to the multiple-response box jump, whereas the rate of force development is higher during the multiple-response version (Ebben et al. 2011).

Provided that the height of the box is adjusted, both box jump variations can also be performed unilaterally. Single-leg box jumps are of higher intensity than bilateral box jumps (Ebben et al. 2011; Jensen and Ebben 2007).

Box jump (single response)

OBJECTIVE

The box jump (single response) is a basic, lower-intensity plyometric exercise. Landing on a box reduces the impact. During this exercise the trainee can improve his/her jumping ability and work on proper landing mechanics. When the player shows proper landing mechanics during this exercise s/he can progress to more reactive jump drills.

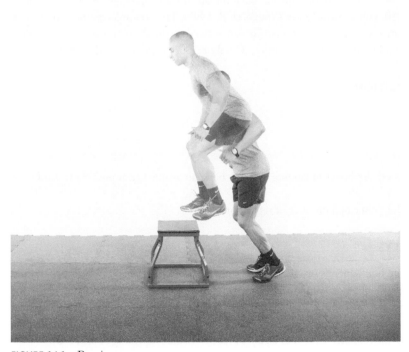

FIGURE 14.1   Box jump

STARTING POSITION

Stand facing a box.

EXECUTION

Jump onto the box.
>   Land softly on the box.
>   Step off the box and repeat for the prescribed number of repetitions.

COACHING KEYS

Land with the knees and hips flexed and the bodyweight centered over the front foot. The knees should point in the same direction as the feet. Do not let the knees sway in.

Box jump (multiple response)

OBJECTIVE

The multiple response box jump is a fast stretch-shortening cycle movement, which can help improve the power output and reactive strength of the leg extensors (Bobbert 1990; Young et al. 1995). Due to the much shorter contact time and decreased amplitude compared to a regular countermovement jump, the mechanical power output is higher during the multiple-response depth jump (Bobbert 1990; Young et al. 1995). The rapid reverse of the downward into an upward movement imposes greater stretch loads on the leg extensor muscles, requiring high eccentric contraction forces (Young et al. 1995). The multiple-response box jump exercise can positively transfer to sprint performance, because the short contact times and high stretch loads resemble those during sprinting (Chelly et al. 2010; Young et al. 1995).

STARTING POSITION

Stand on a box.

EXECUTION

Jump backwards off the box. On landing, bounce back up as quickly as possible to land onto the box again.
>   Repeat for the prescribed number of repetitions.

COACHING KEYS

The height of the box depends on the trainee's jumping ability. The height of the box should challenge the player but not compromise proper landing technique. Contact times increase with higher box heights (Young et al. 1995). Very high boxes, in which heavy heel contact upon landing cannot be prevented, no longer serve the desired training effect of short stretch-shortening cycle movements (Ebben et al. 2011; Taube et al. 2012; Young et al. 1995).

The ground reaction force during the landing progressively increases with the height of the box (Bobbert et al. 1987; Ebben et al. 2011; Jensen and Ebben 2007). As long as the height of the box does not exceed the individual's jumping ability, the multiple response box jump is no more intense than regular jumping drills (Ebben et al. 2011; Jensen and Ebben 2007).

Hurdle jumps

Identical to box jumps, the single-response hurdle jumps depend more on neuromuscular mechanisms, whereas passive elastic force production dominates during the multiple-response variation (Ebben et al. 2011).

The hurdle jumps can be performed bilaterally or unilaterally.

Hurdle jump (single response)

OBJECTIVE

The single-response hurdle jump (Figure 14.2) is a slow, stretch-shortening cycle movement. The player performs repetitive countermovement jumps over a hurdle.

STARTING POSITION

Line up the hurdles. Set the hurdles at a height that is challenging.

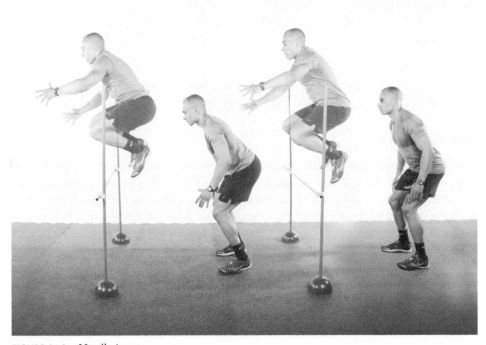

FIGURE 14.2   Hurdle jump

Stand facing the hurdles, with your feet about shoulder–width apart.

EXECUTION

Jump over the first hurdle.
  Land softly between the first and second hurdle.
  Drive your arms backward again, reload, and jump over the next hurdle.
  Continue until all the hurdles are cleared.

COACHING KEYS

Land in balance with the bodyweight centered over the front foot.

Hurdle jump (multiple response)

OBJECTIVE

In the multiple response hurdle jump the player explodes off the ground immediately on landing. Plyometrics that minimize the ground contact time are an excellent way to improve reactive strength. Stretch loads and rate of force development are higher during the multiple response compared to the single-response hurdle jump (Cappa and Behm 2011; Ebben et al. 2011).

STARTING POSITION

Stand facing the hurdles.

EXECUTION

Jump over the first hurdle.
  Land on the balls of the feet, between the first and second hurdle.
  On landing quickly explode off the ground into the next hop.

COACHING KEYS

Increasing the height of the hurdles does not necessarily increase the rate of force production (Cappa and Behm 2011). When the hurdle height is set between 100 percent and 140 percent of the player's vertical jump height, the contact time and ground reaction forces reflect those observed during many explosive sport actions, such as sprinting (Cappa and Behm 2011; Mero and Komi 1986; Weyand et al. 2000). Setting the hurdles higher results in longer contact times and will force the player to tuck in the knees more to pass over the hurdle (Cappa and Behm 2011).

When performing the single-leg hurdle jump (multiple response) it is advisable to use mini hurdles. Lowering the hurdle height will decrease the contact time and enhance the rate of force development (Cappa and Behm 2011). Single-leg jumps over higher hurdles (e.g., a height of 70 percent of the individual's bilateral vertical jump height) produce high amounts of muscle, tendon, ligament, and joint stress and should therefore only be prescribed for highly trained players (Cappa and Behm 2011).

Lateral hurdle jump

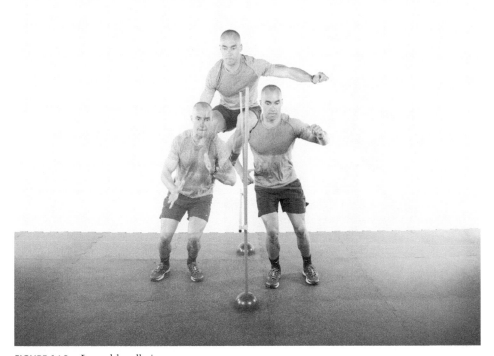

FIGURE 14.3 Lateral hurdle jump

OBJECTIVE

The lateral hurdle jump (Figure 14.3) adds a lateral component to the hurdle jump. This fast stretch-shortening cycle movement can help enhance the ability to change direction.

STARTING POSITION

Stand sideways to the hurdle.

EXECUTION

Jump laterally over the hurdle.
    Land on the forefeet and quickly explode off the ground again.
    Continue jumping side to side over the hurdle for the prescribed number of repetitions.

COACHING KEYS

Minimize the ground contact time. Avoid heavy heel contact.

Step-up jump

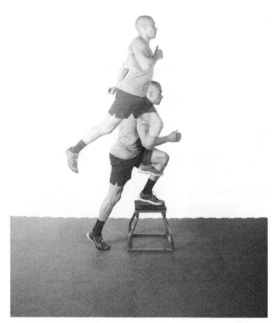

FIGURE 14.4   Step-up jump

OBJECTIVE

The step-up jump (Figure 14.4) is a ballistic step-up motion.

STARTING POSITION

Stand facing a box.
    Place the whole foot on the box.

EXECUTION

Powerfully extend the lead leg and jump up.
    Land again with the same foot on the bench.
    Bounce off the ground with the back foot and explode into your next jump.
    Perform the prescribed number of repetitions and switch sides.

COACHING KEYS

Slightly lean forward with your shoulders over the box to continuously load the lead leg.
    The level of difficulty increases with the height of the box. The height of the box should not exceed knee height.

Bulgarian split squat jump

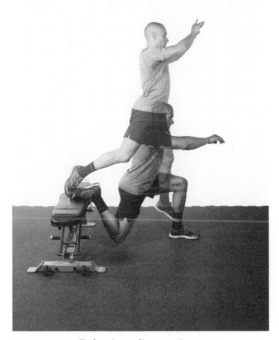

FIGURE 14.5 Bulgarian split squat jump

OBJECTIVE

The Bulgarian split squat jump (Figure 14.5) is an effective exercise to develop single-leg power.

STARTING POSITION

Stand facing away from a bench, with your back foot placed on the bench.

EXECUTION

Squat down until the rear knee almost touches the floor or the thigh is parallel to the floor.
Squat back up as explosively as possible and jump out.
On landing, lower your body back into the squat position.

COACHING KEYS

Keep the torso erect during the whole exercise.
Descend in a controlled manner on landing.
Make sure the knee of the supporting leg stays well aligned between hip and ankle.

Side-to-side box jump

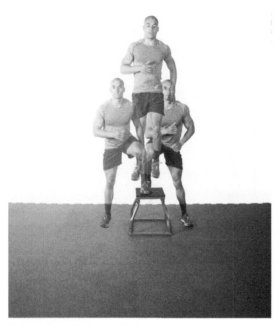

FIGURE 14.6 Side-to-side box jump

OBJECTIVE

The side-to-side box jump (Figure 14.6) adds a lateral component to the step-up jump. Movement occurs in both the sagittal and frontal plane of motion.

STARTING POSITION

Stand to the side of a box.
  Place the whole foot on the box.
  Shift part of your weight to the lead leg.

EXECUTION

Powerfully extend the lead leg and jump up.
  Cross over the box in the air.
  Land with the other foot on the bench.
  Bounce off the ground with the trail foot and explode into the next jump.

COACHING KEYS

Keep the lead leg loaded.

Lateral cone hops

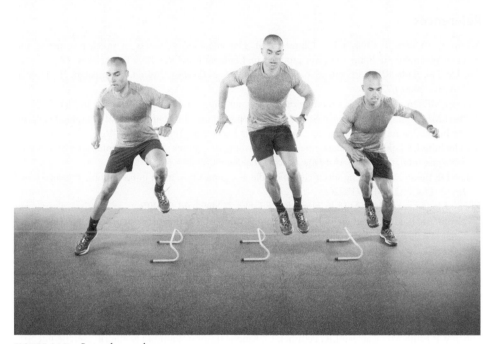

FIGURE 14.7 Lateral cone hops

OBJECTIVE

Lateral cone hops (Figure 14.7) will help develop power in the sagittal and frontal plane to improve cutting ability and the ability to change direction.

STARTING POSITION

Line up three cones or mini hurdles.
    Stand at one end of the cones, facing the cones sideways.
    Assume a single-leg stance, lifting the inside foot off the ground.

EXECUTION

Jump laterally over the first cone.
    Land on both feet between the first and second cone.
    On landing quickly explode off the ground into the next hop.
    Land on both feet between the second and third cone, bouncing up into the next lateral hop.
    Land on the outside leg, next to the third cone.
    Immediately push off in the opposite direction and repeat the jumping pattern.
    Continue jumping for the prescribed number of repetitions.

COACHING KEYS

The difficulty level of this exercise can be increased by placing the cones further apart.

References

Adams K, O'Shea JP, O'Shea KL, Climstein M. The effect of six weeks of squat, plyometric and squat-plyometric training on power production. *J Strength Cond Res*. 1992 Feb;6(1):36–41.

Baechle TR, Earle RW. *Essentials of strength training and conditioning*. 2nd ed. Champaign, IL: Human Kinetics; 2000. 672 pp.

Bobbert MF. Drop jumping as a training method for jumping ability. *Sports Med*. 1990 Jan;9(1):7–22.

Bobbert MF, Huijing PA, van Ingen Schenau GJ. Drop jumping. II. The influence of dropping height on the biomechanics of drop jumping. *Med Sci Sports Exerc*. 1987 Aug;19(4):339–46.

Brandenburg J, Czajka A. The acute effects of performing drop jumps of different intensities on concentric squat strength. *J Sports Med Phys Fitness*. 2010 Sep;50(3):254–61.

Cappa DF, Behm DG. Training specificity of hurdle vs. countermovement jump training. *J Strength Cond Res*. 2011 Oct;25(10):2715–20.

Chelly MS, Ghenem MA, Abid K, Hermassi S, Tabka Z, Shephard RJ. Effects of in-season short-term plyometric training program on leg power, jump- and sprint performance of soccer players. *J Strength Cond Res*. 2010 Oct;24(10):2670–6.

Chimera NJ, Swanik KA, Swanik CB, Straub SJ. Effects of plyometric training on muscle-activation strategies and performance in female athletes. *J Athl Train*. 2004 Mar;39(1):24–31.

Chu D, Plummer L. The language of plyometrics. *Strength Cond J*. 1984 Oct;6(5):30–1.

Cuoco A, Tyler TF. Plyometric training and drills. In: Andrews J, Harrelson G, Wilk K, editors. *Physical rehabilitation of the injured athlete*. 4th ed. Philadelphia: Elsevier Saunders; 2012. pp. 571–95.

Ebben WP. Complex training: a brief review. *J Sports Sci Med*. 2002 Jun;1(2):42–6.

Ebben WP, Fauth ML, Garceau LR, Petushek EJ. Kinetic quantification of plyometric exercise intensity. *J Strength Cond Res*. 2011 Dec;25(12):3288–98.

Fouré A, Nordez A, Cornu C. Plyometric training effects on Achilles tendon stiffness and dissipative properties. *J Appl Physiol (1985)*. 2010 Sep;109(3):849–54.

Fouré A, Nordez A, McNair P, Cornu C. Effects of plyometric training on both active and passive parts of the plantarflexors series elastic component stiffness of muscle-tendon complex. *Eur J Appl Physiol*. 2011 Mar;111(3):539–48.

Fowler NE, Lees A. A comparison of the kinetic and kinematic characteristics of plyometric drop-jump and pendulum exercises. *J Appl Biomechanics*. 1998 Aug;14(3):260–75.

Hewett TE, Stroupe AL, Nance TA, Noyes FR. Plyometric training in female athletes. Decreased impact forces and increased hamstring torques. *Am J Sports Med*. 1996 Nov–Dec;24(6):765–73.

Jensen RL, Ebben WP. Quantifying plyometric intensity via rate of force development, knee joint, and ground reaction forces. *J Strength Cond Res*. 2007 Aug;21(3):763–7.

Kubo K, Morimoto M, Komuro T, Yata H, Tsunoda N, Kanehisa H, Fukunaga T. Effects of plyometric and weight training on muscle-tendon complex and jump performance. *Med Sci Sports Exerc*. 2007 Oct;39(10):1801–10.

Luebbers PE, Potteiger JA, Hulver MW, Thyfault JP, Carper MJ, Lockwood RH. Effects of plyometric training and recovery on vertical jump performance and anaerobic power. *J Strength Cond Res*. 2003 Nov;17(4):704–9.

Macaluso F, Isaacs AW, Myburgh KH. Preferential type II muscle fiber damage from plyometric exercise. *J Athl Train*. 2012 Jul–Aug;47(4):414–20.

Maio Alves JM, Rebelo AN, Abrantes C, Sampaio J. Short-term effects of complex and contrast training in soccer players' vertical jump, sprint, and agility abilities. *J Strength Cond Res*. 2010 Apr;24(4):936–41.

Markovic G, Mikulic P. Neuro-musculoskeletal and performance adaptations to lower-extremity plyometric training. *Sports Med*. 2010 Oct 1;40(10):859–95.

Mero A, Komi PV. Force-, EMG-, and elasticity-velocity relationships at submaximal, maximal and supramaximal running speeds in sprinters. *Eur J Appl Physiol Occup Physiol*. 1986;55(5):553–61.

Meylan C, Malatesta D. Effects of in-season plyometric training within soccer practice on explosive actions of young players. *J Strength Cond Res*. 2009 Dec;23(9):2605–13.

Michailidis Y, Fatouros IG, Primpa E, Michailidis C, Avloniti A, Chatzinikolaou A, Barbero-Álvarez JC, Tsoukas D, Douroudos II, Draganidis D, Leontsini D, Margonis K, Berberidou F, Kambas A. Plyometrics' trainability in preadolescent soccer athletes. *J Strength Cond Res*. 2013 Jan;27(1):38–49.

Moreno SD, Brown LE, Coburn JW, Judelson DA. Effect of cluster sets on plyometric jump power. *J Strength Cond Res*. 2014 Sep;28(9):2424–8.

Morrissey MC, Harman EA, Johnson MJ. Resistance training modes: specificity and effectiveness. *Med Sci Sports Exerc*. 1995 May;27(5):648–60.

Ozbar N, Ates S, Agopyan A. The effect of 8-week plyometric training on leg power, jump and sprint performance in female soccer players. *J Strength Cond Res*. 2014 Oct;28(10):2888–94.

Ramírez-Campillo R, Meylan C, Alvarez C, Henríquez-Olguín C, Martínez C, Cañas-Jamett R, Andrade DC, Izquierdo M. Effects of in-season low-volume high-intensity plyometric training on explosive actions and endurance of young soccer players. *J Strength Cond Res*. 2014 May;28(5):1335–42.

Rimmer E, Sleivert G. Effects of a plyometrics intervention program on sprint performance. *J Strength Cond Res*. 2000 Jul;14(3):295–301.

Sáez-Sáez de Villarreal E, Kellis E, Kraemer WJ, Izquierdo M. Determining variables of plyometric training for improving vertical jump height performance: a meta-analysis. *J Strength Cond Res*. 2009 Mar;23(2):495–506.

Sáez-Sáez de Villarreal E, Requena B, Newton RU. Does plyometric training improve strength performance? A meta-analysis. *J Sci Med Sport*. 2010 Sep;13(5):513–22.

Schmidtbleicher D. Training for power. Presented at the 13th National Strength and Conditioning Association national convention on strength training and conditioning; 1990 June 28–30; San Diego, CA.

Sedano Campo S, Vaeyens R, Philippaerts RM, Redondo JC, de Benito AM, Cuadrado G. Effects of lower-limb plyometric training on body composition, explosive strength, and kicking speed in female soccer players. *J Strength Cond Res*. 2009 Sep;23(6):1714–22.

Siegler J, Gaskill S, Ruby B. Changes evaluated in soccer-specific power endurance either with or without a 10-week, in-season, intermittent, high-intensity training protocol. *J Strength Cond Res*. 2003 May;17(2):379–87.

Taube W, Leukel C, Lauber B, Gollhofer A. The drop height determines neuromuscular adaptations and changes in jump performance in stretch-shortening cycle training. *Scand J Med Sci Sports*. 2012 Oct;22(5):671–83.

Thomas K, French D, Hayes PR. The effect of two plyometric training techniques on muscular power and agility in youth soccer players. *J Strength Cond Res*. 2009 Jan;23(1):332–5.

Tobin DP, Delahunt E. The acute effect of a plyometric stimulus on jump performance in professional rugby players. *J Strength Cond Res*. 2014 Feb;28(2):367–72.

Váczi M, Tollár J, Meszler B, Juhász I, Karsai I. Short-term high intensity plyometric training program improves strength, power and agility in male soccer players. *J Hum Kinet*. 2013 Mar;36:17–26.

Van Soest AJ, Roebroeck ME, Bobbert MF, Huijing PA, van Ingen Schenau GJ. A comparison of one-legged and two-legged countermovement jumps. *Med Sci Sports Exerc*. 1985 Dec;17(6):635–9.

Verkhoshanski Y. Are depth jumps useful? *Sov Sports Rev*. 1968;3:75–6.

Verkhoshanski Y. Perspectives in the improvement of speed-strength preparation of jumpers. *Sov Sports Rev*. 1969;4:28–34.

Vissing K, Brink M, Lønbro S, Sørensen H, Overgaard K, Danborg K, Mortensen J, Elstrøm O, Rosenhøj N, Ringgaard S, Andersen JL, Aagaard P. Muscle adaptations to plyometric vs. resistance training in untrained young men. *J Strength Cond Res*. 2008 Nov;22(6):1799–810.

Weyand PG, Sternlight DB, Bellizzi MJ, Wright S. Faster top running speeds are achieved with greater ground forces not more rapid leg movements. *J Appl Physiol (1985)*. 2000 Nov;89(5):1991–9.

Wilk KE, Voight ML, Keirns MA, Gambetta V, Andrews JR, Dillman CJ. Stretch-shortening drills for the upper extremities: theory and clinical application. *J Orthop Sports Phys Ther.* 1993 May;17(5):225–39.

Wong PL, Chamari K, Wisløff U. Effects of 12-week on-field combined strength and power training on physical performance among U-14 young soccer players. *J Strength Cond Res.* 2010 Mar;24(3):644–52.

Young WB, Pryor JF, Wilson GJ. Effect of instructions on characteristics of countermovement and drop jump performance. *J Strength Cond Res.* 1995 Nov;9(4):232–6.

15

OLYMPIC LIFTS

The SAID principle (specific adaptations to imposed demands) also applies to speed. In order that the soccer player can compete explosively s/he also has to lift explosively. Many studies have shown that with Olympic lifting exercises the highest amount of power can be produced of all human movement (Garhammer 1993; Haff *et al.* 2001; Häkkinen 1989; MacKenzie *et al.* 2014). The Olympic lifts have power outputs far greater than those of the squat or any other exercise (Garhammer 1993; MacKenzie *et al.* 2014). The Olympic lifts have to be integrated into training to bring power performance to a peak (Baker 1996; Tricoli *et al.* 2005).

Because of their biomechanical similarity, Olympic lifts have an excellent carry-over to athletic performance (Canavan *et al.* 1996; Tricoli *et al.* 2005). The same leg and hip actions can be seen in the power snatch and power clean as is used in many athletic actions. Utilizing Olympic lifts as part of the strength training will improve sprint performance, jump height, and leg strength (Hoffman *et al.* 2004; Tricoli *et al.* 2005). All explosive athletic actions that require triple extension carried through to full extension can benefit from the use of Olympic lifts (Miller 1981). Sprinting, changing direction, and jumping all involve an explosive extension of the hip, knee, and ankle.

The Olympic lifts involve complex multiple-joint movements that also require great balance, coordination, stability, and flexibility (Hedrick and Wada 2008; Tricoli *et al.* 2005). Performance in the Olympic lifts is also correlated to 20 m sprint and jumping performance (Hori *et al.* 2008). A high rate of force development, balance, joint, and core stability are paramount in soccer and implementing Olympic lifts into training can improve athletic soccer performance.

15.1 Clean progression (Figure 15.1)

The Olympic lifts are difficult skills to teach and acquire, but this also counts for sport skills. By means of a learning progression any skill can be acquired. The learning progression to teach proper technique in the power clean starts with the high hang clean pull, to focus on the triple extension of the ankle, knee, and hip, the so-called jumping phase (Duba *et al.* 2009; Newton 2002).

If the player masters the high hang clean pull and shows good technique in the front squat, s/he should have little difficulty in racking the bar in the high hang power clean.

Until this step in the learning progression all the lifts were performed from above the knees (high hang position). Lifting from above the knees is relatively easy and can be quickly mastered. The next step is the low hang clean pull to teach the transition phase or scoop (Enoka 1979; Miller 1980; Newton 2002). In the low hang position the bar is lifted from just below the kneecaps. The scoop gets the athlete in a good jumping position. When the scoop is performed properly the hips and knees are driven forward (rotary action of the hips) resulting in a slight hip and knee flexion (Miller 1980; Newton 2002). This imposes a stretch on the knee and hip extensors. The stored elastic energy during the stretch enables the muscles of the legs to react more explosively. The scoop is the key to a productive power clean.

If the scoop is mastered and the player has sufficient flexibility at the hips and low back s/he can start lifting from the floor. The power clean is the last step in the learning progression.

The high and low hang versions are not only a means to get to lifting from the floor, but they can make up a big part of the training program, even when the power clean from the floor is mastered. Until the player has not developed the necessary hip and low back flexibility to lift from the floor, only high hang and low hang versions are used.

High hang clean pull

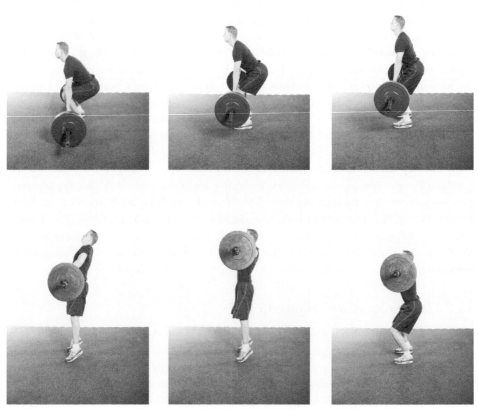

FIGURE 15.1 Clean progression

OBJECTIVE

The logical progression of teaching the power clean starts with the high hang clean pull. The player will learn the power position and the second pulling motion.

The high hang clean pull starts in the power position. This is the position from which the most power can be exerted (Souza *et al.* 2002; Stone *et al.* 1998). The power position is a frequently recurring position in soccer. Because of the favorable leverages in this position, the player can react quickly in response to a stimulus.

STARTING POSITION (PHOTO 3 OF FIGURE 15.1)

Stand with the feet between hip- and shoulder-width apart and toes pointing forward.
   The weight is on the balls of the feet.
   Hold the bar slightly wider than shoulder-width.
   The arms are straight, the elbows are pointing out, and the wrists curled inwards.
   The bar touches the thighs just above the knees.
   Position your shoulders over or slightly in front of the bar.
   The back is arched. Look straight ahead.

EXECUTION (PHOTOS 4 AND 5 OF FIGURE 15.1)

Initiate the movement with an explosive triple extension (extension of the ankle, knee, and hip) like in a vertical jump.
   At the end of the jump shrug your shoulders upward and bend the elbows.
   Do not attempt to hold the bar in this position, but return to the starting position.

COACHING KEYS

Do not allow the torso angle to drop by extending the knees before the hips.
   Do not shrug the shoulders and lift the elbows before explosively jumping upward.
   Do not jump off the platform during the explosive triple extension.
   Pull the bar up close or in contact with the body.

High hang power clean

OBJECTIVE

Before attempting the high hang power clean make sure you master the high hang clean pull and the front squat.

STARTING POSITION (PHOTO 3 OF FIGURE 15.1)

Start with the bar in the high hang position. The chest is pushed forward and the back is extended.

EXECUTION (PHOTOS 4 AND 6 OF FIGURE 15.1)

Initiate the movement with an explosive triple extension (second pull).

At the end of the jump, shrug your shoulders upward and bend the elbows.

At the highest point of the bar, pull yourself under the bar, rotate the elbows forward and catch the bar in the front squat position.

COACHING KEYS

Rotate the elbows around the bar to catch the bar with the elbows high.

Low hang clean pull

OBJECTIVE

In the starting position of the low hang clean pull the bar is positioned just under the knee-caps. In this step of the learning progression focus on getting into a good jumping position after performing the scoop.

Before attempting the low hang clean pull make sure you master the high hang clean pull.

When the scoop (first part of the low hang power clean) is performed properly a stretch will be imposed on the knee and hip extensors, providing for storage and subsequent use of elastic energy. This pre-stretch enables the muscles of the legs to react more explosively. This action is very similar to that found in plyometrics. Olympic lifting from below the knee will develop this reactive ability.

STARTING POSITION (PHOTO 2 OF FIGURE 15.1)

Stand with the feet between hip- and shoulder-width apart and toes pointing forward.

The weight is on the middle of the feet.

Hold the bar slightly wider than shoulder-width.

The arms are straight, the elbows are pointing out.

The bar is held just beneath the kneecaps.

Position your shoulders slightly in front of the bar.

The back is arched. Look straight ahead.

EXECUTION (PHOTOS 3, 4, AND 5 OF FIGURE 15.1)

Raise the bar by extending the hips.

As the bar passes the knees, pull your shoulders straight up while driving your hips forward. This will dorsiflex the ankles and slightly increases the flexion at the knees. This enables the knees to move under the bar so the bar will make contact with the thighs.

At the completion of the scoop the body is in the high hang position to initiate the second pull.

COACHING KEYS

When learning the low hang clean pull perform it slowly. When you master the movement, increase the speed of execution.

Low hang power clean

OBJECTIVE

Before attempting the low hang power clean make sure you master the high hang power clean and the low hang clean pull.

STARTING POSITION (PHOTO 2 OF FIGURE 15.1)

Start with the bar in the low hang position.

EXECUTION (PHOTOS 3, 4, AND 6 OF FIGURE 15.1)

Raise the bar by extending the hips.
   Subsequently perform the scoop.
   At the completion of the scoop the body is in the high hang position to initiate the second pull.
   Catch the bar in the front squat position at the completion of the second pull.

COACHING KEYS

When learning the low hang power clean perform it slowly. Gradually, increase the speed of execution.

Power clean

OBJECTIVE

After mastering the most difficult phase by moving through the learning progression, the athlete can move to the full lift with lifting the barbell from the floor.
   The power clean from the floor has the advantage of a long upward drive and that power is exerted over a long trajectory.
   Lifting a barbell from the floor demands good flexibility at the ankles, hips, and lower back.

STARTING POSITION (PHOTO 1 OF FIGURE 15.1)

Stand with the feet between hip- and shoulder-width apart and toes pointing forward.
   The weight is balanced between the middle and the balls of the feet.
   Hold the bar slightly wider than shoulder-width.
   The arms are straight, the elbows are pointing out, and the wrists are curled inwards.
   Position the bar close to the shins.
   Position your shoulders over or slightly in front of the bar.
   The back is arched. Look straight ahead.
   The shoulder blades are retracted.

EXECUTION (PHOTOS 2, 3, 4, AND 6 OF FIGURE 15.1)

Lift the bar off the floor through a combined knee and hip extension, to a position just below the knees.
   Subsequently perform the scoop and second pull to catch the bar in the front squat position.

COACHING KEYS

During the first pull, pull the bar up as close to the shins as possible.

During the first pull, the weight is shifted from the balls to the middle of the feet.

Drive your chest up and forward during the first pull. Maintain a constant torso position to the floor, by raising your hips and shoulders at the same time.

15.2 Squat clean

OBJECTIVE

The squat clean (Figure 15.2) combines the power clean and the front squat into one exercise. The power clean is followed by a front squat to complete one repetition.

STARTING POSITION

Hold the bar slightly wider than shoulder–width.

The arms are straight, the elbows are pointing out, and the wrists are curled inwards.

Position the bar close to the shins.

Position your shoulders over or slightly in front of the bar.

The back is arched. Look straight ahead.

The shoulder blades are retracted.

EXECUTION

Perform the power clean and catch the bar in the front squat position.

Descend with control until the thighs are parallel to the floor. Keep the body weight centered over the heel and mid-foot. Keep the heels in contact with the floor throughout the descent.

Squat back up by extending the knees and hips.

Return to the starting position and repeat the exercise for the prescribed number of repetitions.

COACHING KEYS

The squat clean can be performed from a high hang position, a low hang position, or from the floor.

15.3 Snatch progression (Figure 15.3)

Identical to the clean progression, the progression to learn the power snatch starts with mastering the second pull. If the player masters the high hang snatch pull and shows good technique in the overhead squat, s/he can progress to the high hang power snatch. Subsequently lifting can start from below the knees to master the scoop. The power snatch from the floor is the last step in the learning progression.

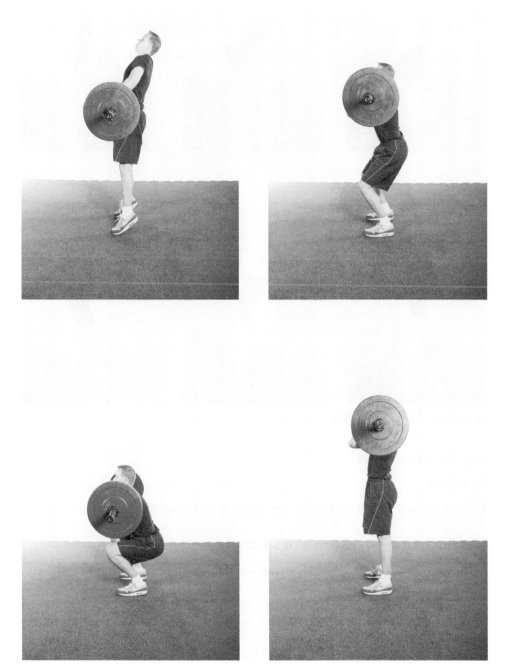

FIGURE 15.2 Squat clean

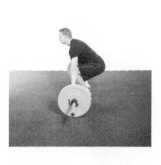 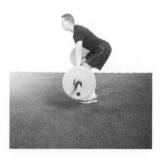 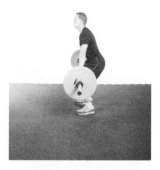

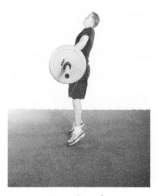 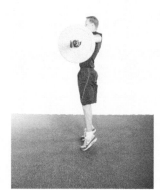 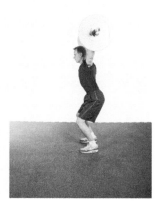

FIGURE 15.3 Snatch progression

High hang snatch pull

OBJECTIVE

The logical progression of teaching the power snatch starts with the high hang snatch pull.

STARTING POSITION (PHOTO 3 OF FIGURE 15.3)

Stand with the feet between hip- and shoulder-width apart and toes pointing forward.
  The weight is on the balls of the feet.
  Hold the bar wider than shoulder-width.
  The arms are straight, the elbows are pointing out.
  The bar touches the thighs just above the knees.
  Position your shoulders over or slightly in front of the bar.
  The back is arched. Look straight ahead.

EXECUTION (PHOTOS 4 AND 5 OF FIGURE 15.3)

Initiate the movement with an explosive triple extension like in a vertical jump.
  At the end of the jump shrug your shoulders upward and bend the elbows.

COACHING KEYS

To determine the appropriate grip width, measure the distance from the outside edge of the shoulder to the knuckles of the opposite arm, which is abducted parallel to the floor. This is the distance between the hands when you grasp the bar for a snatch.

High hang power snatch

OBJECTIVE

Before you move to the high hang power snatch make sure you master the high hang snatch pull and the overhead squat.

STARTING POSITION (PHOTO 3 OF FIGURE 15.3)

Hold the bar in the high hang position.

EXECUTION (PHOTOS 4, 5, AND 6 OF FIGURE 15.3)

Initiate the second pull motion.

When the bar reaches about sternum height, pull the body under the bar by rotating the arms around and under the bar.

Push yourself under the bar until your elbows are extended.

Catch the bar in an overhead squat position. Complete the catch by squatting up.

COACHING KEYS

Proper timing to execute the drop-under is important. Pull the bar high and quickly drop under the bar on completing the second pull to avoid catching the bar overhead with flexed elbows.

Low hang snatch pull

OBJECTIVE

Before attempting the low hang snatch pull make sure you master the high hang snatch pull.

STARTING POSITION (PHOTO 2 OF FIGURE 15.3)

The weight is on the middle of the feet.

The bar is held just beneath the kneecaps.

Position your shoulders over the bar.

EXECUTION (PHOTOS 3, 4, AND 5 OF FIGURE 15.3)

Lift the bar to mid-thigh by extending the hips and driving the knees forward.

At the completion of the scoop the body is in the high hang position to initiate the second pull.

COACHING KEYS

When learning the low hang snatch pull perform it slowly. When you master the movement, increase the speed of execution.

Low hang power snatch

OBJECTIVE

Before attempting the low hang power snatch make sure you master the high hang power snatch and the low hang snatch pull.

STARTING POSITION (PHOTO 2 OF FIGURE 15.3)

Start with the bar in the low hang position.

EXECUTION (PHOTOS 3, 4, 5, AND 6 OF FIGURE 15.3)

Execute the scoop and second pull to catch the bar in the overhead position.

COACHING KEYS

Catch the bar overhead with the arms extended.

Power snatch

OBJECTIVE

The power snatch requires good dynamic flexibility in the ankles, hips, lower and upper back and the shoulders, and optimal stability throughout the spine.

STARTING POSITION (PHOTO 1 OF FIGURE 15.3)

Stand with the feet between hip- and shoulder-width apart and toes pointing forward.
  The weight is balanced towards the balls of the feet.
  Position the bar close to the shins.
  Position your shoulders over the bar.
  The back is arched. Look straight ahead.
  The shoulder blades are retracted.

EXECUTION (PHOTOS 2, 3, 4, 5, AND 6 OF FIGURE 15.3)

Lift the bar off the floor through a combined knee and hip extension, to a position just below the knees.
  Subsequently perform the scoop and second pull to catch the bar in the overhead squat position.

COACHING KEYS

During the first pull, pull the bar up as close to the shins as possible.

During the first pull, the weight is shifted from the balls to the middle of the feet.

Drive your chest up and forward during the first pull. Maintain a constant torso position to the floor, by raising your hips and shoulders at the same time.

15.4 Squat snatch

OBJECTIVE

The squat snatch (Figure 15.4) combines the power snatch and the overhead squat into one exercise. The power snatch is followed by an overhead squat to complete one repetition.

STARTING POSITION

Hold the bar wider than shoulder-width.

The arms are straight and the elbows are pointing out.

Position the bar close to the shins.

Position your shoulders over the bar.

The back is arched. Look straight ahead.

The shoulder blades are retracted.

EXECUTION

Perform the power snatch and catch the bar in the overhead squat position.

Descend with control until the thighs are parallel to the floor. Keep the body weight centered over the heel and mid-foot. Keep the heels in contact with the floor throughout the descent.

Squat back up by extending the knees and hips.

Return to the starting position and repeat the exercise for the prescribed number of repetitions.

COACHING KEYS

The squat snatch can be performed from a high hang position, a low hang position, or from the floor.

15.5 Jerk

The jerk is a less complicated Olympic lift. So unlike the power clean and power snatch, you can learn the jerk without breaking down the movement into parts.

Alternating split jerk (Figure 15.5)

OBJECTIVE

Make sure you master the overhead press, so you feel comfortable with pressing weights overhead.

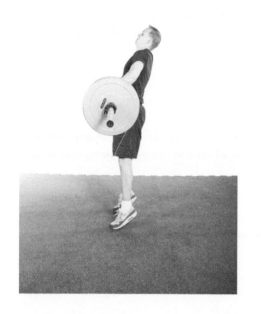 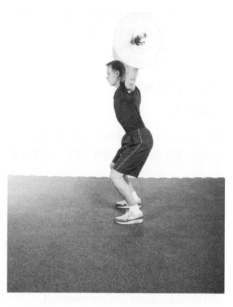

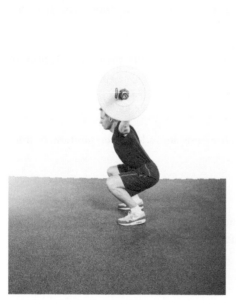 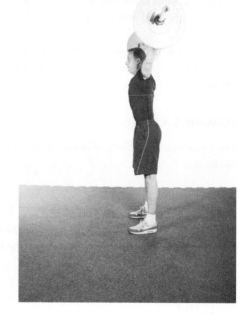

FIGURE 15.4   Squat snatch

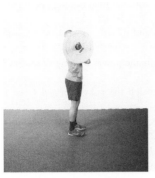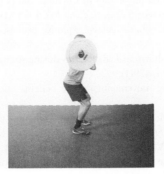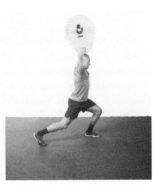

FIGURE 15.5 Alternating split jerk

STARTING POSITION

Stand with the feet between hip- and shoulder-width apart and toes pointing forward.

Position the barbell on the front of the shoulders. Place the hands slightly wider than shoulder-width. Lift the elbows up and forward.

Keep the torso erect and the core tight. Look straight ahead.

EXECUTION

Descend with control into the power position. Keep the heels in contact with the floor throughout the descent.

Explode back up by forcefully extending the legs, using this momentum to lift the barbell overhead.

When the bar moves overhead, explosively shift one foot backward and the other forward.

Push yourself under the bar by extending your elbows.

Catch the bar in the split stance with the arms extended.

Complete the lift by bringing the front leg back.

Perform for the prescribed number of repetitions alternating the forward leg during the split stance.

COACHING KEYS

Push the barbell or dumbbells up as vertically as possible, while maintaining a straight body position. Avoid leaning back.

References

Baker D. Improving vertical jump performance through general, special, and specific strength training: a brief review. *J Strength Cond Res.* 1996 May;10(2):131–6.

Canavan PK, Garrett GE, Armstrong LE. Kinematic and kinetic relationships between an Olympic-style lift and the vertical jump. *J Strength Cond Res.* 1996 May;10(2):127–30.

Duba J, Kraemer W, Martin G. Progressing from the hang power clean to the power clean: a 4-step model. *Strength Cond J.* 2009 June;31(3):58–66.

Enoka RM. The pull in Olympic weightlifting. *Med Sci Sports.* 1979;11(2):131–7.

Garhammer J. A review of power output studies of Olympic and powerlifting: methodology, performance prediction, and evaluation tests. *J Strength Cond Res.* 1993 May 7(2):76–89.

Haff GG, Whitley A, Potteiger JA. A brief review: explosive exercises and sports performance. *Strength Cond J.* 2001 Jun;23(3):13–20.

Häkkinen K. Neuromuscular and hormonal adaptations during strength and power training. A review. *J Sports Med Phys Fitness.* 1989 Mar;29(1):9–26.

Hedrick A, Wada H. Weightlifting movements: do the benefits outweigh the risks? *Strength Cond J.* 2008;Dec:30(6):26–35.

Hoffman JR, Cooper J, Wendell M, Kang J. Comparison of Olympic vs. traditional power lifting training programs in football players. *J Strength Cond Res.* 2004 Feb;18(1):129–35.

Hori N, Newton RU, Andrews WA, Kawamori N, McGuigan MR, Nosaka K. Does performance of hang power clean differentiate performance of jumping, sprinting, and changing of direction? *J Strength Cond Res.* 2008 Mar;22(2):412–18.

MacKenzie SJ, Lavers RJ, Wallace BB. A biomechanical comparison of the vertical jump, power clean, and jump squat. *J Sports Sci.* 2014 Aug;32(16):1576–85.

Miller C. Sequence exercise to learn the rotary, action of the legs and hips common to many sports. *Strength Cond J.* 1980 June;2(3):38–9.

Miller C. Rotary jerk-hip and leg action common to many sports. *Strength Cond J.* 1981 Apr;3(2):30–1.

Newton HS. *Explosive lifting for sports.* Champaign, IL: Human Kinetics; 2002. 191 pp.

Souza AL, Shimada SD, Koontz A. Ground reaction forces during the power clean. *J Strength Cond Res.* 2002 Aug;16(3):423–7.

Stone MH, O'Bryant HS, Williams FE, Johnson RL, Pierce KC. Analysis of bar paths during the snatch in elite male weightlifters. *Strength Cond J.* 1998 Aug;20(4):30–8.

Tricoli V, Lamas L, Carnevale R, Ugrinowitsch C. Short-term effects on lower-body functional power development: weightlifting vs. vertical jump training programs. *J Strength Cond Res.* 2005 May;19(2):433–7.

PART V
Blood flow restriction training

16
BLOOD FLOW RESTRICTION TRAINING

The traditional training paradigm suggests that high-intensity loads of over 65 percent of the 1RM are required to optimize strength and hypertrophy gains (Campos *et al.* 2002; Kraemer and Ratamess 2004; McDonagh *et al.* 1984). However, a growing body of evidence reports on the effectiveness of low-load resistance training (20–50 percent of 1RM) combined with blood flow restriction to increase muscular hypertrophy and strength (Loenneke *et al.* 2012c; Pope *et al.* 2013).

Blood flow restriction training originated in Japan and involves wrapping a cuff or an elastic knee wrap around the trained limb to occlude the venous blood flow while the arterial inflow is maintained. Research on this topic was initiated in the 1990s and shows that blood flow restriction training, performed in isolation or in combination with traditional resistance training, is effective at increasing hypertrophy, strength, and muscular endurance (Loenneke *et al.* 2012c; Pope *et al.* 2013). Low-intensity strength training in combination with blood flow restriction can induce strength and hypertrophy gains similar to those observed with high-intensity strength training, without increasing indices of muscle damage nor resulting in prolonged decrements in torque (Laurentino *et al.* 2012; Loenneke *et al.* 2013a, 2014; Wilson *et al.* 2013).

During the soccer competition, prolonged periods of bi-weekly games occur, during which it is not possible to plan higher-intensity strength training to maintain strength levels. Two or three weeks without strength training will result in decreases of strength and power levels and negatively affects performance (Hortobágyi *et al.* 1993; Izquierdo *et al.* 2007; Koutedakis 1995). Blood flow restriction can induce hypertrophy and strength gains despite the low exercise intensity, while minimal to no muscle damage occurs (Loenneke *et al.* 2014; Wilson *et al.* 2013). Research shows that torque decrements following blood flow restriction training quickly recover by 1 hour post exercise and return to baseline within 24 hours after training (Loenneke *et al.* 2013a). Due to the minimal neuromuscular, psychological, and mechanical joint stress, blood flow restriction training can provide an effective training stimulus to maintain or increase strength levels during competition periods that require unloading.

16.1 Practical application

The objective of blood flow restriction training is to occlude venous blood outflow from the muscles without seriously affecting arterial blood flow. Blood will circulate into the working muscles but cannot escape, resulting in venous pooling. While research is carried out with pneumatic cuffs, training can be performed using elastic knee wraps. These need to be applied as high as possible on the limbs being trained. When applied on the arms they should be wrapped just below the deltoids and for lower body exercises they should be wrapped around the top of the thighs, just below the gluteal fold. It is impossible to occlude the venous blood flow of the gluteal, shoulder, or trunk muscles, but research shows that low-load resistance training in combination with blood flow restriction elicits hypertrophy in both occluded and non-occluded muscles (Abe *et al.* 2005, 2012).

The pressure that is applied when pneumatic cuffs are used is based on systolic blood pressure. When applying pneumatic cuffs a pressure between 160 and 200 mmHg was used in most studies (Loenneke *et al.* 2012c). Ratings of perceived exertion and discomfort are higher and elevations in heart rate and blood pressure are greater when wide cuffs are used compared to narrow cuffs (Rossow *et al.* 2012). Loenneke *et al.* (2013b) therefore advise to base the pressure on cuff width and the individual's limb circumference in order to provide a more optimal training stimulus. When elastic knee wraps are used they should be wrapped around the limb at approximately 70 percent of maximal tightness. This means they are applied tightly around the limb without a feeling of excessive discomfort during rest. Check the pulse at the wrist or ankle after the wraps are applied to make sure the arterial blood flow is not cut off. A slight change of color and mild swelling of the trained limb upon termination of the exercise protocol are indications of venous pooling.

The cuffs are applied right before the start of the exercise and removed upon termination of the final set. The cuffs need to be maintained throughout the entire exercise. Taking the wraps off between sets reduces the intramuscular metabolic stress and will not enhance fast-twitch muscle fiber recruitment (Suga *et al.* 2012). Keeping the cuffs on for a prolonged time after terminating the exercise has not been proven to bring additional benefits.

Low-load blood flow restriction training, using approximately 20–30 percent of the 1RM is most supported by research (Loenneke *et al.* 2012c, 2013a; Luebbers *et al.* 2014; Ohta *et al.* 2003; Sata 2005; Wilson *et al.* 2013; Yamanaka *et al.* 2012). Several low-load resistance training protocols in combination with blood flow restriction have been shown to increase strength and hypertrophy (Table 16.1).

TABLE 16.1 Exercise protocols in progressive load order

Reps/set	% of 1RM	Rest interval between sets
15 – 15 – 15	20	30 seconds
30 – 15 – 15 – 15	20	45 seconds
30 – 20 – 20 – 20	20	45 seconds
15 – 12 – 12 – 12	30	30–60 seconds
15 – 15 – 15 – 15	30	30–60 seconds
30 – 15 – 15 – 15	30	45–60 seconds
3 sets until failure	50 (set 1 & 2) – 30 (set 3)	60 seconds

16.2 Blood flow restriction training in rehabilitation and sports

Blood flow restriction training has also been used successfully in rehabilitation (Ohta *et al.* 2003; Sata 2005; Takarada *et al.* 2000c). Low-load resistance training in combination with venous blood flow occlusion has been shown to reduce pain and swelling in patients with patella tendonitis and can speed up the recovery following anterior cruciate ligament recon-struction (Ohta *et al.* 2003; Sata 2005; Takarada *et al.* 2000c).

Immobilization following surgery results in a significant decrease of strength and muscle mass (Kubota *et al.* 2008, 2011; Takarada *et al.* 2000c). In the first stage following surgery blood flow restriction without any form of exercise is effective to attenuate post operative disuse atrophy and strength loss (Takarada *et al.* 2000c; Figure 16.1). The application of a compressive force (50–238 mmHg) for five minutes, followed by three minutes of rest, repeated five times, twice a day significantly reduces disuse atrophy and muscular weakness (Kubota *et al.* 2008, 2011; Takarada *et al.* 2000c).

The supine rehabilitation exercises during this early phase following surgery can also be performed with blood flow restriction in order to increase strength and exercise capacity (Sumide *et al.* 2009). Once the player is ambulatory, treadmill walking in combination with blood flow restriction (5 x 2 minutes walk – 1 minute rest) will further facilitate the recupera-tion of strength and muscle mass (Abe *et al.* 2006). Also low-intensity cycling with restricted leg blood flow can elicit improvements in strength, muscle mass, and endurance capacity (Abe *et al.* 2010). In the next phase of rehabilitation, cycling and walking with blood flow restric-tion can be phased out to progressively incorporate low-load functional exercises combined with vascular occlusion to increase strength and hypertrophy (Lejkowski and Pajaczkowski 2011; Loenneke *et al.* 2012a; Ohta *et al.* 2003).

In rehabilitation and sports conditioning, blood flow restriction training is not a replace-ment for higher-intensity strength training, but can be used in combination. In early phases of rehabilitation or when time is limited between games to allow sufficient recuperation from

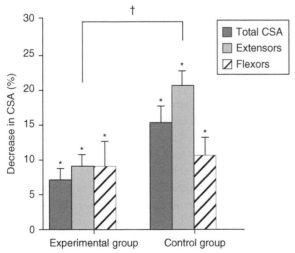

FIGURE 16.1   Blood flow restriction without any form of exercise diminishes post operative disuse atrophy (Takarada *et al.* 2000c)

TABLE 16.2 Highly trained athletes can benefit from blood flow restriction training

Variable	Blood flow restriction	Control group
1RM Squat	+ 30 lbs	+ 15 lbs
1RM Bench press	+ 20 lbs	+ 9 lbs
Thigh circumference	+ 0.5 inches	+ 0.3 inches
Upper chest circumference	+ 1.5 inches	+ 0.3 inches

Athletes performed four sets of squat and bench press, with or without blood flow restriction, after the completion of their high-load strength training.
Protocol: 30 reps – 20 reps – 20 reps – 20 reps with 20 percent of 1RM and 45" rest interval between sets. 3x/week for 4 weeks.
Increases in strength and hypertrophy were significantly greater in blood flow restriction group (Yamanaka et al. 2012).

higher-intensity resistance training, low-intensity strength training in combination with blood flow restriction can be beneficial. Strength gains are in par with high-load strength training while the neuromuscular stress is reduced.

Also with highly trained athletes it has been shown that low-intensity strength training combined with vascular occlusion can increase muscle size, strength, and endurance (Takarada et al. 2002; Yamanaka et al. 2012; Table 16.2). Adding one or two low-load blood flow restriction exercises at the end of a high-load strength training routine will result in a greater increase of strength and muscle mass (Yamanaka et al. 2012; Yasuda et al. 2011).

16.3 Mechanisms

The exact mechanisms by which blood flow restriction induces hypertrophy are not fully known, but several mechanisms appear to be present throughout most studies. Blood flow restriction training stimulates muscle hypertrophy through an enhanced accumulation of metabolites, muscle cell swelling, myogenic stem cell proliferation, and the decreased expression of protein breakdown markers (Loenneke et al. 2012a, 2012b; Nielsen et al. 2012).

Accumulation of metabolites: The accumulation of metabolites enhances the recruitment of higher-threshold (fast-twitch) muscle fibers (Takarada et al. 2000b). Muscle activation levels during the exercise with occlusion are significantly elevated compared to the exercise without occlusion although the same amount of mechanical work is produced (Manini et al. 2011; Moritani et al. 1992; Takarada et al. 2000a, 2000b). The increased accumulation of metabolites plays an important role in motor unit recruitment and rate coding patterns (Moritani et al. 1992). The hypoxic intramuscular environment during blood flow restriction exercise makes the metabolism more anaerobic and may elicit the elevated motor unit activation of more glycolytic (fast-twitch) fibers (Moritani et al. 1992). Due to local hypoxia and suppressed lactate clearance, lactate levels are higher during training with occlusion compared to training without occlusion (Takarada et al. 2000a). The higher accumulation of lactate may further promote additional motor unit recruitment (Miller et al. 1996). Elevated lactate concentrations will also trigger the release of growth hormone through feedback from chemoreceptors (Gosselink et al. 1998; Takarada et al. 2000a).

Muscle cell swelling: Restricted blood flow training induces cell swelling through a combination of venous blood pooling, the accumulation of metabolites, and reactive hyperemia following the removal of the venous blood flow occlusion (Fahs *et al.* 2012; Hoffmann *et al.* 2009; Loenneke *et al.* 2012b). Cellular hydration plays an important role in the regulation of protein turnover (Häussinger *et al.* 1993). Cell swelling (hydration) acts as an anabolic signal, augmenting protein synthesis, while cell shrinkage will trigger protein degradation (Häussinger *et al.* 1993).

Myogenic stem cell proliferation: Myogenic stem cells are precursors of muscle cells. These cells are quiescent, but upon activation can proliferate, differentiate, and fuse with existing muscle fibers (Petrella *et al.* 2008). This process plays an important role in muscle repair and growth. The number of myonuclei may impose a ceiling effect on muscle fiber hypertrophy (Kadi *et al.* 2004; Petrella *et al.* 2008). There is extensive evidence of myogenic stem cell proliferation following long-term high-intensity strength training (Kadi *et al.* 2004; Mackey *et al.* 2011; Olsen *et al.* 2006; Petrella *et al.* 2008). Low-intensity strength training performed with venous blood flow occlusion also results in the proliferation of myogenic stem cells and addition of myonuclei (Nielsen *et al.* 2012).

Decreased expression of protein breakdown markers: Myostatin is a growth factor that regulates muscle mass. Myostatin overexpression has been shown to reduce muscle mass and the number of mononuclei (Laurentino *et al.* 2012). There is evidence that myostatin gene expression is reduced in response to prolonged heavy-resistance strength training (Roth *et al.* 2003). Myostatin gene expression has also been shown to diminish following low-load strength training in combination with blood flow restriction (Laurentino *et al.* 2012). When low-intensity strength training is combined with blood flow restriction, the effect on hypertrophy and strength also seems to be augmented through the deregulation of protein breakdown markers (MuRF-1), depressed protein synthesis markers (Atrogin-1), and the increased expression of cell growth markers (mTOR, MAPK) (Fry *et al.* 2010; Fujita *et al.* 2007; Loenneke *et al.* 2012a; Manini *et al.* 2011).

References

Abe T, Yasuda Midorikawa TT, Sato Y, Kearns CF, Inoue K, Koizumi K, Ishii N. Skeletal muscle size and circulating IGF-1 are increased after two weeks of twice daily Kaatsu resistance training. *Int J Kaatsu Training Res.* 2005 Jul;1(1):6–12.

Abe T, Kearns CF, Sato Y. Muscle size and strength are increased following walk training with restricted venous blood flow from the leg muscle, Kaatsu-walk training. *J Appl Physiol (1985).* 2006 May;100(5):1460–6.

Abe T, Fujita S, Nakajima T, Sakamaki M, Ozaki H, Ogasawara R, Sugaya M, Kudo M, Kurano M, Yasuda T, Sato Y, Ohshima H, Mukai C, Ishii N. Effects of low-intensity cycle training with restricted leg blood flow on thigh muscle volume and VO2MAX in young men. *J Sports Sci Med.* 2010 Sep;9(3):452–8.

Abe T, Loenneke JP, Fahs CA, Rossow LM, Thiebaud RS, Bemben MG. Exercise intensity and muscle hypertrophy in blood flow-restricted limbs and non-restricted muscles: a brief review. *Clin Physiol Funct Imaging.* 2012 Jul;32(4):247–52.

Campos GER, Luecke TJ, Wendeln HK, Toma K, Hagerman FC, Murray TF, Ragg KE, Ratamess NA, Kraemer WJ, Staron RS. Muscular adaptation in response to three different resistance-training regimens: specificity of repetition maximum training zones. *Eur J Appl Physiol.* 2002 Nov;88(1–2):50–60.

Fahs CA, Rossow LM, Loenneke JP, Thiebaud RS, Kim D, Bemben DA, Bemben MG. Effect of different types of lower body resistance training on arterial compliance and calf blood flow. *Clin Physiol Funct Imaging.* 2012 Jan;32(1):45–51.

Fry CS, Glynn EL, Drummond MJ, Timmerman KL, Fujita S, Abe T, Dhanani S, Volpi E, Rasmussen BB. Blood flow restriction exercise stimulates mTORC1 signaling and muscle protein synthesis in older men. *J Appl Physiol (1985).* 2010 May;108(5):1199–209.

Fujita S, Abe T, Drummond MJ, Cadenas JG, Dreyer HC, Sato Y, Volpi E, Rasmussen BB. Blood flow restriction during low-intensity resistance exercise increases S6K1 phosphorylation and muscle protein synthesis. *J Appl Physiol (1985)*. 2007 Sep;103(3):903–10.

Gosselink KL, Grindeland RE, Roy RR, Zhong H, Bigbee AJ, Grossman EJ, Edgerton VR. Skeletal muscle afferent regulation of bioassayable growth hormone in the rat pituitary. *J Appl Physiol (1985)*. 1998 Apr;84(4):1425–30.

Häussinger D, Roth E, Lang F, Gerok W. Cellular hydration state: an important determinant of protein catabolism in health and disease. *Lancet*. 1993 May 22;341(8856):1330–2.

Hoffmann EK, Lambert IH, Pedersen SF. Physiology of cell volume regulation in vertebrates. *Physiol Rev*. 2009 Jan;89(1):193–277.

Hortobágyi T, Houmard JA, Stevenson JR, Fraser DD, Johns RA, Israel RG. The effects of detraining on power athletes. *Med Sci Sports Exerc*. 1993 Aug;25(8):929–35.

Izquierdo M, Ibañez J, González-Badillo JJ, Ratamess NA, Kraemer WJ, Häkkinen K, Bonnabau H, Granados C, French DN, Gorostiaga EM. Detraining and tapering effects on hormonal responses and strength performance. *J Strength Cond Res*. 2007 Aug;21(3):768–75.

Kadi F, Schjerling P, Andersen LL, Charifi N, Madsen JL, Christensen LR, Andersen JL. The effects of heavy resistance training and detraining on satellite cells in human skeletal muscles. *J Physiol*. 2004 Aug 1;558(Pt 3):1005–12.

Koutedakis Y. Seasonal variation in fitness parameters in competitive athletes. *Sports Med*. 1995 Jun;19(6):373–92.

Kraemer WJ, Ratamess NA. Fundamentals of resistance training: progression and exercise prescription. *Med Sci Sports Exerc*. 2004 Apr;36(4):674–88.

Kubota A, Sakuraba K, Sawaki K, Sumide T, Tamura Y. Prevention of disuse muscular weakness by restriction of blood flow. *Med Sci Sports Exerc*. 2008 Mar;40(3):529–34.

Kubota A, Sakuraba K, Koh S, Ogura Y, Tamura Y. Blood flow restriction by low compressive force prevents disuse muscular weakness. *J Sci Med Sport*. 2011 Mar;14(2):95–9.

Laurentino GC, Ugrinowitsch C, Roschel H, Aoki MS, Soares AG, Neves M Jr, Aihara AY, Fernandes Ada R, Tricoli V. Strength training with blood flow restriction diminishes myostatin gene expression. *Med Sci Sports Exerc*. 2012 Mar;44(3):406–12.

Lejkowski PM, Pajaczkowski JA. Utilization of vascular restriction training in post-surgical knee rehabilitation: a case report and introduction to an under-reported training technique. *J Can Chiropr Assoc*. 2011 Dec;55(4):280–7.

Loenneke JP, Abe T, Wilson JM, Thiebaud RS, Fahs CA, Rossow LM, Bemben MG. Blood flow restriction: an evidence based progressive model (review). *Acta Physiol Hung*. 2012a Sep;99(3):235–50.

Loenneke JP, Fahs CA, Rossow LM, Abe T, Bemben MG. The anabolic benefits of venous blood flow restriction training may be induced by muscle cell swelling. *Med Hypotheses*. 2012b Jan;78(1):151–4.

Loenneke JP, Wilson JM, Marín PJ, Zourdos MC, Bemben MG. Low intensity blood flow restriction training: a meta-analysis. *Eur J Appl Physiol*. 2012c May;112(5):1849–59.

Loenneke JP, Thiebaud RS, Fahs CA, Rossow LM, Abe T, Bemben MG. Blood flow restriction does not result in prolonged decrements in torque. *Eur J Appl Physiol*. 2013a Apr;113(4):923–31.

Loenneke JP, Fahs CA, Rossow LM, Thiebaud RS, Mattocks KT, Abe T, Bemben MG. Blood flow restriction pressure recommendations: a tale of two cuffs. *Front Physiol*. 2013b Sep;10(4):249.

Loenneke JP, Thiebaud RS, Abe T. Does blood flow restriction result in skeletal muscle damage? A critical review of available evidence. *Scand J Med Sci Sports*. 2014 Dec;24(6):e415–22.

Luebbers PE, Fry AC, Kriley LM, Butler MS. The effects of a seven-week practical blood flow restriction program on well-trained collegiate athletes. *J Strength Cond Res*. 2014 Aug;28(8):2270–80.

McDonagh MJ, Davies CT. Adaptive response of mammalian skeletal muscle to exercise with high loads. *Eur J Appl Physiol Occup Physiol*. 1984;52(2):139–55.

Mackey AL, Holm L, Reitelseder S, Pedersen TG, Doessing S, Kadi F, Kjaer M. Myogenic response of human skeletal muscle to 12 weeks of resistance training at light loading intensity. *Scand J Med Sci Sports*. 2011 Dec;21(6):773–82.

Manini TM, Vincent KR, Leeuwenburgh CL, Lees HA, Kavazis AN, Borst SE, Clark BC. Myogenic and proteolytic mRNA expression following blood flow restricted exercise. *Acta Physiol (Oxf)*. 2011 Feb;201(2):255–63.

Miller KJ, Garland SJ, Ivanova T, Ohtsuki T. Motor-unit behavior in humans during fatiguing arm movements. *J Neurophysiol*. 1996 Apr;75:1629–36.

Moritani T, Michael-Sherman W, Shibata M, Matsumoto T, Shinohara M. Oxygen availability and motor unit activity in humans. *Eur J Appl Physiol Occup Physiol*. 1992;64(6):552–6.

Nielsen JL, Aagaard P, Bech RD, Nygaard T, Hvid LG, Wernbom M, Suetta C, Frandsen U. Proliferation of myogenic stem cells in human skeletal muscle in response to low-load resistance training with blood flow restriction. *J Physiol*. 2012 Sep 1;590(Pt 17):4351–61.

Ohta H, Kurosawa H, Ikeda H, Iwase Y, Satou N, Nakamura S. Low-load resistance muscular training with moderate restriction of blood flow after anterior cruciate ligament reconstruction. *Acta Orthop Scand*. 2003 Feb;74(1):62–8.

Olsen S, Aagaard P, Kadi F, Tufekovic G, Verney J, Olesen JL, Suetta C, Kjaer M. Creatine supplementation augments the increase in satellite cell and myonuclei number in human skeletal muscle induced by strength training. *J Physiol*. 2006 Jun 1;573(Pt 2):525–34.

Petrella JK, Kim JS, Mayhew DL, Cross JM, Bamman MM. Potent myofiber hypertrophy during resistance training in humans is associated with satellite cell-mediated myonuclear addition: a cluster analysis. *J Appl Physiol (1985)*. 2008 Jun;104(6):1736–42.

Pope ZK, Willardson JM, Schoenfeld BJ. Exercise and blood flow restriction. *J Strength Cond Res*. 2013 Oct;27(10):2914–26.

Rossow LM, Fahs CA, Loenneke JP, Thiebaud RS, Sherk VD, Abe T, Bemben MG. Cardiovascular and perceptual responses to blood-flow-restricted resistance exercise with differing restrictive cuffs. *Clin Physiol Funct Imaging*. 2012 Sep;32(5):331–7.

Roth SM, Martel GF, Ferrell RE, Metter EJ, Hurley BF, Rogers MA. Myostatin gene expression is reduced in humans with heavy-resistance strength training: a brief communication. *Exp Biol Med (Maywood)*. 2003 Jun;228(6):706–9.

Sata S. Kaatsu training for patella tendonitis patient. *Int J Kaatsu Training Res*. 2005 Jul;1(1):29–32.

Suga T, Okita K, Takada S, Omokawa M, Kadoguchi T, Yokota T, Hirabayashi K, Takahashi M, Morita N, Horiuchi M, Kinugawa S, Tsutsui H. Effect of multiple set on intramuscular metabolic stress during low-intensity resistance exercise with blood flow restriction. *Eur J Appl Physiol*. 2012 Nov;112(11):3915–20.

Sumide T, Sakuraba K, Sawaki K, Ohmura H, Tamura Y. Effect of resistance exercise training combined with relatively low vascular occlusion. *J Sci Med Sport*. 2009 Jan;12(1):107–12.

Takarada Y, Nakamura Y, Aruga S, Onda T, Miyazaki S, Ishii N. Rapid increase in plasma growth hormone after low-intensity resistance exercise with vascular occlusion. *J Appl Physiol (1985)*. 2000a Jan;88(1):61–5.

Takarada Y, Takazawa H, Sato Y, Takebayashi S, Tanaka Y, Ishii N. Effects of resistance exercise combined with moderate vascular occlusion on muscular function in humans. *J Appl Physiol (1985)*. 2000b Jun;88(6):2097–106.

Takarada Y, Takazawa H, Ishii N. Applications of vascular occlusion diminish disuse atrophy of knee extensor muscles. *Med Sci Sports Exerc*. 2000c Dec;32(12):2035–9.

Takarada Y, Sato Y, Ishii N. Effects of resistance exercise combined with vascular occlusion on muscle function in athletes. *Eur J Appl Physiol*. 2002 Feb;86(4):308–14.

Wilson JM, Lowery RP, Joy JM, Loenneke JP, Naimo MA. Practical blood flow restriction training increases acute determinants of hypertrophy without increasing indices of muscle damage. *J Strength Cond Res*. 2013 Nov;27(11):3068–75.

Yamanaka T, Farley RS, Caputo JL. Occlusion training increases muscular strength in division IA football players. *J Strength Cond Res*. 2012 Sep;26(9):2523–9.

Yasuda T, Ogasawara R, Sakamaki M, Ozaki H, Sato Y, Abe T. Combined effects of low-intensity blood flow restriction training and high-intensity resistance training on muscle strength and size. *Eur J Appl Physiol*. 2011 Oct;111(10):2525–33.

PART VI

Program design

17

PERIODIZATION

Training variation is paramount for long-term improvement of endurance, strength, power, and speed. When an athlete is exposed for a prolonged period of time to the same training stimulus, this stimulus will fail to elicit further physiological adaptations and performance will reach a plateau (Gamble 2013; Wathen et al. 2000). Training variation keeps the training interesting and enhances the athlete's motivation. Training monotony also places the same kind of strain on the body during consecutive workouts and will result in overuse injury (Anderson et al. 2003). All the different training parameters – choice of exercise, exercise order, number of sets, amount of reps per set, rest interval – can be modified to provide training variation (Kraemer and Fleck 2007).

Periodization is the methodical planning and structuring of variation in training content, volume, and intensity to optimize performance at predetermined time points (Gamble 2006; Haff 2013; Naclerio et al. 2013). The critical aims of periodization in soccer are fatigue management and to consistently maintain a high level of performance throughout the entire competitive season.

Periodization was first used and researched in the former Soviet Union, but has since been optimized and a variety of periodization models were introduced (Issurin 2010).

17.1 Training cycles

In any periodization model three different cycles are distinguished: the macrocycle, mesocycles, and microcycles (Bompa 1999; Naclerio et al. 2013). In soccer the annual plan comprises a whole season, starting from the first day of active recovery following the end of the season until the last game of the next season. The annual plan is divided into smaller units that can each have their own training goals. The annual plan in soccer is typically divided into three macrocycles: the off-season, pre-season, and the in-season. A macrocycle consists of several mesocycles. A mesocycle can be composed of two to five microcycles (Plisk and Stone 2003; Siff 2003; Stone et al. 2007). A microcycle refers to the weekly training plan and its structure and content determine the quality of the training program (Bompa 1999).

17.2 Linear periodization

In the classic linear periodization model, the training year is divided into different phases (Bompa 1999). During the general preparation phase, volume and intensity are progressively increased to develop general physical qualities like muscle hypertrophy, basic metabolic conditioning, strength endurance, and connective tissue strength (Bompa 1999). The specific preparation phase follows the general preparation phase. The goal of this phase is to transfer the general fitness gains made early in the training year to more sport-specific fitness and performance characteristics (Haff 2013). During the specific preparation, phase volume decreases while intensity further increases to develop maximal strength, power, and intensify the metabolic conditioning (Bompa 1999). The competitive phase emphasizes sport-specific skill development and technical, tactical readiness for competition (Haff 2013). During the competitive phase training is highly specific and training frequency and volume are tapered to eliminate all training fatigue and allow supercompensation and optimal performance during the competition (Bompa 1999). The transition phase starts immediately following the main competition period and links two annual cycles. The goal of the transition phase is active recovery (Bompa 1999).

For several reasons however, the classic linear periodization paradigm is less suited to soccer:

- Linear periodization is intended for sports that have their major annual competition during the summer (Plisk and Stone 2003). In sports like track and field and swimming, the competition period only lasts a few months and athletes have a long period to prepare. The soccer season on the other hand is characterized by a long competition period and short pre-season. Soccer players are required to maintain their form close to their peak over a prolonged period of time (Gamble 2013). In linear periodization peaking for competition is achieved through tapering. Tapering during a competition period that can even exceed 35 weeks would result in a considerable loss of muscle mass, strength, and power and a deterioration of performance towards the end of the season (Allerheiligen 2003; Baker 1998; Hoffman and Kang 2003).
- The different phases of linear periodization emphasize different goals and elicit specific physiological adaptations. In the linear periodization model a progressive shift takes place from general to increasingly specific training modes (Bompa 1999). For strength there is a progress from strength endurance, to hypertrophy, to maximal strength, to power (Bompa 1999). With this coherent progression, physiological adaptations from a previous phase will facilitate adaptations in the subsequent phase (Prestes et al. 2009; Rhea et al. 2002). Soccer players cannot afford to emphasize the development of power only towards the end of the competitive season and compromise a good seasonal debut.
- During a phase in linear periodization only two or three training goals can be effectively emphasized (Zatsiorsky and Kraemer 2006). Soccer is multi factorial (physical, technical, tactical) and requires various goals, which also involve opposite hormonal responses and neuromuscular fatigue, to be stressed at any time (Gamble 2004).

17.3 Nonlinear periodization

Nonlinear (undulating) periodization may originate from the late 1970s or early 1980s when football strength coaches started using two different strength-training sessions within a training week (Kraemer and Fleck 2007). One session was oriented towards hypertrophy, consisting mainly of single-joint lifts, while the second session was aimed at developing strength and consisted mainly out of functional multi-joint lifts (Kraemer and Fleck 2007).

Nonlinear periodization involves session-by-session variation of volume and intensity in addition to variation between mesocycles (Wathen et al. 2000). Both daily and weekly undulating periodization schemes exist (Buford et al. 2007). In daily undulating periodization there is a daily alteration in training volume and intensity so that each session within the week provides a different training stimulus, whereas weekly undulating periodization adapts volume and intensity on a weekly basis (Rhea et al. 2002).

Nonlinear periodization has been shown to be effective in maintaining or even increasing strength, power, speed, endurance, and muscle mass over the course of the long competitive season in soccer (Silvestre et al. 2006).

Applied to the situation of soccer, nonlinear periodization offers several advantages over classic linear periodization:

- Nonlinear periodization allows for the various qualities of soccer to be addressed concurrently (Zatsiorsky and Kraemer 2006).
- Nonlinear periodization offers the advantage of flexibility. The alteration of volume and intensity does not necessarily have to follow a strict pattern and can be adapted more easily to the stress of games (Gamble 2013; Wathen et al. 2000).
- Not adhering to a linear increase in intensity and decrease of volume also allows more flexibility when peaking and to keep the players close to their peak over an extended time period (Gamble 2013).
- The enhanced versatility of undulating periodization also allows to adapt the training to diverse situations: minutes played during a game, muscle soreness, minor trauma from tackle.
- Session-by-session variation in training intensity also diminishes neuromuscular fatigue and allows greater strength increases (Baker et al. 1994; Rhea et al. 2002).

17.4 Periodization for soccer: practical application

Off- and pre-season

The two different periodization models have their practical application during different phases of the soccer season. The linear periodization model can help the player progressively prepare for the higher intensity of more specific strength workouts.

At the end of the competition phase, players require a period of active rest to recover from the physiological and psychological fatigue (Bompa 1999; Wathen et al. 2000). After this transition period the player enters the off-season, which is a period of training that in the vast majority of soccer teams does not occur in a team setting. Due to the length of the competitive season, most teams and players will only have a short off-season. After the off-season the pre-season starts, which is the offset of the organized technical and tactical team practices.

Training intensity and volume during the pre- and off-season can still follow a pattern of linear periodization (Gamble 2013). Programming during the off-season corresponds to the general preparation phase of classic linear periodization in which general exercises have a high priority, training intensity is low, and volume is relatively higher (Gamble 2013). Strength training during this phase starts with an emphasis on connective tissue strength and strength endurance. The goal of the off-season is to develop general athleticism and to form a general foundation prior to more soccer-specific conditioning (Gamble 2013). Next to a linear periodization, off-season programming may also comprise elements of undulating periodization. Elite athletes will benefit from additional workout-to-workout alterations in intensity and volume (Monteiro et al. 2009). For young and less experienced athletes however, a strictly linear periodization is sufficient (Bompa 1999; Kraemer and Fleck 2007; Plisk and Stone 2003).

During the pre-season, training progressively becomes more specific while intensity increases and volume decreases (Gamble 2013). The emphasis of strength training shifts to development of strength and power.

The implementation of practice games during pre-season forces the strength and conditioning coach to integrate daily undulating periodization in addition to linear programming, in order to allow recovery from and for games. The incidence of injury in soccer is highest during the pre-season and beginning of the competition period (Agel and Schisel 2013; Mallo and Dellal 2012). Adding daily volume and intensity undulation in pre-season will better help control the training workload and can reduce the incidence of injury (Mallo and Dellal 2012).

According to the length of the off- and pre-season and the date of scheduled practice games, an appropriate loading paradigm can be applied. Several loading patterns with different ratios of loading:unloading weeks are prescribed in the literature (Plisk and Stone 2003; Siff 2003; Stone et al. 2007). A period of loading is always concluded by a recovery week, which allows the players to recover and supercompensation to occur (Stone et al. 2007).

The incidence of injury is remarkably higher during games compared to practices (Eirale et al. 2013; Vanlommel et al. 2013). It should therefore be avoided that players compete in a state of fatigue (Kujala et al. 1997; Worrell 1994). A week in which a practice game against a stronger opponent or more than one practice game is scheduled requires unloading and preferably coincides with an unloading week. Ratios of 1:1, 2:1, 3:1 and 4:1 of loading:unloading weeks are possible (Plisk and Stone 2003; Siff 2003; Stone et al. 2007).

In-season

From the start of the in-season a predominantly nonlinear approach is more appropriate. This will allow the use of higher intensity during the in-season strength training sessions in order to maintain the player's strength, power, and muscle mass (Baker et al. 1994; Rhea et al. 2002). It will also allow the multiple tasks of soccer to be addressed concurrently and to adapt training to the stress of games (Gamble 2013; Wathen et al. 2000; Zatsiorsky and Kraemer 2006). In addition to nonlinear periodization, exercise specificity, volume, and intensity can also follow a linear pattern to meet the demands of the extended competition period. The average intensity and volume can differ between the early, middle, and final competitive phases (Gambetta 2007). The early competitive period can still consist of a higher amount of general work to provide sufficient overload, compared to the advanced phases of competition in which specificity prevails (Gambetta 2007). In addition to daily undulation, this transition from moderately general to predominantly specific will follow a linear pattern.

International breaks or other breaks during the competition can also be used to plan some extra strength work (Gamble 2013).

During the off- and pre-season a minimum of two strength workouts a week should be implemented to elicit strength and power improvements (McMaster et al. 2013). During the in-season strength training frequency can range between one and three times per week, according to the game schedule (Gamble 2013). Strength improvements during the in-season are more related to training intensity than to volume (Hoffman and Kang 2003). Average training intensities ranging from 70 percent to 88 percent of 1RM have been shown to maintain power and develop strength over the course of the competitive season (McMaster *et al*. 2013).

References

Agel J, Schisel J. Practice injury rates in collegiate sports. *Clin J Sport Med*. 2013 Jan;23(1):33–8.

Allerheiligen B. In-season strength training for power athletes. *Strength Cond J*. 2003 Jun;25(3):23–8.

Anderson L, Triplett-McBride T, Foster C, Doberstein S, Brice G. Impact of training patterns on incidence of illness and injury during a women's collegiate basketball season. *J Strength Cond Res*. 2003 Nov;17(4):734–8.

Baker D. Applying the in-season periodization of strength and power training to football. *Strength Cond J*. 1998 Apr;20(2):18–27.

Baker D, Wilson G, Carlyon R. Periodization: the effect on strength of manipulating volume and intensity. *J Strength Cond Res*. 1994 Nov;8(4):235–42.

Bompa T. *Periodization training: theory and methodology*. 4th ed. Champaign, IL: Human Kinetics; 1999. 424 pp.

Buford TW, Rossi SJ, Smith DB, Warren AJ. A comparison of periodization models during nine weeks with equated volume and intensity for strength. *J Strength Cond Res*. 2007 Nov;21(4):1245–50.

Eirale C, Farooq A, Smiley FA, Tol JL, Chalabi H. Epidemiology of football injuries in Asia: a prospective study in Qatar. *J Sci Med Sport*. 2013 Mar;16(2):113–17.

Gambetta V. *Athletic development: the art and science of functional sports conditioning*. Champaign, IL: Human Kinetics; 2007. Chapter 6, Program planning and fine-tuning; pp. 81–117.

Gamble P. Physical preparation of elite level rugby union football players. *Strength Cond J*. 2004 Aug;26(4):10–23.

Gamble P. Periodization of training for team sport athletes. *Strength Cond J*. 2006 Oct;28(5):55–6.

Gamble P. *Strength and conditioning for team sports: sport-specific physical preparation for high performance*. 2nd ed. New York: Routledge; 2013. 304 pp.

Haff G. Periodization of training. In: Chandler TJ, Brown LE, editors. *Conditioning for strength and human performance*. Baltimore, MD: Lippincott Williams & Wilkins; 2013. pp. 326–45.

Hoffman JR, Kang J. Strength changes during an in-season resistance-training program for football. *J Strength Cond Res*. 2003 Feb;17(1):109–14.

Issurin VB. New horizons for the methodology and physiology of training periodization. *Sports Med*. 2010 Mar 1;40(3):189–206.

Kraemer WJ, Fleck SJ. *Optimizing strength training: designing nonlinear periodization workouts*. Champaign, IL: Human Kinetics; 2007. 256 pp.

Kujala UM, Orava S, Järvinen M. Hamstring injuries. Current trends in treatment and prevention. *Sports Med*. 1997 Jun;23(6):397–404.

McMaster DT, Gill N, Cronin J, McGuigan M. The development, retention and decay rates of strength and power in elite rugby union, rugby league and American football: a systematic review. *Sports Med*. 2013 May;43(5):367–84.

Mallo J, Dellal A. Injury risk in professional football players with special reference to the playing position and training periodization. *J Sports Med Phys Fitness*. 2012 Dec;52(6):631–8.

Monteiro AG, Aoki MS, Evangelista AL, Alveno DA, Monteiro GA, Piçarro Ida C, Ugrinowitsch C. Nonlinear periodization maximizes strength gains in split resistance training routines. *J Strength Cond Res*. 2009 Jul;23(4):1321–6.

Naclerio F, Moody J, Chapman M. Applied periodization: a methodological approach. *J Hum Sport Exerc*. 2013;8(2):350–66.

Plisk SS, Stone MH. Periodization strategies. *Strength Cond J*. 2003 Dec;25(6):19–37.

Prestes J, De Lima C, Frollini AB, Donatto FF, Conte M. Comparison of linear and reverse linear periodization effects on maximal strength and body composition. *J Strength Cond Res*. 2009 Jan;23(1):266–74.

Rhea MR, Ball SD, Phillips WT, Burkett LN. A comparison of linear and daily undulating periodized programs with equated volume and intensity for strength. *J Strength Cond Res*. 2002 May;16(2):250–5.

Siff MC. *Supertraining*. 6th ed. Denver, CO: Supertraining Institute; 2003. 496 pp.

Silvestre R, Kraemer WJ, West C, Judelson DA, Spiering BA, Vingren JL, Hatfield DL, Anderson JM, Maresh CM. Body composition and physical performance during a National Collegiate Athletic Association Division I men's soccer season. *J Strength Cond Res*. 2006 Nov;20(4):962–70.

Stone MH, Stone M, Sands WA. *Principles and practice of resistance training*. Champaign, IL: Human Kinetics; 2007. Chapter 13, The concept of periodization; pp. 259–86.

Vanlommel L, Vanlommel J, Bollars P, Quisquater L, Van Crombrugge K, Corten K, Bellemans J. Incidence and risk factors of lower leg fractures in Belgian soccer players. *Injury*. 2013 Dec;44(12):1847–50.

Wathen D, Baechle TR, Earle RW. Training variation: periodization. In: Baechle TR, Earle RW, editors. *Essentials of strength training and conditioning*. 2nd ed. Champaign, IL: Human Kinetics; 2000. pp. 513–28.

Worrell TW. Factors associated with hamstring injuries: an approach to treatment and preventative measures. *Sports Med*. 1994;17(5):338–45.

Zatsiorsky VW, Kraemer WJ. *Science and practice of strength training*. 2nd ed. Champaign, IL: Human Kinetics; 2006. Chapter 5, Timing in strength training; pp. 89–108.

18

PROGRAM DESIGN

This chapter addresses the different variables involved in the design of a strength training workout. The effectiveness to achieve specific physiological adaptations to a strength training program depends on five training variables (Kraemer 1983; Kraemer and Fleck 2007):

1. Intensity.
2. Number of sets.
3. Exercise choice.
4. Exercise order.
5. Rest periods between sets and exercises.

The manipulation of these variables reflects the goal of the strength training session and determines the neural, hypertrophic, and hormonal response to the workout (Bird *et al.* 2005). A good understanding of these training variables is therefore essential to provide optimal training stimuli and control the training load (Bird *et al.* 2005; Kraemer 1983). The gradual manipulation of these variables also enables the coach to better individualize workouts (Kraemer 1983).

18.1 Intensity

The intensity determines the amount of resistance being lifted and is together with the exercise selection the most important training variable in strength training (McDonagh and Davies 1984; Stoppani 2006).

The intensity and amount of resistance used can be determined by two different methods. The intensity is typically expressed as a percentage of the 1RM (repetition maximum), which is the amount of weight the trainee is able to lift for one repetition. Based on the percentage of 1RM, a lot of useful information about training intensity is gathered from training logs of elite athletes. Elite athletes use a wide variety of training percentages. The vast majority of sets are performed with a load between 60 percent and 90 percent of 1RM and the highest proportion of lifts (35 percent) are performed with weights ranging from 70 percent to 80 percent of 1RM

TABLE 18.1 Prilepin's table for optimal strength and power development

Intensity: % 1RM	Rep range	Reps total	Optimal reps
<70%	3–6	18–30	24
70–79%	3–6	12–24	18
80–89%	2–4	10–20	15
>89%	1–2	4–10	7

(Zatsiorsky 1995; Table 18.1). It has been shown that experienced lifters need to train with a mean intensity of 85 percent of 1RM to enhance strength (Petersen *et al.* 2004). In order for athletes to be able to maintain strength levels over the course of the competitive season, weights of 80 percent of 1RM and above have to be lifted weekly (Hoffman and Kang 2003).

Alexander Prilepin studied the training logs of more than a thousand world champions of various age categories. His table gives recommendations about the optimal number of repetitions that should be performed within each intensity zone to maximize strength and power development.

The downside of prescribing intensity as a percentage of the 1RM is that it requires regular 1RM testing. In a sport like football in which various training goals need to be addressed simultaneously, applying a percentage-based intensity prescription for all strength training exercises is probably too time-consuming. The percentage-based method can be used to prescribe the intensity for the main exercises, while a repetition-based approach can be applied for the other exercises.

In the repetition-based method the prescribed load can be depicted by an RM range, for example a 6–8RM range. This means the lifter uses a load he can maximally lift 6–8 times. The use of a target RM range ensures the lifter does not lift to failure during each set. As the lifter gets stronger, the load is progressively increased, so he can continue to work within the prescribed RM ranges.

Based on empirical evidence and research it is well established that certain RM ranges provide corresponding training effects (Fleck and Kraemer 2004). Training with RM ranges between 1 and 6 has the greatest effect on maximal strength and power output, hypertrophy is enhanced most with a 7–12RM range, and ranges above 12RM are most effective to improve local muscular endurance (Campos *et al.* 2002; Fleck and Kraemer 2004; McDonagh and Davies 1984; Stoppani 2006).

The use of a percentage-based prescription of training intensity is warranted for exercises with complex intermuscular coordination or that require the load to be moved with high speed (Fleck and Kraemer 1987). Lifting to failure during these exercises results in deterioration of technique and a decrease of power output. Performing these movements to a true repetition maximum results in momentary failure. This does not benefit the training outcome and the possible deterioration of technique places the lifter at higher risk of injury.

The number of repetitions and training intensity within a workout varies by exercise. For exercises with complex intermuscular coordination and exercises with high biomechanical, kinematic, and kinetic similarity with the main sport movements, a lower number of repetitions is applied. A higher training intensity elicits the maximal activation of motor units with optimal discharge frequency (Zatsiorsky 1995). The enhanced intra- and intermuscular coordination in sport-specific exercises will transfer to similar movement patterns in soccer (Bosch

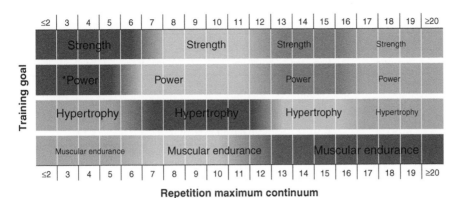

FIGURE 18.1 Repetition-per-set continuum (Baechle et al. 2008)

2012; Zatsiorsky 1995). Acquiring and mastering proper exercise technique is of utmost importance before the soccer player can start lifting with higher intensity.

Movements in which the intermuscular coordination is less complex and deviates more from sport-specific skills the number of repetitions will be higher (Zatsiorsky 1995).

18.2 Number of sets

Similar to training intensity, the number of sets per exercise can vary between the different exercises of the strength workout (Figure 18.1). A range of 3–6 sets per exercise is considered optimal to enhance strength (Fleck and Kraemer 1987; Stoppani 2006). Training goal and status affect how many sets will be performed per exercise. If the goal of training is to focus on a certain movement pattern or muscle group, a higher amount of sets can be prescribed for the corresponding exercises. To improve general muscular fitness, beginners can benefit from a one-set method, while more experienced athletes require multiple sets to elicit strength and muscle size gains (Kraemer *et al.* 2002).

Only considering the number of sets is an oversimplification however, because the different training parameters interact (Fleck and Kraemer 2014). Performing six sets of squats requires a lot more energy than six sets of leg press or biceps curl. Studies that draw conclusions based on a comparison of the number of sets regardless of training intensity and exercise selection have therefore limited relevance to training. Several meta-analyses quantified a dose–response relationship for training intensities, volume, and frequency (Petersen *et al.* 2004, 2005; Rhea *et al.* 2003). A mean training intensity of 60 percent of 1RM, a mean training volume of four sets per muscle group, and three training sessions per week elicit maximal strength gains in untrained individuals (Petersen *et al.* 2005; Rhea *et al.* 2003). Recreationally trained individuals maximally enhance strength training two times per week, using a mean volume of four sets per muscle group at a mean training intensity of 80 percent of 1RM (Petersen *et al.* 2005; Rhea *et al.* 2003). Trained athletes exhibit maximal strength improvements training two days per week with a mean training intensity of 85 percent of 1RM and a mean volume of eight sets per muscle group (Petersen *et al.* 2004, 2005).

A dose–response relationship is also inherent to Prilepin's table. Each intensity bracket comprises a repetition range and the optimal number of repetitions. More experienced lifters rarely stick to a single intensity per exercise. In most training methods to enhance strength

TABLE 18.2 INOL formula applied on Prilepin's table

Intensity: % 1RM	100 − average intensity	Reps total	INOL rep range	Optimal reps	INOL optimal reps
<70%	37.5	18–30	0.48–0.8	24	0.64
70–79%	25	12–24	0.48–0.96	18	0.72
80–89%	15	10–20	0.67–1.33	15	1
>89%	6.25	4–10	0.64–1.6	7	1.12

TABLE 18.3 INOL score for an exercise during 3:1 ratio of loading:unloading microcycles

Set	Microcycle 1 Reps (% 1RM)	Microcycle 2 Reps (% 1RM)	Microcycle 3 Reps (% 1RM)	Microcycle 4 Reps (% 1RM)
Set 1	6 (65%)	6 (67.5%)	6 (70%)	6 (60%)
Set 2	5 (75%)	5 (77.5%)	4 (80%)	6 (70%)
Set 3	4 (80%)	3 (82.5%)	3 (85%)	5 (80%)
Set 4	2 (85%)	2 (85%)	2 (87.5%)	
Set 5		2 (87.5%)	2 (90%)	

INOL microcycle 1 = 6/(100 − 65) + 5/(100 − 75) + 4/(100 − 80) + 2/(100 − 85)
= 0.17 + 0.2 + 0.2 + 0.13 = 0.70
INOL microcycle 2 = 0.18 + 0.22 + 0.17 + 0.13 + 0.16 = 0.87
INOL microcycle 3 = 0.2 + 0.2 + 0.2 + 0.16 + 0.2 = 0.96
INOL microcycle 4 = 0.15 + 0.2 + 0.25 = 0.6

the intensity is progressively increased or decreased through the course of sets performed per exercise. In periodization for soccer it is important to properly distribute the training load over the various microcycles. A simple formula quantifies the relationship between volume and intensity (Hristov 2005):

INOL= Number of lifts at a given intensity/(100 − intensity)

Applying the INOL formula on Prilepin's table and dividing the average intensity per intensity bracket by the optimal number of reps provides a range of INOL scores that reflect the dose–response continuum for intensity and number of sets per exercise (Tables 18.2 and 18.3).

The dose–response continuum based on Prilepin's table provides useful information to design and quantify the load of strength-training workouts. The INOL score for a single exercise should range between 0.48 and 1.6. In accordance to Prilepin's chart, an INOL score lower than 0.48 means the training stimulus provided by the exercises is insufficient to elicit adaptation. An INOL score of more than 1.6 is very taxing on the central nervous system and induces fatigue.

Imagine this example for the front squat exercise during a 3:1 ratio of loading:unloading microcycles.

18.3 Exercise choice

Multiple-joint vs. single-joint exercises: Resistance training for soccer should focus on multiple-joint exercises and movement, not on single muscles or muscle groups. Athletic movement is multiple-joint in nature. Body control, whole-body force, and power production determine success in soccer. Sprinting, jumping, kicking the ball, playing the ball while being challenged by the opponent require all total-body strength and power. Multiple-joint movements require complex intermuscular coordination and are associated with similar plastic changes in the central nervous system as skill training (see Chapter 4, Strength training considered as skill training with resistance). Training with multiple-joint exercises will hence result in higher carry-over to sports performance.

General vs. sport-specific exercises: A good balance should exist between more general exercises that provide sufficient overload and sport-specific exercises with biomechanical, kinematic, and kinetic similarity to soccer (Siff 2002). Kinetic and kinematic specificity refers to the velocity, timing, and relative force aspects of the movement (Gamble 2013). The back squat and jump squat have similar biomechanical characteristics, but have a different impact on the force–velocity curve and result in different training outcomes (Newton *et al.* 1999). During the off-, pre-season, and periods without games, strength workouts can comprise a higher percentage of general exercises, while training sessions during the competition period contain more sport-specific exercises to optimize transfer. General exercises and variation in exercise selection will help develop a solid base of training to achieve optimal performance in the future, while training with sport-specific exercises results in the greatest short-term effects (Bondarchuk 2007).

Variety of exercises in all three planes of motion: During soccer a great amount of different movements are performed in all planes of motion. The soccer player has to be powerful in a great variety of movements and be able to stabilize and control various joint angles. Strength training for soccer should therefore include a wide variety of movements and address all three planes of motion.

Ground-based exercises: Because most forces during soccer are applied to the ground, a large percentage of exercises (approximately 75 percent) should be ground-based (Kenn 2003). The more force and power the player can apply to the ground the faster s/he will be able to run and change direction and the higher s/he can jump.

Unilateral vs. bilateral exercises: Soccer is a single-leg dominant sport. During running and sprinting the body is propelled forward through powerful single-leg actions (McCurdy and Conner 2003). Single-leg strength and stability play an important role in athletic performance and injury prevention (McCurdy and Conner 2003; Myer *et al.* 2006). During single-leg strengthening exercises the gluteal and external hip rotator muscles are engaged more to prevent internal thigh rotation and knee valgus (Beardsley and Contreras 2014; Ekstrom *et al.* 2007). Unilateral training has also been shown to elicit greater activation of the core muscles and can therefore be considered as a valuable means to strengthen the core (Behm *et al.* 2005; Tarnanen *et al.* 2012). Unilateral training is sport-specific in nature and will also result in more balanced strength development (Sale 1988). A strength training routine for soccer should next to bilateral exercises also implement a significant amount of unilateral movements.

Balance between opposing movement patterns: Equally emphasizing opposing movement patterns in strength training plays an important role in injury prevention and the development of a balanced body (Table 18.4). Soccer players with a hamstring/quadriceps strength imbalance are more prone to hamstring and knee injuries (Aagaard *et al.* 1997, 1998; Croisier *et al.* 2008; Zebis *et al.* 2011). An overemphasis of upper body pressing strength with insufficient attention for upper body pulling movements can result in a slouched posture, abnormal scapular kinematics, and decreased upper limb power (Cools *et al.* 2003).

TABLE 18.4 Opposing movement patterns

Opposing movement pattern	
Knee dominant exercises	Hip dominant exercises
Upper body horizontal press	Upper body horizontal pull (Rowing)
Upper body vertical press	Upper body vertical pull (Pull-up)

18.4 Exercise order

The exercise order influences the load that can be lifted, the number of repetitions that can be performed, and the amount of power that can be exerted during each exercise and plays an important role in maximizing power, strength, and even hypertrophy (Simão et al. 2010; Spineti et al. 2010).

Exercises that require complex neuromuscular coordination and power-oriented exercises are sequenced first in the workout. The absence of fatigue at the beginning of the workout will allow greater neural drive, force, and power production. It has been shown that when major multiple-joint exercises are performed later in the workout, the weight lifted or the number of repetitions that can be performed with a particular weight, is reduced (Miranda et al. 2010; Sforzo and Touey 1996; Simão et al. 2005, 2007; Spreuwenberg et al. 2006). Performing the exercises without prior fatigue will provide a superior training stimulus.

When the strength workout emphasizes a certain movement pattern, the focus exercises will be programmed at the beginning of the workout. This allows the trainee to use heavier resistance and exert more power when performing the priority exercises.

Training goals and the implementation of certain training methods will also influence the exercise sequence. In the Russian or complex training method a set of heavy resistance training is followed by a set of a biomechanically similar plyometric exercises. Lifting a near maximal load stimulates the central nervous system and enhances the power output in the subsequent plyometric set (Docherty et al. 2004; Hilfiker et al. 2007).

The order of exercises also plays a role during circuit training in which the exercises are performed in an alternating sequence. Alternating lower and upper body exercises gives the muscles recruited in the exercise more time to recover and will enhance the neural drive.

When new exercises with complex neuromuscular coordination are introduced, they need to be sequenced early in the workout. Movement quality is better when fatigue is limited, which will reinforce the acquisition and perfection of new movement patterns.

Sequence exercises to provide a superior training stimulus:

- total-body exercises before exercises in which fewer muscle groups are recruited;
- multiple-joint before single-joint exercises;
- power-oriented exercises before strength exercises (unless complex training method is applied);
- higher-intensity exercises before lower-intensity exercises;
- alternate pushing and pulling movements;
- alternate lower and upper body movements;
- priority exercises at the beginning of the workout;
- new exercises that require the mastering of complex movement patterns first.

18.5 Rest periods between sets and exercises

When the training goal is to increase power and maximal strength using maximal or near-maximal loads and multiple-joint exercises, a rest interval of 2–3 minutes between sets is recommended (Kraemer *et al.* 2002). Shorter rest periods of 1–2 minutes can be used for exercises in which less muscle mass is recruited or when the intensity is lower (Kraemer *et al.* 2002). Shorter rest periods can also be used in circuit strength training in which different movements are alternated, because this form of training does not result in as high blood lactate concentrations and level of fatigue as regular short-rest training sessions (Fleck and Kraemer 2014).

Shorter rest periods between sets increase the metabolic, hormonal, and cardiovascular response to the strength workout. Due to the fatigue induced by short rest periods, the number of repetitions that can be performed during the first set progressively decreases during each subsequent set (Miranda *et al.* 2007, 2009; Willardson and Burkett 2006). The total number of repetitions that can be performed and the workout volume is hence lower compared to longer rest periods (Miranda *et al.* 2007). Rest periods of one minute result in higher blood lactate and growth hormone levels compared to strength training using three-minute rest periods (de Salles *et al.* 2009; Kraemer *et al.* 1990, 1993; Robinson *et al.* 1995). Adenosine triphosphate-phosphocreatine (ATP-PC) provides the immediate energy to lift high resistances. This energy system requires at least three minutes to completely replenish (Takahashi *et al.* 1995; Tesch and Wright 1983). Short rest intervals therefore result in a progressive reduction in ATP and phosphocreatine and force production will predominantly rely on the glycolytic lactate metabolic pathway (Takahashi *et al.* 1995; Tesch and Wright 1983). The strong relationship between blood lactate and anabolic hormones explains the enhanced anabolic response to short-rest, high-volume (e.g., three sets of 10RM with one-minute rest interval) strength training protocols (Hakkinen and Pakarinen 1993; Kraemer *et al.* 1993).

Short rest periods appear to be beneficial for muscle growth but longer rest periods result in significantly greater increases of strength and power (de Salles *et al.* 2009, 2010; Pincivero *et al.* 1997; Robinson *et al.* 1995). Good movement quality, power production, and enhanced fast-twitch motor recruitment require longer rest periods between sets (de Salles *et al.* 2009; Fleck and Kraemer 2014; Willardson and Burkett 2006).

When training to enhance strength, power, and athletic ability, longer rest intervals are recommended to allow greater recovery and maintenance of intensity, power output, and movement quality (Kraemer *et al.* 2002). Few additional strength gains are derived however from very long rest periods between sets (more than three minutes) (Willardson and Burkett 2008). In training for soccer, where multiple training goals need to be addressed simultaneously, rest periods between two and three minutes will optimize strength and power development and limit the duration of the strength workout, leaving sufficient time and energy for other conditioning priorities. Rest intervals between sets can also be altered in a periodized manner over different workouts. This will alter the metabolic demand of the training and create a different training stimulus. Shorter rest periods can enhance the muscle's buffering capacity to better tolerate high blood lactate levels (Mohr *et al.* 2007; Tallon *et al.* 2005). But remember that soccer-specific practices already address this need and that the main goal of strength training for soccer is to increase athletic performance through enhanced strength and power.

References

Aagaard P, Simonsen EB, Beyer N, Larsson B, Magnusson P, Kjaer M. Isokinetic muscle strength and capacity for muscular knee joint stabilization in elite sailors. *Int J Sports Med.* 1997 Oct;18(7):521–5.

Aagaard P, Simonsen EB, Magnusson SP, Larsson B, Dyhre-Poulsen P. A new concept for isokinetic hamstring: quadriceps muscle strength ratio. *Am J Sports Med.* 1998 Mar–Apr;26(2):231–7.

Baechle TR, Earle RW, Wathen D. *Essentials of strength training and conditioning.* 3rd ed. Champaign, IL: Human Kinetics; 2008. 641 pp.

Beardsley C, Contreras B. The increasing role of the hip extensor musculature with heavier compound lower-body movements and more explosive sport actions. *Strength Cond J.* 2014 Apr;36(2):49–55.

Behm DG, Leonard A, Young W, Bonsey A, MacKinnon S. Trunk muscle EMG activity with unstable and unilateral exercises. *J Strength Cond Res.* 2005 Feb;19(1):193–201.

Bird SP, Tarpenning KM, Marino FE. Designing resistance training programmes to enhance muscular fitness: a review of the acute programme variables. *Sports Med.* 2005;35(10):841–51.

Bondarchuk A. *Transfer of training in sports.* Grand Rapids, MI: Ultimate Athlete Concepts; 2007. 218 pp.

Bosch F. *Krachttraining en coördinatie, een integratieve benadering.* Rotterdam: 2010 Uitgevers; 2012. 352 pp.

Campos GE, Luecke TJ, Wendeln HK, Toma K, Hagerman FC, Murray TF, Ragg KE, Ratamess NA, Kraemer WJ, Staron RS. Muscular adaptations in response to three different resistance-training regimens: specificity of repetition maximum training zones. *Eur J Appl Physiol.* 2002 Nov;88(1–2):50–60.

Cools AM, Witvrouw EE, Declercq GA, Danneels LA, Cambier DC. Scapular muscle recruitment patterns: trapezius muscle latency with and without impingement symptoms. *Am J Sports Med.* 2003 Jul–Aug;31(4):542–9.

Croisier JL, Ganteaume S, Binet J, Genty M, Ferret JM. Strength imbalances and prevention of hamstring injury in professional soccer players: a prospective study. *Am J Sports Med.* 2008 Aug;36(8):1469–75.

de Salles BF, Simão R, Miranda F, Novaes Jda S, Lemos A, Willardson JM. Rest interval between sets in strength training. *Sports Med.* 2009;39(9):765–77.

de Salles BF, Simão R, Miranda H, Bottaro M, Fontana F, Willardson JM. Strength increases in upper and lower body are larger with longer inter-set rest intervals in trained men. *J Sci Med Sport.* 2010 Jul;13(4):429–33.

Docherty D, Robbins D, Hodgson M. Complex training revisited: a review of its current status as a viable training approach. *Strength Cond J.* 2004 Dec;26(6):52–7.

Ekstrom R, Donatelli R, Carp K. Electromyographical analysis of core trunk, hip, and thigh muscles during 9 rehabilitation exercises. *J Orthop Sports Phys Ther.* 2007 Dec;37(12):754–62.

Fleck SJ, Kraemer WJ. *Designing resistance training programs.* 2nd ed. Champaign, IL: Human Kinetics; 1987. 275 pp.

Fleck SJ, Kraemer WJ. *Designing resistance training programs.* 3rd ed. Champaign, IL: Human Kinetics; 2004. 392 pp.

Fleck SJ, Kraemer WJ. *Designing resistance training programs.* 4th ed. Champaign, IL: Human Kinetics; 2014. 520 pp.

Gamble P. *Strength and conditioning for team sports: sport-specific physical preparation for high performance.* 2nd ed. New York: Routledge; 2013. 304 pp.

Häkkinen K, Pakarinen A. Acute hormonal responses to two different fatiguing heavy-resistance protocols in male athletes. *J Appl Physiol (1985).* 1993 Feb;74(2):882–7.

Hilfiker R, Hübner K, Lorenz T, Marti B. Effects of drop jumps added to the warm-up of elite sport athletes with a high capacity for explosive force development. *J Strength Cond Res.* 2007 May;21(2):550–5.

Hoffman JR, Kang J. Strength changes during an in-season resistance-training program for football. *J Strength Cond Res.* 2003 Feb;17(1):109–14.

Hristov H. How to design strength training programs using Prilepin's table [Internet]. [place unknown: publisher unknown]; 2005 Oct 2 [updated 2005 Oct 2; cited 2015 Feb 17]. Available from: www.powerliftingwatch.com/files/prelipins.pdf/.

Kenn J. *The coach's strength training playbook.* Monterey, CA: Coaches Choice; 2003. 160 pp.

Kraemer WJ. Exercise prescription in weight training: manipulating program variables. *Strength Cond J.* 1983 Jun;5(3):58–9.

Kraemer WJ, Fleck SJ. *Optimizing strength training: designing nonlinear periodization workouts.* Champaign, IL: Human Kinetics; 2007. Chapter 3, Acute program variables; pp. 41–64.

Kraemer WJ, Marchitelli L, Gordon SE, Harman E, Dziados JE, Mello R, Frykman P, McCurry D, Fleck SJ. Hormonal and growth factor responses to heavy resistance exercise protocols. *J Appl Physiol (1985).* 1990 Oct;69(4):1442–50.

Kraemer WJ, Fleck SJ, Dziados JE, Harman EA, Marchitelli LJ, Gordon SE, Mello R, Frykman PN, Koziris LP, Triplett NT. Changes in hormonal concentrations after different heavy-resistance exercise protocols in women. *J Appl Physiol (1985).* 1993 Aug;75(2):594–604.

Kraemer WJ, Adams K, Cafarelli E, Dudley GA, Dooly C, Feigenbaum MS, Fleck SJ, Franklin B, Fry AC, Hoffman JR, Newton RU, Potteiger J, Stone MH, Ratamess NA, Triplett-McBride T; American College of Sports Medicine. American College of Sports Medicine position stand. Progression models in resistance training for healthy adults. *Med Sci Sports Exerc.* 2002 Feb;34(2):364–80.

McCurdy K, Conner C. Unilateral support resistance training incorporating the hip and knee. *Strength Cond J.* 2003 Apr;25(2):45–51.

McDonagh MJ, Davies CT. Adaptive response of mammalian skeletal muscle to exercise with high loads. *Eur J Appl Physiol Occup Physiol.* 1984;52(2):139–55.

Miranda H, Fleck SJ, Simão R, Barreto AC, Dantas EH, Novaes J. Effect of two different rest period lengths on the number of repetitions performed during resistance training. *J Strength Cond Res.* 2007 Nov;21(4):1032–6.

Miranda H, Simão R, Moreira LM, de Souza RA, de Souza JA, de Salles BF, Willardson JM. Effect of rest interval length on the volume completed during upper body resistance exercise. *J Sports Sci Med.* 2009 Sep 1;8(3):388–92.

Miranda H, Simão R, dos Santos Vigário P, de Salles BF, Pacheco MT, Willardson JM. Exercise order interacts with rest interval during upper-body resistance exercise. *J Strength Cond Res.* 2010 Jun;24(6):1573–7.

Mohr M, Krustrup P, Nielsen JJ, Nybo L, Rasmussen MK, Juel C, Bangsbo J. Effect of two different intense training regimens on skeletal muscle ion transport proteins and fatigue development. *Am J Physiol Regul Integr Comp Physiol.* 2007 Apr;292(4):R1594–602.

Myer GD, Ford KR, Brent JL, Hewett TE. The effects of plyometric vs. dynamic stabilization and balance training on power, balance, and landing force in female athletes. *J Strength Cond Res.* 2006 May;20(2):345–53.

Newton RU, Kraemer WJ, Häkkinen K. Effects of ballistic training on preseason preparation of elite volleyball players. *Med Sci Sports Exerc.* 1999 Feb;31(2):323–30.

Peterson MD, Rhea MR, Alvar BA. Maximizing strength development in athletes: a meta-analysis to determine the dose-response relationship. *J Strength Cond Res.* 2004 May;18(2):377–82.

Peterson MD, Rhea MR, Alvar BA. Applications of the dose-response for muscular strength development: a review of meta-analytic efficacy and reliability for designing training prescription. *J Strength Cond Res.* 2005 Nov;19(4):950–8.

Pincivero DM, Lephart SM, Karunakara RG. Effects of rest interval on isokinetic strength and functional performance after short-term high intensity training. *Br J Sports Med.* 1997 Sep;31(3):229–34.

Rhea MR, Alvar BA, Burkett LN, Ball SD. A meta-analysis to determine the dose response for strength development. *Med Sci Sports Exerc.* 2003 Mar;35(3):456–64.

Robinson JM, Stone MH, Johnson RL, Penland CM, Warren BJ, Lewis RD. Effects of different weight training exercise/rest intervals on strength, power, and high intensity exercise endurance. *J Strength Cond Res.* 1995 Nov;9(4):216–21.

Sale DG. Neural adaptation to resistance training. *Med Sci Sports Exerc.* 1988 Oct;20(5 Suppl):S135–45.

Sforzo GA, Touey PR. Manipulating exercise order affects muscular performance during a resistance exercise training session. *J Strength Cond Res.* 1996 Feb;10(1):20–4.

Siff MC. Functional training revisited. *Strength Cond J.* 2002 Oct;24(5):42–6.

Simão R, Farinatti Pde T, Polito MD, Maior AS, Fleck SJ. Influence of exercise order on the number of repetitions performed and perceived exertion during resistance exercises. *J Strength Cond Res.* 2005 Feb;19(1):152–6.

Simão R, Farinatti Pde T, Polito MD, Viveiros L, Fleck SJ. Influence of exercise order on the number of repetitions performed and perceived exertion during resistance exercise in women. *J Strength Cond Res.* 2007 Feb;21(1):23–8.

Simão R, Spineti J, de Salles BF, Oliveira LF, Matta T, Miranda F, Miranda H, Costa PB. Influence of exercise order on maximum strength and muscle thickness in untrained men. *J Sports Sci Med.* 2010 Mar;9(1):1–7.

Spineti J, de Salles BF, Rhea MR, Lavigne D, Matta T, Miranda F, Fernandes L, Simão R. Influence of exercise order on maximum strength and muscle volume in nonlinear periodized resistance training. *J Strength Cond Res.* 2010 Nov;24(11):2962–9.

Spreuwenberg LP, Kraemer WJ, Spiering BA, Volek JS, Hatfield DL, Silvestre R, Vingren JL, Fragala MS, Häkkinen K, Newton RU, Maresh CM, Fleck SJ. Influence of exercise order in a resistance-training exercise session. *J Strength Cond Res.* 2006 Feb;20(1):141–4.

Stoppani J. *Encyclopedia of muscle & strength.* Champaign, IL: Human Kinetics; 2006. 408 pp.

Takahashi H, Inaki M, Fujimoto K, Katsuta S, Anno I, Niitsu M, Itai Y. Control of the rate of phosphocreatine resynthesis after exercise in trained and untrained human quadriceps muscles. *Eur J Appl Physiol Occup Physiol.* 1995;71(5):396–404.

Tallon MJ, Harris RC, Boobis LH, Fallowfield JL, Wise JA. The carnosine content of vastus lateralis is elevated in resistance-trained bodybuilders. *J Strength Cond Res.* 2005 Nov;19(4):725–9.

Tarnanen SP, Siekkinen KM, Häkkinen AH, Mälkiä EA, Kautiainen HJ, Ylinen JJ. Core muscle activation during dynamic upper limb exercises in women. *J Strength Cond Res.* 2012 Dec;26(12):3217–24.

Tesch PA, Wright JE. Recovery from short term intense exercise: its relation to capillary supply and blood lactate concentration. *Eur J Appl Physiol Occup Physiol.* 1983;52(1):98–103.

Willardson JM, Burkett LN. The effect of rest interval length on the sustainability of squat and bench press repetitions. *J Strength Cond Res.* 2006 May;20(2):400–3.

Zatsiorsky VM. *Science and practice of strength training.* Champaign, IL: Human Kinetics; 1995. 243 pp.

Zebis MK, Andersen LL, Ellingsgaard H, Aagaard P. Rapid hamstring/quadriceps force capacity in male vs. female elite soccer players. *J Strength Cond Res.* 2011 Jul;25(7):1989–93.

19

SAMPLE TRAINING PROGRAMS

The main purpose of strength training is not the development of strength per se, but to maximize athletic performance through improved movement quality, power, and strength endurance. The sequencing of various strength training sessions that induce distinct physiological adaptations is the best way to achieve this goal (Bompa and Haff 2009).

This chapter presents sample training programs for different levels of soccer players. A soccer team contains a broad mix of players of varying training background, age, and level of athletic ability. There is no one-size-fits-all training program when it comes to soccer. Designing a diverse strength training session for the beginner, intermediate, and advanced levels is a first step to address the needs of each player. The intermuscular coordination of the programmed exercises becomes more complex and the load of the training session progressively augments from the beginner to the advanced workouts. The advanced sessions, for players with a more extensive strength training experience, have also a more sport-specific character compared to beginner workouts that encompass a somewhat higher proportion of more general work to develop a sound foundation. For soccer players with a more advanced training status, program design must become more specific to induce the desired training adaptations when a particular aspect of performance is addressed (Gamble 2013).

Dividing each strength training session into three different intensity levels will further enable the coach to take the difference in recovery time between players into account and to adapt the intensity level of the workout to emerging conditions. The three intensity levels are associated with differences in timing for recovery and supercompensation. Olbrecht states that according to the intensity of the strength training, the maximal supercompensation will occur between 40 and 72 hours after the strength workout (Olbrecht 2007). According to the two-factor model, supercompensation (called training effect in the two-factor model) is the result of the interaction between the fitness gains and induced fatigue as a result of the training stimulus. While the fitness effect of training is long lasting, the fatigue effect is greater in magnitude, but shorter in duration (Zatsiorsky 1995). Recovery time following strength training varies between individuals and depends to a great extent on the training status and experience. The force output of experienced athletes can recover and even overshoot the initial level within 48 hours following a strenuous eccentric workout, while a more prolonged force reduction was reported for individuals with less training experience (Ebbeling and Clarkson 1990; Michaut *et al.* 1998).

Nine possible combinations (3 training levels × 3 intensity levels) means training can be tailored to the needs and constraints of each player. Last-minute changes can be made without overly deviating from meso- and macrocycle periodization. The difference in training status and recovery time between players can be accounted for and strength training can be easily fitted to the game schedule.

19.1 Strength training sessions

Strength endurance

The strength endurance session has various objectives:

- Enhance strength endurance: During soccer, short bouts of high-intensity actions and sprints are performed repeatedly with a short rest in between actions. Accelerating, stopping, changing direction, decelerating, and jumping require a high amount of force production. A proper level of strength endurance enables the player to repeatedly perform high-intensity actions over the course of the entire game. Strength endurance training has been reported to improve repeated-sprint ability (Edge *et al.* 2006).
- Injury prevention: The strength endurance training session can also be considered as an injury-prevention session. Training intensity is lower to progressively prepare the tendons, ligaments, and muscle tissue for the increased load of more intense strength workouts and the high demands of soccer. The strength endurance sessions incorporate various different movements and movement variations, which will develop a balance between opposing movement patterns and lay a strong neuromuscular foundation (Bompa and Haff 2009). The enhanced short-term work capacity, connective tissue strength, and balance will improve the player's ability to recover and reduce the risk of injury (Bompa and Haff 2009).
- Movement skill training: One of the main goals of strength training besides enhancing strength and power is to improve movement quality. When lifting high loads the training is more sterile from a movement perspective because of safety considerations. Movements cannot mimic the joint angles experienced in soccer. The load during strength endurance workouts is lower. Because the load is lower it is possible to integrate alterations in the environment (unstable surface) or movement variations that address various planes of motion to reinforce the differentiation between variable and invariable movement components.
- Metabolic conditioning and enhance body composition: Strength training is a burst activity that mainly strains anaerobic energy pathways and may therefore be considered a more intense form of training, despite a lower heart rate response (Elliot *et al.* 1992). Strength endurance sessions, characterized by short rest periods in between sets, enable the player to lift a considerable amount of total weight in a short time period (Murphy and Schwarzkopf 1992). Especially incorporating multiple-joint, ground-based exercises into the strength endurance workout maximizes the workload. Strength endurance training can therefore help maintain optimal fitness levels during the off-season.

- An additional benefit of strength endurance training is the increased metabolic rate during and after the training (Elliot *et al.* 1992; Gillette *et al.* 1994; Murphy and Schwarzkopf 1992; Pichon *et al.* 1996). Performing a strength or other strenuous workout increases the rate of oxygen intake leading to a higher resting metabolism for the next hours (Brown *et al.* 2006; Da Silva *et al.* 2010). This increased energy expenditure following exercise has been termed excess post-exercise oxygen consumption (EPOC) (Brown *et al.* 2006). Studies have shown that the EPOC increment can last up to 48 hours after the conclusion of the workout and accounts for 10–25 percent of the total energy cost of the exercise, playing a contributing role in weight management (Børsheim and Bahr 2003; Brown *et al.* 2006; Da Silva *et al.* 2010; Murphy and Schwarzkopf 1992; Schuenke *et al.* 2002; Sedlock *et al.* 1989). The magnitude of EPOC clearly increases with the amount of activated muscle mass and the intensity and duration of the exercises and is inversely related with the rest time between sets (Da Silva *et al.* 2010; Elliot *et al.* 1992; Haddock and Wilkin 2006; Thornton and Potteiger 2002). Research has shown that a larger and longer EPOC effect can be obtained through circuit strength training in comparison to standard strength training methods or aerobic training (Gillette *et al.* 1994; Murphy and Schwarzkopf 1992). The enhanced energy requirements of strength endurance training can help players that strive to decrease their body fat percentage. Coaches can therefore opt to frequently schedule a strength endurance workout for players whose performances would benefit from a reduction of body fat.

Strength endurance training parameters

- Organization: During the strength endurance training session, the sets are performed in a circuit manner. The exercises are performed in a vertical progression, meaning one set of each exercise is completed before the second set is performed. Because a higher amount of repetitions are performed, a big part of the energy is provided by the glycolytic system (lactic energy system), resulting in a rapid lactic acid accumulation. A high level of lactic acid build-up will impair movement quality (Bompa and Carrera 2005). The main purpose of strength training is not to enhance lactic acid tolerance, but to improve strength and movement quality. Lactic acid tolerance is also addressed more sport-specifically during soccer practices. Circuit training does not result in as high blood lactate concentrations as regular training sessions and is therefore better suited to develop strength endurance (Fleck and Kraemer 2014). Setting up the circuit so that different movement patterns are alternated will further enable the players to lift at a higher percentage of their maximum. The circuit organization, especially when it is well planned, maximizes lifting quality despite the shorter rest times associated with strength endurance training. Circuit training is also superior for movement skill acquisition and perfection, one of the major objectives of the strength endurance session. Performing different exercises or movement patterns in an alternating fashion increases the number of times a motor pattern has to be recalled from the long-term memory and therefore results in better long-term retention of the trained motor pattern (see Chapter 4, Strength training considered as skill training with resistance).
- Exercise selection: Because the load is lower the selected exercises and movement patterns can be more complex, comprising multiple planes of motion and mimicking the more extreme joint angles that are encountered during soccer. A variety of different movement

patterns will maximally enhance the differentiation between the variable and invariable movement components. The integration of some low to moderate unstable surface exercises and exercises with accommodating resistance can further improve movement robustness (see Chapter 4, Strength training considered as skill training with resistance). Because soccer is a single-leg dominant sport, the strength endurance training session will for a big part consist of unilateral exercises. Unilateral training elicits greater activation of the core muscles and results in a more balanced strength development. Furthermore the strength endurance session can comprise one or more exercise complexes. An exercise complex is a combination of two or more exercises merged together or performed back to back. This will increase the volume and energy expenditure of the workout and will help promote muscular endurance. Also, some eccentric exercises should be incorporated into the strength endurance workouts. The majority of injuries occur during the deceleration phase of movement when the muscles contract while lengthening (Alentorn-Geli et al. 2009). When the forces required to decelerate the movement exceed the forces of the muscle-tendon unit, injury can occur to the muscle or tendon (LaStayo et al. 2003). Muscle strain injuries are very common in soccer, especially the hamstring and adductor strains (Dvorak et al. 2011; Woods et al. 2004). Soccer players with a history of recurring hamstring or adductor muscle injuries have greater impairment of eccentric strength compared to concentric strength (Croisier et al. 2002; Thorborg et al. 2014). Increasing the eccentric strength of the hamstrings and hip adductors will enhance their energy-absorbing capacity and can reduce the risk of injury (Croisier et al. 2002, 2008; Thorborg 2012). Eccentric exercise has also an effect on the mechanical and morphological tendon properties (LaStayo et al. 2003; Obst et al. 2013). Sub maximal eccentric exercise increases the collagen fiber content and tendon cross-sectional area and has been shown to be beneficial in the prevention and rehabilitation of tendinosis (Alfredson et al. 1998; Grigg et al. 2009; LaStayo et al. 2003; Stanish et al. 1986; Zarins and Ciullo 1983).

• Load: The intensity is lower, approximately 50–70 percent of 1RM. Because a greater variety of exercises are used during the strength endurance session compared to other workouts, the repetition-based method is used predominantly to prescribe exercise intensity. An exercise intensity of 50–70 percent of 1RM corresponds to a 12–20RM range (Table 19.1).

TABLE 19.1 Strength endurance training parameters

Training parameter	Work
Exercise selection	Variety of movement patterns that comprise multiple planes of motion
	Exercise complexes
	Sub maximal eccentric exercises
Organization	Circuit
Load	50–70% of 1RM or 12–20RM
Number of reps/set	5–15 (exercise complex: 4–10)
Number of sets/exercise	2–3
Rest interval	60–90 seconds

Hypertrophy

A muscle with a larger cross-sectional area can generate more force due to the higher number of sarcomeres in parallel. Hypertrophy will therefore increase the player's potential to produce greater force and enhance strength and power. In contrast to bodybuilders, the goal of a hypertrophy training session is not to gain as much muscle mass as possible but to selectively increase the cross-sectional area of the fast-twitch muscle fibers, which can generate more force at higher velocities and produce more power.

Zatsiorsky states that the hypertrophy stimulus is a function of the protein breakdown and the total amount of work performed (total weight lifted). High-intensity loads will result in more muscle fiber damage and protein breakdown (Zatsiorsky 1995). The number of lifts that can be performed using a high percentage of the 1RM is limited however, and training volume is lower. At the other extreme, using light loads, the total amount of work will be great due to the high number of reps that can be performed, but protein degradation is low. Loads between 7RM and 12RM provide an optimal balance between training intensity (protein degradation) and produced mechanical work and seem therefore optimal for hypertrophy purposes.

Muscle fibers are recruited according to the size principle. As the intensity of contraction increases progressively more motor units of increasing size are recruited. The smaller motor units consist of slow-twitch fibers, while larger motor units are typically composed of fast-twitch fibers. Lifting heavier loads will maximally recruit the larger high-threshold motor units and results in preferential fast-twitch fiber hypertrophy (Fry 2004). Recruiting muscle fibers is not enough to elicit growth. In order to be trained and grow, muscle fibers need to be fatigued (Zatsiorsky 1995). Slow-twitch muscle fibers are resistant to fatigue and therefore require higher volume to elicit growth, while evidence indicates that heavier loads are required to maximally induce fast-twitch fiber hypertrophy (Fry 2004; Schuenke et al. 2013). This is in accordance with the study by Fry, that showed that weightlifters and powerlifters exhibit preferential hypertrophy of type II fibers compared to bodybuilders that show hypertrophy in both type I and II fibers (Fry 2004). Bodybuilders generally train with moderate loads and shorter rest intervals while weightlifters and powerlifters on the other hand generally train with higher loads and longer rest intervals (Schoenfeld 2010).

The fast-twitch fibers are preferentially recruited during fast and explosive movements such as sprinting, a soccer kick, change of direction, etc. (Cormie et al. 2011). Preferential fast-twitch fiber hypertrophy will therefore not only improve the soccer player's body composition but will also enhance their athletic potential. This stands in contrast with traditional hypertrophy methods of body-builders, which may increase the amount of muscle mass without a concurrent improvement of athleticism. The increased muscle mass may even lead to reduced relative strength and power values.

Hypertrophy training parameters

Power, strength, and a high strength to body weight ratio (relative strength) are paramount in soccer. Due to the limited available time for strength training in soccer, multiple training goals also have to be addressed simultaneously in a single training session. Lifting moderate to higher loads, longer rest periods, full range of motion training, a back-off set, and lifting to failure during the last set will induce hypertrophy and will at the same time boost the soccer player's strength and power potential.

- Higher loads: Lifting heavier loads will maximally recruit the larger high-threshold motor units (Fry 2004; Schuenke *et al.* 2013). Fast-twitch fibers can generate high amounts of strength and power and they are bigger, which means they have a greater growth potential. For beginners both heavier (3–6RM) and moderate loads (7–12RM) are effective to develop strength and produce hypertrophy (Berger 1962; Campos *et al.* 2002; Chestnut and Docherty 1999; Schuenke *et al.* 2012; Tanimoto *et al.* 2008). Soccer players that have more strength training experience need to use higher intensity (>80 percent 1RM) for the main exercises to achieve strength gains while moderate loads (6–12RM) can be planned for the assistance exercises to augment the volume of the hypertrophy workout.
- Longer rest periods: Bodybuilding methodology consists for a big part of performing higher repetitions with shorter rest time in between sets. Short rest periods (one-minute rest intervals between sets) tax the glycolytic lactate metabolic pathway more and result in higher lactate levels. Strength workouts that are highly glycolytic in nature may enhance the anabolic response, due to the strong relationship between blood lactate and growth hormone. Recent insight indicates however, that the effect of designing the strength workout in function of maximizing the surge in anabolic hormones might be overrated (Schoenfeld 2013). Due to the fatigue induced by short rest periods, the number of repetitions that can be performed during the first set progressively decreases during each subsequent set (Miranda *et al.* 2007, 2009; Willardson and Burkett 2006). Shorter rest periods can even prejudice training volume to an extent that it compromises muscular hypertrophy. Shorter rest periods also mainly tax and train the slow-twitch fibers and result in significantly less strength and power gains compared to longer rest periods (de Salles *et al.* 2009, 2010; Pincivero *et al.* 1997; Robinson *et al.* 1995). Reducing rest time at the expense of movement quality and volume compromises the development of strength and power and should therefore be avoided in strength training for soccer. Research is also conflictive as to whether shorter rest periods elicit more hypertrophy.
- Full range of motion: Full range of motion training induces significantly greater hypertrophy compared to shorter range of motion training (Bloomquist *et al.* 2013; McMahon *et al.* 2014). Full range of motion squats not only result in greater gains in cross-sectional area of the thigh muscles but also elicit greater increases in strength and jump performance (Bloomquist *et al.* 2013; McMahon *et al.* 2014). Full range of motion strength training has been shown to increase the number of sarcomeres in series. An increased amount of sarcomeres in series means that there are more elements that simultaneously contract, resulting in a higher total contraction speed and higher levels of muscular power (McMahon *et al.* 2014). Strength losses from detraining also seem to be slower following full range of motion compared to limited range of motion training (McMahon *et al.* 2014). Full range of motion training is beneficial for increasing muscle mass, strength, and power. Range of motion should not be compromised for lifting greater loads (McMahon *et al.* 2014).
- Back-off set: A back-off set is the addition of a single higher rep set at the end of an exercise. Adding a hypertrophy stimulus to a workout that is primarily designed to increase strength has some advantages. The higher rep set increases the mechanical work and metabolic stress of the workout and provides an additional hypertrophy stimulus. A study by Goto *et al.* showed that adding a single back-off set of 25–30 reps with 50 percent

TABLE 19.2 Weeks 1–3 of Magnusson/Ortmayer template

Week 1		Week 2		Week 3	
Sets/Reps	% of 1RM	Sets/Reps	% of 1RM	Sets/Reps	% of 1RM
4 × 4	70%	4 × 4	70%	4 × 4	70% + 5 kg
2 × 2	80%	1 × 2	80%	1 × 2	80% + 5 kg
1 × 8+	70%	1 × 2	90%	1 × 2	90% + 5 kg
		1 × 8+	70%	1 × 8+	70% + 5 kg

TABLE 19.3 Hypertrophy training parameters

Training parameter	Work
Exercise selection	Multiple-joint exercises executed in full range of motion + some eccentric exercises
Organization	Traditional
Load	Focus exercises: 70–90% of 1RM Assistance exercises: 6–12 RM
Number of reps/set	Focus exercises: 4–8 Assistance exercises: 6–12
Number of sets/exercise	3–6
Rest interval	2–3 minutes

of 1RM to a strength routine of 5 sets of 3–5 reps with 90 percent of 1RM not only increased the gains in muscle size, but also enhanced measures of strength and power (Goto et al. 2004). The researchers were unsure of the exact mechanisms for the higher strength and power gains. The speed of lifting is higher during the back-off set with lighter weights. Training further along the force–velocity curve (higher speed end compared to high-force/low-speed end of traditional strength training) might explain the increased power measurements. The higher mechanical loading, accumulation of metabolites, and growth hormone release accompanying this higher rep set may also have affected muscle fiber adaptation (Goto et al. 2004; Stoppani 2006). The enhanced blood circulation and concentration of metabolites result in a bigger muscle pump effect, which augments the anabolic response and potentially maximizes strength gains. There are also several other examples of renowned strength training routines that incorporate a back-off set or combine high and moderate to low intensity within the same workout. The Magnusson/Ortmayer routine, a popular routine in power lifting that is known for its effectiveness to develop lower body strength, includes a back-off set with moderate weight (Table 19.2). During the last set of the exercise the trainee tries to perform as many reps as possible with 70 percent of 1RM (Table 19.3). In the Westside barbell and Jim Wendler's 5/3/1 routine, higher intensity is programmed for the main exercises followed by moderate-intensity work for the assistance exercises. Elite athletes can also benefit from the combination of higher and moderate to light intensity within a training session. Adding one or two low-intensity blood flow restriction exercises at the end of a high-intensity strength training routine has been shown to result in a greater increase of strength and muscle mass (Yamanaka *et al.* 2012; Yasuda *et al.* 2011).

- Failure: Taking this back-off set to failure may provide an additional training stimulus that can affect hypertrophy and strength gains (Stoppani 2006). Soccer players should be careful with training to failure due to the high neuromuscular stress. Periodically taking the last set of the exercise to failure can boost hypertrophy and even strength gains (Drinkwater *et al.* 2005; Goto *et al.* 2005; Rooney *et al.* 1994).

Maximal strength

Maximal strength is a basic and important factor to enhance the soccer player's physical performance:

- A high and positive correlation exists between peak power and maximum strength ($r=0.77–0.94$) in both the upper body and lower body (see Chapter 13, Training principles to develop power).
- Improving maximal strength will also enhance strength endurance. Strong players can repeat a vigorous action more times before fatigue sets in, compromising movement quality, compared to players with less strength (Bompa and Carrera 2005; Zatsiorsky and Kraemer 2006).
- Maximal strength training enhances athletic performance as a result of an improved intra- and intermuscular coordination (Table 19.4). The better coordination and increased recruitment of fast-twitch muscle fibers will transfer to similar movements in soccer.

Maximal strength training parameters

- Load: Zatsiorsky states that lifting above 90 percent of your 1RM leads to very slow bar speeds and low power outputs. Loads of 90 percent of 1RM and below are better suited to enhance the rate of force development (Zatsiorsky 1995). Increasing the rate of force development allows the player to produce higher forces during fast movements and is crucial in soccer where time is critical (see Chapter 13, Training principles to develop power). The statement of Zatsiorky is in accordance with L.S. Dvorkin, who carried out

TABLE 19.4 Improvements in intra- and intermuscular coordination following maximal strength training

	Improvements as a result of maximal strength training
Intramuscular	Increased motor unit activation: more fast-twitch fibers are recruited
	Increased motor unit synchronization: More motor units can be activated simultaneously, resulting in higher force production
	Enhanced rate coding: The motor units are activated with a higher neural firing frequency. Through increasing the frequency at which the neural impulses are sent to the motor units, the force output of muscle fibers is increased.
Intermuscular	Better synchronization between synergists
	Decreased antagonist activation: antagonist muscles relax while agonists contract

research with weightlifters of all qualifications over a prolonged period of time to determine the effect of training load. He concluded that all levels of lifters made the highest gains in back squat strength with 3–4 reps/set at 70–80 percent of 1RM (Dvorkin 2005). Also the Sheiko method, a multi-year training plan developed by Boris Sheiko (coach of the Russian powerlifting team since the 1990s) that can take a powerlifter from novice to elite, requires lifting loads that range most of the time between 70 percent and 80 percent of 1RM. Explosively lifting loads of 70–80 percent of 1RM with perfect technique and no sticking point results in the highest gains in 1RM loads, especially in the medium and long term (Dvorkin 2005). Also the meta-analysis from Rhea *et al.* of 140 studies and Peterson *et al.* of 32 studies confirm that competitive athletes and experienced lifters experience maximal strength gains when training at an intensity range of 75–85 percent (Peterson *et al.* 2004; Rhea *et al.* 2003). Athletes do not train at the same intensity, but use different intensities across exercises and sets. According to empirical and research evidence, the highest proportion of weights lifted during the maximal strength workout consists of 70–90 percent of 1RM (Zatsiorsky 1995). Soccer players without lifting experience can even gain strength with weights as low as 60 percent of 1RM (Rhea *et al.* 2003).

- Lifting speed: Moving the load as fast as possible during the concentric phase of movement is a major objective for the development of athletic strength (Kenn 2003). Grinding out repetitions at very slow speed for the sake of quantity not only compromises speed and power performance, but will also result in decreased strength gains (Padulo *et al.* 2012). Pushing the bar as fast as possible during the concentric phase of the repetition leads to the recruitment of more fast-twitch fibers and superior strength gains (Liow and Hopkins 2003; Padulo *et al.* 2012; Rana *et al.* 2008).
- Rest interval: It is generally accepted that when training to enhance speed and power, quality should be stressed at all times. Like power and speed, strength also relies to a great extent on efficient neuromuscular processes. The effectiveness of a program to increase strength is related to the quality of the strength workout. Longer rest periods (≥2 minutes) will enable the player to maintain movement quality throughout the various sets and entire workout.

Strength-speed/speed-strength

Explosive strength and maximal strength training elicit distinct neural changes (Tillin and Folland 2014; Table 19.5). Where maximal strength training increases the number of motor

TABLE 19.5 Maximal strength training parameters

Training parameter	Work
Exercise selection	Multiple-joint exercises executed in full range of motion
Organization	Traditional (circuit when time is limited)
Load	>70% of 1RM
Number of reps/set	Focus exercises: 1–6
	Assistance exercises: 5–10
Number of sets/exercise	3–8
Rest interval	2–3 minutes

units that can be recruited, explosive strength training increases the rate at which these motor units are activated (Moritani 1993; Tillin and Folland 2014).

The activation threshold of the fast-twitch type II motor units is lower for explosive high-speed movements than for slower contractions (Cormie *et al.* 2011). Zatsiorsky also states that a set of motor units can have a low threshold for one motion and a higher threshold for another (Zatsiorsky and Kraemer 2006). Explosive strength training enhances the ability to rapidly recruit the fast-twitch muscle fibers (Bompa and Carrera 2005; Gamble 2013).

Strength training is also velocity-specific, which means that the strength gains are greatest at the trained velocity (Morrissey *et al.* 1995). This velocity specificity seems to be even greater at faster contraction speeds (Morrissey *et al.* 1995). While a high correlation exists between strength and vertical jump or measures of agility, strength gains in trained athletes have limited or no impact on sprinting speed. To improve the entire spectrum of athletic movements in soccer the whole force–velocity curve needs to be addressed (see Chapter 13, Training principles to develop power).

Explosive low-load/high-velocity strength training also elicits architectural muscle changes (Alegre *et al.* 2006). The increased fascicle length as a result of explosive strength training improves the capacity to develop higher velocities of contraction (Alegre *et al.* 2006). Furthermore explosive strength training induces preferential fast-twitch fiber hypertrophy (Stone 1993).

Recent research also highlights the important role that the ability to rapidly produce force may play in joint stabilization and the prevention of injuries. Soccer players with a low hamstring/quadriceps strength ratio are at increased risk of hamstring strain and knee injury. Cruciate ligament injuries have been shown to occur within 50 ms after initial ground contact (Krosshaug *et al.* 2007). The ability to rapidly produce force can therefore play a more important role in joint stabilization and the prevention of injuries than the maximal contraction force. The hamstring/quadriceps ratio at the initial phase of contraction (within 50 ms) is lower than the hamstring/quadriceps ratio during maximal voluntary contraction (Zebis *et al.* 2011). This shows that the potential to stabilize the knee is reduced during the initial phase of contraction. The study from Zebis *et al.* also indicates that rate of force development hamstring/quadriceps strength ratios can be more relevant in relation to fast dynamic actions that are typical for soccer, compared to maximal strength ratios (Zebis *et al.* 2011). Explosive strength training of the hamstring muscles enhances the ability to rapidly produce force and stabilize the knee joint at the initial phase of contraction and can play an important role in the prevention of injuries (see Chapter 12, Muscle anatomy and function).

Strength-speed/speed-strength training parameters (Table 19.6)

* Organization: Research shows that concurrent strength and explosiveness training enhances power and motor performance more than when either is trained in isolation. Addressing various training goals in one workout requires a good organization. The speed/strength or strength/speed workouts can be organized in a traditional horizontal or a vertical circuit manner. Both methods are equally effective at increasing strength and power (Alcaraz *et al.* 2011). The Bulgarian method is a good example of how a circuit can be structured to optimize strength, power, and speed. By composing the circuit of exercises that all occupy a different position along the force–velocity curve, the whole curve can be addressed. A third form of organization called complex training, involving

TABLE 19.6 Strength-speed/speed-strength training parameters

Training parameter	
Exercise selection	Sport-specific strength exercises, Olympic lifts, ballistics, plyometrics, and resisted sport-specific tasks
Organization	Traditional or circuit
Load	Variety of loads that span entire F–V curve:
	>70% of 1RM +
	50–70% of 1RM
	Lighter load ballistics, plyometrics, and resisted sport-specific tasks
	Load that produces peak power output results in greatest increase in power → Load of peak power output varies between exercises
Number of reps/set	>70% of 1RM: 1–6
	50–70% of 1RM & <50% of 1RM: 4–10 (4–6 for focus exercises with complex intermuscular coordination)
	Olympic lifts: 1–6
	Plyometrics: 6–15
	Sport-specific resisted drills: 2–8 seconds
Number of sets/exercise	3–6
Rest interval	Traditional: 2–3 minutes
	Circuit: 90 seconds

both horizontal and vertical organizational characteristics, is also beneficial for the development of speed, power, and strength. During complex training a set of heavy resistance training is followed by a set of a biomechanically similar plyometric exercises. Due to the post-activation potentiation phenomenon, explosiveness is enhanced during the subsequent explosive set. Heavy-resistance training/ballistics, heavy-resistance training/ sport-specific task, and ballistics/sport-specific task are other combinations that can be used to optimize athletic performance.

- Load: Resistance training is velocity-specific. This means the greatest increases in power output are experienced at or near the trained load. Soccer involves dynamic actions that span the entire force–velocity curve. Explosive strength training for soccer should therefore address all the different modalities of the force–velocity curve in a single workout or in a periodized manner. High-intensity strength training (≥ 80 percent 1RM) induces the recruitment of the greatest amount of fast-twitch muscle fibers, which can produce more power (Kawamori and Haff 2004). Integrating some high-intensity strength exercises is also vital to maintain strength levels over the course of the competition period (Hoffman and Kang 2003). Lifting relatively lighter loads will contribute to development of explosive strength and power. The peak force output is still high, while the movement velocity is closer to the velocity of athletic skills performed during soccer (Cormie *et al.* 2007). Lifting loads between 50 and 70 percent of 1RM in an explosive manner results in a higher power output and a high rate of force development (Cronin *et al.* 2001; Häkkinen *et al.* 1985; Harris *et al.* 2000; Jones *et al.* 2001; Kawamori and Haff 2004; Newton and Kraemer 1994).
- Exercise type: A high movement speed and the intention to move the load as fast as possible are paramount to improve explosive power. Preferably a high quantity of ballistic

exercises or exercises that can be performed ballistically should be integrated into the explosive strength training. During exercises in which the load is not released, the movement has to be decelerated towards the end of the trajectory to avoid joint damage. This results in reduced agonist and increased antagonist activation, especially during the final phase (see Chapter 13, Training principles to develop power). Average force, average and peak velocity and power are therefore significantly higher during ballistic exercises, compared to exercises in which the load is not released (squat jump vs. speed squat, plyometric push-up vs. regular push-up) (Cronin *et al.* 2001; Kawamori and Haff 2004). A lot of unilateral strength exercises enable the lifter to manage moderately high loads (50–70 percent of 1RM) and still safely accelerate throughout the entire range of motion (step-up, split squat, Bulgarian split squat, lunge variations). When the front rack position or dumbbells is used during these explosive lifts the weight can still be dropped in case the player loses balance. Exercises with pulley machines provide another safe and effective option. During the Olympic lifts the trainee also has to accelerate the bar through the entire range of motion. The high amount of power that can be produced during Olympic lifts and their movement and velocity specificity to athletic activities (running, jumping) makes these lifts a valuable tool to enhance dynamic athletic performance. To address the speed-end of the curve, fast (<250 ms) and slow (>250 ms) stretch-shortening plyometric exercises and resisted sport-specific tasks can be integrated into workout.

- Rest interval: Because the determining factor to increase explosiveness is the speed of performance, rest intervals should be longer to preserve a high quality of movement during the entire workout. This means the rest between sets amounts to at least two minutes when a traditional training organization is used. In a circuit organization in which different movement patterns are alternated, the duration of rest between sets can be reduced (90 seconds).
- Neuromuscular specificity: Because intra- and intermuscular coordination are important factors contributing to power output, explosive strength training should have a highly sport-specific character. The training should consist of a high level of movements that are kinetically and kinematically similar to athletic movement patterns seen in soccer. The explosive strength workout is considered to be the fine tuning of strength training.

Blood flow restriction

Low-intensity strength training in combination with blood flow restriction can induce strength and hypertrophy gains similar to those observed with high-intensity strength training. Despite the low exercise intensity, the activation of the more glycolytic fast-twitch fibers is enhanced due to the hypoxic intramuscular environment. Blood flow restriction training has been shown to cause minimal to no muscle damage and full recovery occurs within 24 hours after training. Due to the minimal neuromuscular, psychological, and mechanical joint stress, low-intensity strength training combined with vascular occlusion can provide an effective training stimulus to maintain or increase strength levels during competition periods that require unloading (Table 19.7).

19.2 Annual training plans

Ahead of the soccer season an annual plan should be made for the whole season. Nothing is written in stone however. The annual plan serves as guidance, but changes will have to

TABLE 19.7 Blood flow restriction training parameters

Training parameter	Work
Exercise selection	Multiple-joint exercises that are performed in the full range of motion are emphasized
Organization	Traditional
Load	20–50% of 1RM
	20–30% of 1RM is most supported by research
Number of reps/set	12–30
Number of sets/exercise	3–4
Rest interval	30–60 seconds

be made according to the emerging conditions. Minutes played during the game, number of high-intensity bouts during a game (game effort), physical discomfort from the tackles received, muscle soreness, and suspensions are just a few examples that may require adaptations of the weekly plan. In professional teams the weekly planning may also be adapted to Omega wave analyses that register central nervous system fatigue.

Failing to plan is planning to fail. The annual plan will determine how the load is progressed and divided over the several micro-, meso-, and macrocycles and greatly improves training effectiveness. A logical progression or balance of the training load over the strength training sessions will also minimize muscle soreness and neuromuscular fatigue (Bompa and Haff 2009).

Annual plan for team with a regular bi-weekly match schedule

Table 19.8 gives an example of a macro-, mesocycle periodization for a team that regularly plays two games per week, such as one that competes in the Champions League. The annual plan is divided into three macrocycles: off-season, pre-season, and in-season. The in-season is further divided into four mesocycles.

The off-season in soccer is very important so the player can develop a strength foundation before starting the pre-season. Most soccer teams start playing practice games within 10 days after the start of the pre-season. A strength foundation will speed up recovery and minimizes muscle soreness during the pre-season (Johnston *et al.* 2014).

The off- and pre-seasons follow a linear training approach. This means there is a progression from strength endurance to hypertrophy, to maximal strength, to speed-strength training sessions. This logical sequencing of training sessions will progressively prepare the player to lift higher loads. This is especially important for players that have less experience with strength training. The gradual load progression minimizes muscle soreness.

During the in-season an undulating periodization model is followed, meaning there is a weekly variation of the strength training emphasis. In soccer it is not the goal to peak towards certain games, but to keep the players close to their peak over the course of the entire season. Based on the competition calendar the in-season can be divided into three to five mesocycles. In this example of an annual periodization paradigm for a team that plays in both national and European competitions, the in-season is broken up into four mesocycles.

Mesocycle one forms a transition from the pre- to the in-season. During this mesocycle the focus is balanced between the different training goals, while the periodization shifts from linear to undulating. Because only one game a week is played during this period, half of the strength workouts consist of hypertrophy and maximal strength sessions, to further increase strength and muscle mass. Also during the international breaks more general work and higher load is planned for the non-international players.

The European games are played during mesocycles two and four. These mesocycles mainly consist of more specific training sessions and sessions that cause less neural load. During the strength-speed and speed-strength training sessions a sport-specific training stimulus is provided to enhance explosiveness and transfer strength and power to soccer performance. Because strength-speed and speed-strength sessions integrate plyometrics and speed work, multiple tasks are addressed concurrently. Sport-specific training maximally facilitates short-term performance enhancement. The integration of multiple skills into one training session will also help maintain strength, power, and speed levels during this predominantly bi-weekly game period in which training time is limited. During this busy competition period that requires unloading, low-intensity strength training in combination with blood flow restriction will also help maintain strength levels and muscle mass with limited neuromuscular, psychological, and mechanical joint stress.

Mesocycle three consists again of a higher percentage of general work and a higher percentage of hypertrophy and maximal-strength training sessions.

Player rotations, suspensions, physical discomfort, fatigue, and other reasons will force the coaches to make adaptations to the annual plan. If for example an intense maximal strength session is planned three days after a game, this might have to be substituted by a low-intensity strength endurance session or a blood flow restriction training in case of a player that still struggles with physical discomfort. For the players that did not come off the bench or played a limited amount of minutes, a planned lower-intensity session can be replaced by a moderate or higher-load session. If a maximal-strength session needed to be substituted for a strength endurance session, a few weeks later it might be appropriate to perform a maximal-strength training instead of a strength-endurance training, so the original balance within a mesocycle is maintained. The coaches can plan as they go and adapt according to the daily situation with the annual periodization paradigm as a guideline.

The players that do not form part of the squad for a game normally carry out a training session on the day of the game. Part of the training can consist of a strength session. Which session is chosen will depend on the player's profile. For a strong player that is less explosive, speed-strength will be more adequate. A player with an extensive injury history may benefit more from a speed endurance training. The choice will also vary according to the mesocycle and can intend to maintain or restore the balance between the different sessions. In mesocycle one, a hypertrophy session may be more adequate, in mesocycle two a strength-speed session, in mesocycle three a maximum strength session, and in mesocycle four a speed-strength session. Especially when extra strength workouts are planned frequently, for a player that repeatedly does not make the squad for example, the choice of extra sessions should intend to maintain the planned equilibrium between sessions within the mesocycle.

Annual plan for team with an occasional bi-weekly match schedule

The annual plan for a team that only occasionally plays two matches a week is also divided into three macrocycles (Table 19.9), while Tables 19.10–12 show sample training programs for the beginner, intermediate, and advanced levels respectively. During the off- and pre-seasons a linear periodization model is used with a logical sequence, from strength endurance to hypertrophy, to maximal strength, to explosive-strength training.

TABLE 19.8 Annual plan for team with a regular bi-weekly match schedule (weekend and midweek matches)

MACRO/MESO	MONTH	Monday	Tuesday	Wednesday	Thursday	Friday	Saturday	Sunday
OFF-SEASON	JUNE	10 SE L	11	12 HY L	13	14 SE L	15	16
		17 SE M	18	19 HY M	20	21 SE M	22	23
		24 SE M	25	26 HY L	27	28 SE M	29	30
	JULY	1 HY M	2	3 SE M	4	5 HY M	6	7
PRE-SEASON		8 SE M	9	10 HY L	11	12 HY M	13 DAY OFF	14 DAY OFF
		15 MxS L	16	17 HY H	18	19 SE M	20	21 Friendly match
		22 DAY OFF	23 DAY OFF	24 MxS M	25	26	27 Friendly match	28 DAY OFF
		29	30 MxS M	31	1 Friendly match	2	3 Friendly match	4 DAY OFF
	AUGUST	5 SE L	6	7 Friendly match	8	9	10 Friendly match	11 DAY OFF
IN-SEASON MESO 1		12 DAY OFF	13 SE M	14	15 STR-SP M	16	17	18 League match

TABLE 19.8 (cont.)

MACRO/MESO	MONTH	Monday	Tuesday	Wednesday	Thursday	Friday	Saturday	Sunday
IN-SEASON **MESO 1**	AUGUST	19 DAY OFF	20	21 **HY H**	22 DAY OFF	23 **SE H**	24	25
		26 League match	27 DAY OFF	28	29 **MxS H**	30	31	
	SEPTEMBER							1 League match
		2 DAY OFF	3 DAY OFF	4 **HY H**	5	6 **SP-STR H**	7	8
		9 **HY M**	10	11 **MxS M**	12	13	14 League match	15 DAY OFF
IN-SEASON **MESO 2**		16	17 CL group stage	18	19	20 **BFR M**	21	22 League match
		23	24	25 League match	26	27	28 League match	29 DAY OFF
		30 **BFR L**						
	OCTOBER		1	2 CL group stage	3	4	5 League match	6 DAY OFF

MACRO/MESO	MONTH	Monday	Tuesday	Wednesday	Thursday	Friday	Saturday	Sunday
IN-SEASON **MESO 2**	OCTOBER	7 DAY OFF	8	9 **MxS H**	10	11 **STR-SP H**	12 DAY OFF	13 DAY OFF
		14	15 **STR-SP M**	16	17 **SE L**	18	19 League match	20 DAY OFF
		21 **BFR L**	22	23 CL group stage	24	25	26 League match	27 DAY OFF
		28 **SE L**	29	30 League match	31			
	NOVEMBER					1	2 League match	3
		4	5 CL group stage	6 DAY OFF	7 **BFR M**	8	9 League match	10 DAY OFF
		11 DAY OFF	12 **MxS H**	13	14	15 **SP-STR H**	16 DAY OFF	17 DAY OFF
		18 **MxS M**	19	20 **STR-SP M**	21	22	23 League match	24 DAY OFF
		25 **BFR L**	26	27 CL group stage	28	29	30 League match	
	DECEMBER							1 DAY OFF
		2	3 **SP-STR H**	4 DAY OFF	5 **SE L**	6	7 Cup match	8
		9	10 CL group stage	11 DAY OFF	12 **BFR L**	13	14 League match	15 DAY OFF

TABLE 19.8 (cont.)

MACRO/MESO	MONTH	Monday	Tuesday	Wednesday	Thursday	Friday	Saturday	Sunday
IN-SEASON **MESO 3**	DECEMBER	16 **SE L**	17	18 Cup match	19	20 **BFR L**	21	22 League match
		23 DAY OFF	24 DAY OFF	25 DAY OFF	26 DAY OFF	27 **SE M**	28	29 **HY H**
		30	31 **MxS M**					
	JANUARY			1	2 Friendly match	3 DAY OFF	4 **SE L**	5
		6 League match	7	8	9 Cup match	10	11	12 League match
		13	14	15 Cup match	16	17	18 League match	19
		20	21 Cup match	22 DAY OFF	23 **BFR L**	24	25 League match	26
		27	28 Cup match	29 DAY OFF	30	31 **HY M**		

MACRO/MESO	MONTH	Monday	Tuesday	Wednesday	Thursday	Friday	Saturday	Sunday
IN-SEASON MESO 3	**FEBRUARY**						1	2 League match
		3	4	5 Cup match	6	7	8 League match	9
		10	11 Cup match	12	13	14 **BFR M**	15	16 League match
		17 DAY OFF	18	19 **MxS H**	20	21	22 League match	23 DAY OFF
IN-SEASON MESO 4		24	25	26 CL 1/8 final	27 DAY OFF	28 **SE L**		
	MARCH						1	2 League match
		3 DAY OFF	4	5 **STR-SP H**	6	7 **SE L**	8	9 League match
		10 DAY OFF	11	12 **SP-STR H**	13	14	15 League match	16
		17	18 CL 1/8 final	19 DAY OFF	20	21 **MxS L**	22	23 League match
		24	25	26 League match	27	28	29	30 DAY OFF
		31						
	APRIL		1	2 CL 1/4 final	3	4	5 League match	6
		7	8 CL 1/4 final	9	10 **BFR L**	11	12 League match	13 DAY OFF
		14	15	16 Cup final	17	18	19 **SP-STR H**	20

TABLE 19.8 (cont.)

MACRO/MESO	MONTH	Monday	Tuesday	Wednesday	Thursday	Friday	Saturday	Sunday
IN-SEASON **MESO 4**	APRIL	21 **SE L**	22	23 CL 1/2 final	24	25	26 League match	27
		28	29 CL 1/2 final	30 DAY OFF				
	MAY				1	2 **STR–SP L**	3	4 League match
		5	6	7 League match	8 DAY OFF	9	10	11 League match
		12 DAY OFF	13	14 **SP–STR L**	15 DAY OFF	16	17	18 League match
		19 DAY OFF	20	21 **(SP–STR L)**	22	23	24 CL final	25

SE = strength endurance workout; HY = hypertrophy workout; MxS = maximal-strength workout; STR–SP = strength–speed workout; SP–STR = speed–strength workout; BFR = blood flow restriction; L = low intensity; M = medium intensity; H = high intensity; CL = Champions League match.

TABLE 19.9 Annual plan for team that occasionally plays two matches a week (weekend and midweek matches)

MACRO/MESO	MONTH	Monday	Tuesday	Wednesday	Thursday	Friday	Saturday	Sunday
OFF-SEASON	JUNE	17 SE L	18	19 HY L	20	21 SE L	22	23
		24 SE M	25	26 HY M	27	28 SE L	29	30
	JULY	1 SE M	2	3 HY M	4	5 SE M	6	7
PRE-SEASON		8 SE M	9	10 MxS L	11	12 HY L	13	14 Friendly match
		15 DAY OFF	16 SE L	17	18 HY M	19	20 Friendly match	21 DAY OFF
		22 HY L	23	24 MxS M	25	26 Friendly match	27 DAY OFF	28 DAY OFF
IN-SEASON MESO 1		29 HY M	30	31 STR-SP L	1	2	3	4 Cup match
	AUGUST	5 DAY OFF	6	7 MxS M	8	9	10 League match	11 DAY OFF
		12	13 STR/SP M	14	15 SE L	16	17 League match	18 DAY OFF
		19	20 HY H	21	22	23 League match	24 DAY OFF	25 League match
		26 SE M	27	28 MxS H	29	30	31 League match	

TABLE 19.9 (cont.)

MACRO/MESO	MONTH	Monday	Tuesday	Wednesday	Thursday	Friday	Saturday	Sunday
IN-SEASON MESO 1	SEPTEMBER							1 DAY OFF
		2 SE L	3	4 SP/STR H	5	6 HY M	7 DAY OFF	8 DAY OFF
		9 SE M	10	11 MxS H	12	13	14 League match	15 DAY OFF
		16	17 HY H	18	19 SE L	20	21 League match	22
		23	24 Cup match	25	26	27 MxS L	28	29 League match
		30						
	OCTOBER		1	2 SP/STR H	3	4	5 League match	6 DAY OFF
		7 SE L	8	9 MxS M	10	11 HY H	12 DAY OFF	13 DAY OFF
		14 SE M	15	16 STR-SP M	17	18	19 League match	20 DAY OFF
		21	22 SE H	23	24 HY L	25	26 League match	27 DAY OFF
IN-SEASON MESO 2		28	29 MxS H	30 DAY OFF	31 SE H			

MACRO/MESO	MONTH	Monday	Tuesday	Wednesday	Thursday	Friday	Saturday	Sunday
IN-SEASON MESO 2	NOVEMBER					1	2	3 League match
		4 DAY OFF	5	6 **STR/SP H**	7	8	9 League match	10 DAY OFF
		11 **SE L**	12	13 **MxS M**	14	15 **HY H**	16 DAY OFF	17 DAY OFF
		18 **MxS M**	19	20 DAY OFF	21 **SP/STR M**	22	23	24 League match
		25 DAY OFF	26	27 **HY H**	28	29	30 League match	
	DECEMBER							1 DAY OFF
		2 **SE L**	3	4 Cup match	5	6	7 League match	8 DAY OFF
		9	10	11	12	13	14	15
		16	17 **MxS H**	18	19	20 League match	21 DAY OFF	22
		23 **MxS L**	24 DAY OFF	25 **STR/SP H**	26 DAY OFF	27 **SE M**	28 League match	29
		30 **HY H**	31					

TABLE 19.9 (cont.)

MACRO/MESO	MONTH	Monday	Tuesday	Wednesday	Thursday	Friday	Saturday	Sunday
IN-SEASON MESO 2	JANUARY			1	2 **SE M**	3	4 **HY H**	5
		6 **SE M**	7	8 **SP/STR M**	9	10 **MxS H**	11 DAY OFF	12 DAY OFF
		13 **HY H**	14	15	16 Friendly match	17	18 Friendly match	19 DAY OFF
		20	21 **MxS M**	22 DAY OFF	23 **STR/SP H**	24	25	26 League match
		27	28	29 **MxS H**	30	31		
		DAY OFF						
	FEBRUARY						1 League match	2 DAY OFF
IN-SEASON MESO3		3	4 **MxS M**	5	6 **STR/SP L**	7	8	9 DAY OFF
		10 **SE L**	11	12 Cup match	13	14	15 League match	16 DAY OFF
		17	18 **MxS L**	19	20 **SP/STR H**	21	22	23 League match
		24	25	26 **MxS H**	27	28		
		DAY OFF						

MACRO/MESO	MONTH	Monday	Tuesday	Wednesday	Thursday	Friday	Saturday	Sunday
IN-SEASON **MESO3**	MARCH	3 **SE L**	4	5 **STR/SP H**	6	7	1 League match	2 DAY OFF
		10 **SE L**	11	12 **SP/STR M**	13	14	8 League match	9 DAY OFF
		17	18 **MxS M**	19	20	21 League match	15 League match	16 DAY OFF
		24	25 League match	26 DAY OFF	27	28 **STR/SP L**	22 DAY OFF	23
		31 DAY OFF					29	30 League match
	APRIL		1 DAY OFF	2	3 **STR/SP L**	4	5 League match	6 DAY OFF
		7	8 **SP/STR H**	9	10	11	12 League match	13
		14	15 Cup match	16 DAY OFF	17 **SE L**	18	19 League match	20 DAY OFF
		21 **SE L**	22	23 **STR/SP H**	24	25	26 League match	27
		28	29 **MxS M**	30				DAY OFF

TABLE 19.9 (cont.)

MACRO/MESO	MONTH	Monday	Tuesday	Wednesday	Thursday	Friday	Saturday	Sunday
IN-SEASON **MESO3**	MAY				1 **SE L**	2	3 League match	4 DAY OFF
		5	6 **SP/STR L**	7	8	9	10 League match	11 DAY OFF
		12	13 **SP/STR L**	14	15	16	17 Cup final	18

SE = strength endurance workout; HY = hypertrophy workout; MxS = maximal-strength workout; STR–SP = strength-speed workout; SP-STR = speed-strength workout; BFR = blood flow restriction; L = low intensity; M = medium intensity; H = high intensity.

TABLE 19.10 Sample training program for beginner level

Strength endurance		High			Medium			Low		
		Intensity	Reps	RI	Intensity	Reps	RI	Intensity	Reps	RI
CIRCUIT	Back lunge and one-arm press		×10–12@	90"		×12–15@	90"		×12–15@	90"
			×10–12@	90"		×12–15@	90"		×12–15@	90"
			×10–12@	90"		×12–15@	90"			
	Push–up progression		×12–15	60"		×12–15	60"		×12–15	90"
			×12–15	60"		×12–15	60"		×12–15	90"
			×12–15	60"		×12–15	60"			
	Crossover and lateral step–up		×5–6@	90"		×6–8@	90"		×6–8@	90"
			×5–6@	90"		×6–8@	90"		×6–8@	90"
			×5–6@	90"		×6–8@	90"			
	Eccentric stability ball hamstring combination		×6–8@	90"		×5–6@	90"			
			×6–8@	90"		×5–6@	90"			
			×6–8@	90"		×5–6@	90"			
	Back extension								×10–12	90"
									×10–12	90"
	Single–leg squat and reach around the clock		×10–12@	90"		×12–15@	90"		×12–15@	90"
			×10–12@	90"		×12–15@	90"		×12–15@	90"
			×10–12@	90"		×12–15@	90"			
	Inverse row		×10–12	60"		×10–12	60"		×12–15	90"
			×10–12	60"		×10–12	60"		×12–15	90"
			×10–12	60"		×10–12	60"		×12–15	90"
	Single–leg Romanian deadlift and row		×10–12@	90"		×10–12@	90"		×10–12@	90"
			×10–12@	90"		×10–12@	90"		×10–12@	90"
			×10–12@	90"		×10–12@	90"			

TABLE 19.10 (cont.)

Hypertrophy	High			Medium			Low		
	Intensity	Reps	RI	Intensity	Reps	RI	Intensity	Reps	RI
1 Single-leg squat and row		×6–8@	2'		×8–10@	2'		×8–10@	2'
		×6–8@	2'		×8–10@	2'		×8–10@	2'
		×6–8@	2'		×8–10@	2'		×8–10@	
		×6–8@			×8–10@				
2 Back lunge and one-arm press		×8–10@	2'		×8–10@	2'		×10–12@	2'
		×8–10@	2'		×8–10@	2'		×10–12@	2'
		×8–10@	2'		×8–10@	2'		×10–12@	
		×8–10@			×8–10@				
3 Push–pull combination		×8–10@	2'		×10–12@	2'		×10–12@	2'
		×8–10@	2'		×10–12@	2'		×10–12@	2'
		×8–10@			×10–12@			×10–12@	
4 Crossover and lateral step-up		×4–5@	2'		×5–6@	2'		×6–8@	2'
		×4–5@	2'		×5–6@	2'		×6–8@	2'
		×4–5@			×5–6@			×6–8@	
5a Eccentric stability ball hamstring combination		×6–8@	2'		×5–6@	2'			
		×6–8@	2'		×5–6@	2'			
		×6–8@			×5–6@				
5b Stability ball hamstring combination								×8–12	90"
								×8–12	

Maximum strength		High			Medium			Low		
		Intensity	Reps	RI	Intensity	Reps	RI	Intensity	Reps	RI
1	Front squat	65%	×6	2'	60%	×6	2'	55%	×6	2'
		75%	×4	2'	70%	×5	2'	65%	×6	2'
		80%	×3	2'	70%	×5	2'	70%	×5	2'
		70%	×5	2'	80%	×3	2'	75%	×4	2'
		80%	×3	2'	80%	×3	2'	80%	×3	
		85%	×3		85%	×2				
2	Bench press (barbell/dumbbells)	65%	×5	2'	60%	×6	2'	55%	×6	2'
		75%	×4	2'	70%	×4	2'	65%	×4	2'
		75%	×4	2'	80%	×3	2'	65%	×4	2'
		85%	×3	2'	80%	×3	2'	75%	×3	
		90%	×2		85%	×3				
3	Slide-board lateral lunge		×6–8@	2'		×8–10@	2'		×8–10@	2'
			×6–8@	2'		×8–10@	2'		×8–10@	2'
			×6–8@	2'		×8–10@	2'		×8–10@	
			×6–8@			×8–10@				
4	Chin-up/Pull-up		×5–6	2'		×6–8	2'		×6–8	2'
			×5–6	2'		×6–8	2'		×6–8	2'
			×5–6			×6–8			×6–8	
5	(Single-leg) back extension		×6–8	2'		×6–8	2'		×8–10	2'
			×6–8	2'		×6–8	2'		×8–10	2'
			×6–8			×6–8			×8–10	

TABLE 19.10 (cont.)

Strength-speed	High			Medium			Low		
	Intensity	Reps	RI	Intensity	Reps	RI	Intensity	Reps	RI
1 COMPLEX Front squat	75%	×4	2'	70%	×5	2'	70%	×4	2'
	75%	×4	2'	75%	×4	2'	75%	×4	2'
	80%	×3	2'	80%	×3	2'	80%	×3	2'
	85%	×3	2'	85%	×3	2'	80%	×3	2'
Box jump (SR)		2×4	2×45"		2×4	2×45"		2×3	2×45"
		2×4	2×45"		2×4	2×45"		2×3	2×45"
		2×4	2×45"		2×4	2×45"		2×3	2×45"
		2×4	45"		2×4	45"		2×3	45"
2 Slide–board lateral slide		20"	90"		20"	90"		20"	90"
		20"	90"		20"	90"		20"	90"
		20"	90"		20"	90"		20"	
		20"			20"				
3 Clapping push–up		×8–10	2'		×6–8	2'		×6–8	2'
		×8–10	2'		×6–8	2'		×6–8	2'
		×8–10			×6–8			×6–8	
4 Plyometric inverse row		×8–10	2'		×6–8	2'		×6–8	2'
		×8–10	2'		×6–8	2'		×6–8	2'
		×8–10			×6–8			×6–8	
5 Single–leg Romanian deadlift and row		×8–10@	90"		×8–10@	90"		×8–10@	90"
		×8–10@	90"		×8–10@	90"		×8–10@	90"
		×8–10@			×8–10@			×8–10@	

Speed-strength

	High			Medium			Low		
	Intensity	Reps	RI	Intensity	Reps	RI	Intensity	Reps	RI
CIRCUIT									
Forward step-up (ballistic)	55%	×5@	90"	50%	×5@	90"	50%	×5@	90"
	62.5%	×5@	90"	60%	×5@	90"	57.5%	×5@	90"
	70%	×5@	90"	70%	×5@	90"	65%	×5@	90"
Battling ropes waves		20"	90"		20"	90"		20"	90"
		20"	90"		20"	90"		20"	90"
		20"	90"		20"	90"		20"	90"
Step-up jump		2×4@	2×45"		2×4@	2×45"		2×3@	2×45"
		2×4@	2×45"		2×4@	2×45"		2×3@	2×45"
		2×4@	2×45"		2×4@	2×45"		2×3@	2×45"
Clapping push-up		×8–10	90"		×6–8	90"		×6–8	90"
		×8–10	90"		×6–8	90"		×6–8	90"
		×8–10	90"		×6–8	90"		×6–8	90"
Resisted sprint	5% BW	30m	2'	10% BW	30m	2'	10% BW	30m	2'
	5% BW	30m	2'	10% BW	30m	2'	10% BW	30m	2'
	5% BW	30m	2'	10% BW	30m	2'	10% BW	30m	2'
Box jumps (MR)		2×4	2×45"		2×4	2×45"		2×3	2×45"
		2×4	2×45"		2×4	2×45"		2×3	2×45"
		2×4	2×45"		2×4	2×45"		2×3	2×45"
Stability ball hamstring combination		×8–12	2'		×8–12	2'		×8–12	2'
		×8–12	2'		×8–12	2'		×8–12	
		×8–12			×8–12				

TABLE 19.10 (cont.)

Blood flow restriction	High			Medium			Low		
	Intensity	Reps	RI	Intensity	Reps	RI	Intensity	Reps	RI
1 Front squat				30%	×15	60"	20%	×30	45"
				30%	×12	60"	20%	×15	45"
				30%	×12	60"	20%	×15	45"
				30%	×12		20%	×15	
2 Bench press (barbell/ dumbbells)				30%	×15	60"	20%	×30	45"
				30%	×12	60"	20%	×15	45"
				30%	×12	60"	20%	×15	45"
				30%	×12		20%	×15	
3 Romanian deadlift				30%	×15	60"	20%	×30	45"
				30%	×12	60"	20%	×15	45"
				30%	×12	60"	20%	×15	45"
				30%	×12		20%	×15	
4 Barbell row				30%	×15	60"	20%	×30	45"
				30%	×12	60"	20%	×15	45"
				30%	×12	60"	20%	×15	45"
				30%	×12		20%	×15	

@ denote for each side.
Eccentric stability ball hamstring combination: This is the hamstring combination, with the sole exception that the concentric movement is performed with both legs while the eccentric contraction is a single-leg movement.

TABLE 19.11 Sample training program for intermediate level

Strength endurance	High			Medium			Low		
	Intensity	Reps	RI	Intensity	Reps	RI	Intensity	Reps	RI
CIRCUIT Lateral lunge		×8–10@	90"		×6–8@	90"		×6–8@	90"
		×8–10@	90"		×6–8@	90"		×6–8@	90"
		×8–10@	90"		×6–8@	60"			
Staggered-stance, one-arm cable press		×8–10@	60"		×10–12@	60"		×12–15@	90"
		×8–10@	60"		×10–12@	60"		×12–15@	90"
		×8–10@	60"		×10–12@	60"			
Crossover and lateral step-up		×6–8@	90"		×6–8@	90"		×5–6@	90"
		×6–8@	90"		×6–8@	90"		×5–6@	90"
		×6–8@	90"		×6–8@	90"			
Assisted Nordic hamstring exercise		×10–12	90"		×8–10	90"			
		×10–12	90"		×8–10	90"			
		×10–12	90"		×8–10	90"			
(Single-leg) back extension								×10–12	90"
								×10–12	90"
Single-leg squat and row		×6–8@	90"		×4–6@	90"		×4–6@	90"
		×6–8@	90"		×4–6@	90"		×4–6@	90"
		×6–8@	90"		×4–6@	90"			
Push-up progression		×12–15	60"		×10–12	60"		×10–12	90"
		×12–15	60"		×10–12	60"		×10–12	90"
		×12–15	60"		×10–12	60"			
Single-leg squat and reach around the clock		×10–12@	60"		×10–12@	60"		×12–15@	90"
		×10–12@	60"		×10–12@	60"		×12–15@	90"
		×10–12@	60"		×10–12@	60"			
Stability ball hamstring combination		×8–12	60"		×8–12	60"		×8–12	90"
		×8–12	60"		×8–12	60"		×8–12	
		×8–12			×8–12				

TABLE 19.11 (cont.)

Hypertrophy	High			Medium			Low		
	Intensity	Reps	RI	Intensity	Reps	RI	Intensity	Reps	RI
1 Bulgarian split squat	62.5%	×6@	2'	60%	×6@	2'	65%	×6@	2'
	70%	×4@	2'	67.5%	×4@	2'	65%	×6@	2'
	70%	×4@	2'	67.5%	×4@	2'	75%	×4@	2'
	80%	×4@	2'	77.5%	×4@	2'	75%	×4@	2'
	80%	×4@		77.5%	×4@		65%	×8@	
	70%	×8@		67.5%	×8@				
2 Weight plate push-up	72.5%	×6	2'	70%	×6	2'	67.5%	×6	2'
	72.5%	×6	2'	80%	×4	2'	72.5%	×6	2'
	82.5%	×4	2'	80%	×4	2'	77.5%	×5	2'
	82.5%	×4	2'	70%	×8		67.5%	×8	
	72.5%	×8							
3 Resisted slide-board back lunge		×6–8@	2'		×8–10@	2'		×8–10@	2'
		×6–8@	2'		×8–10@	2'		×8–10@	2'
		×6–8@			×8–10@			×8–10@	
4 Inverse row		×6–8	2'		×8–10	2'		×8–10	2'
		×6–8	2'		×8–10	2'		×8–10	2'
		×6–8			×8–10			×8–10	
5a Assisted Nordic hamstring exercise		×10–12	2'		×8–10	2'			
		×10–12	2'		×8–10	2'			
		×10–12			×8–10				
5b Stability ball hamstring combination								×8–12	90"
								×8–12	

Maximum strength		High			Medium			Low		
		Intensity	Reps	RI	Intensity	Reps	RI	Intensity	Reps	RI
1a	Front squat	65%	x6	2'	60%	x6	2'			
		75%	x4	2'	70%	x4	2'			
		85%	x2	2'	70%	x3	2'			
		70%	x5	2'	80%	x3	2'			
		80%	x3	2'-3'	80%	x3	2'-3'			
		90%	x2		85%	x2				
1b	Squat and press							55%	x6	2'
								55%	x6	2'
								65%	x4	2'
								65%	x4	2'
								70%	x3	
2	Alternating split jerk	65%	x5	2'	60%	x6	2'	55%	x6	2'
		75%	x4	2'	70%	x4	2'	65%	x4	2'
		75%	x4	2'	80%	x3	2'	65%	x4	2'
		85%	x3	2'	80%	x3	2'	75%	x3	
		90%	x2		85%	x3				
3	Bench press (barbell/dumbbells)	70%	x6	2'	70%	x6	2'	65%	x6	2'
		75%	x6	2'	80%	x5	2'	75%	x6	2'
		80%	x4	2'	85%	x4	2'	80%	x4	2'
		85%	x4	2'	85%	x4		85%	x3	
		90%	x3							
4	Sternum chin-up		x5-6	2'		x6-8	2'		x6-8	2'
			x5-6	2'		x6-8	2'		x6-8	2'
			x5-6			x6-8			x6-8	
5	Single-leg Romanian deadlift and row		x6-8@	90"		x6-8@	90"		x8-10@	90"
			x6-8@	90"		x6-8@	90"		x8-10@	90"
			x6-8@			x6-8@			x8-10@	

TABLE 19.11 (cont.)

Strength-speed		High			Medium			Low		
		Intensity	Reps	RI	Intensity	Reps	RI	Intensity	Reps	RI
1 COMPLEX	Front squat	75%	×5	2'	70%	×5	2'	70%	×5	2'
		75%	×5	2'	75%	×5	2'	75%	×5	2'
		80%	×4	2'	80%	×4	2'	80%	×4	2'
		85%	×4		85%	×3		80%	×4	
	Jump squat	30%	×6	2'	30%	×5	2'	Barbell	×5	2'
		30%	×6	2'	30%	×5	2'	Barbell	×5	2'
		40%	×5	2'	30%	×5	2'	Barbell	×5	2'
		40%	×5		30%	×5		Barbell	×5	
	Box jump (MR)		2×5	2×45"		2×4	2×45"		2×4	2×45"
			2×5	2×45"		2×4	2×45"		2×4	2×45"
			2×5	2×45"		2×4	2×45"		2×4	2×45"
			2×5	45"		2×4	45"		2×4	45"
2	(Dumbbell) alternating split jerk	70%	×4	2'	65%	×4	2'	65%	×4	2'
		70%	×4	2'	70%	×4	2'	70%	×4	2'
		80%	×3		75%	×3		75%	×3	
3	Battling ropes waves		20"	90"		20"	90"		20"	90"
			20"	90"		20"	90"		20"	90"
			20"	90"		20"	90"		20"	90"
4	Single-leg Romanian deadlift and row		×6–8@	90"		×6–8@	90"		×8–10@	90"
			×6–8@	90"		×6–8@	90"		×8–10@	90"
			×6–8@			×6–8@			×8–10@	

Speed-strength

		High			Medium			Low		
		Intensity	Reps	RI	Intensity	Reps	RI	Intensity	Reps	RI
C I R C U I T	Bulgarian split squat	55%	×5@	90"	50%	×5@	90"	50%	×5@	90"
		62.5%	×5@	90"	60%	×5@	90"	57.5%	×5@	90"
		70%	×5@	90"	70%	×5@	90"	65%	×5@	90"
	Plyometric inverse row		×6–8	90"		×6–8	90"		×6–8	90"
			×6–8	90"		×6–8	90"		×6–8	90"
			×6–8	90"		×6–8	90"		×6–8	90"
	Bulgarian split squat jump	30%	×6@	90"	30%	×6@	90"	30%	×5@	90"
		30%	×6@	90"	30%	×5@	90"	30%	×5@	90"
		30%	×6@	90"	30%	×5@	90"	30%	×5@	90"
	Depth jump push-up		×8–10	90"		×6–8	90"		×6–8	90"
			×8–10	90"		×6–8	90"		×6–8	90"
			×8–10	90"		×6–8	90"		×6–8	90"
	Resisted sprint	5% BW	30–40 m	2'	10% BW	30 m	2'	10% BW	30 m	2'
		5% BW	30–40 m	2'	10% BW	30 m	2'	10% BW	30 m	2'
		5% BW	30–40 m	2'	10% BW	30 m	2'	10% BW	30 m	2'
	Lateral cone hops (MR)		2×3	2×45"		2×3	2×45"		2×2	2×45"
			2×3	2×45"		2×3	2×45"		2×2	2×45"
			2×3	2×45"		2×3	2×45"		2×2	2×45"
	Stability ball combination		×8–12	2'		×8–12	2'		×8–12	2'
			×8–12	2'		×8–12	2'		×8–12	2'
			×8–12			×8–12				

TABLE 19.11 (cont.)

Blood flow restriction	High			Medium			Low		
	Intensity	Reps	RI	Intensity	Reps	RI	Intensity	Reps	RI
1 Front squat				30%	x15	60"	20%	x30	45"
				30%	x15	60"	20%	x20	45"
				30%	x15	60"	20%	x20	45"
				30%	x15		20%	x20	
2 Bench press (barbell/dumbbells)				30%	x15	60"	20%	x30	45"
				30%	x15	60"	20%	x20	45"
				30%	x15	60"	20%	x20	45"
				30%	x15		20%	x20	
3 Back lunge				30%	x15@	60"	30%	x15@	60"
				30%	x15@	60"	30%	x12@	60"
				30%	x15@	60"	30%	x12@	60"
				30%	x15@		30%	x12@	
4 Barbell row				30%	x15	60"	20%	x30	45"
				30%	x15	60"	20%	x20	45"
				30%	x15	60"	20%	x20	45"
				30%	x15		20%	x20	

@ denote for each side.

TABLE 19.12 Sample training program for advanced level

Strength endurance	High			Medium			Low		
	Intensity	Reps	RI	Intensity	Reps	RI	Intensity	Reps	RI
C I R C U I T Side-to-side box jump	70%	×10	90"	60%	×10	90"	50%	×10	90"
	70%	×10	90"	60%	×10	90"	50%	×10	90"
	70%	×10	90"	60%	×10	90"			
Staggered-stance, one-arm cable press		×8–10@	60"		×10–12@	60"		×12–15@	60"
		×8–10@	60"		×10–12@	60"		×12–15@	60"
		×8–10@	60"		×10–12@	60"			
Single-leg squat and row		×8–10@	60"		×6–8@	90"		×6–8@	90"
		×8–10@	60"		×6–8@	90"		×6–8@	90"
		×8–10@	60"		×6–8@	90"			
Slide-board front lever push-up		×12–15	60"		×10–12	60"		×10–12	60"
		×12–15	60"		×10–12	60"		×10–12	60"
		×12–15	60"		×10–12	60"			
Crossover and lateral step-up		×6–8@	60"		×6–8@	60"		×6–8@	90"
		×6–8@	60"		×6–8@	60"		×6–8@	90"
		×6–8@	60"		×6–8@	60"			
Inverse row		×8–10	60"		×10–12	60"		×12–15	60"
		×8–10	60"		×10–12	60"		×12–15	60"
		×8–10	60"		×10–12	60"			
Nordic hamstrings		×8–10	60"		×6–8	60"			
		×8–10	60"		×6–8	60"			
		×8–10	60"		×6–8	60"			
Stability ball hamstring combination								×12–15	60"
								×12–15	60"
Barbell torque		×12	90"		×12	90"		×15	60"
		×12	90"		×12			×15	90"
		×12							

TABLE 19.12 (*cont.*)

Hypertrophy	High			Medium			Low		
	Intensity	*Reps*	*RI*	*Intensity*	*Reps*	*RI*	*Intensity*	*Reps*	*RI*
1a Squat clean	62.5%	×6	2'	60%	×6	2'			
	72.5%	×4	2'	70%	×4	2'			
	72.5%	×4	2'	70%	×4	2'			
	82.5%	×4	2'	80%	×4	2'			
	82.5%	×4	2'	80%	×4	2'			
Front squat	72.5%	×8		70%	×8				
1b Squat clean and press							55%	×6	2'
							65%	×4	2'
							70%	×4	2'
							70%	×4	2'
Front squat							65%	×8	
2 Weight plate push–up	75%	×6	2'	72.5%	×6	2'	70%	×6	2'
	75%	×6	2'	82.5%	×4	2'	75%	×6	2'
	85%	×4	2'	82.5%	×4	2'	80%	×5	2'
	85%	×4	2'	72.5%	×8		70%	×8	
	75%	×8							
3 Slide–board lateral lunge		×6–8@	2'		×6–8@	2'		×8–10@	2'
		×6–8@	2'		×6–8@	2'		×8–10@	2'
		×6–8@			×6–8@			×8–10@	
4 Pull-up		×6–8	2'		×6–8	2'		×8–10	2'
		×6–8	2'		×6–8	2'		×8–10	2'
		×6–8			×6–8			×8–10	
5a Nordic hamstring exercise		×8–10	2'		×6–8	2'			
		×8–10	2'		×6–8	2'			
		×8–10			×6–8				
5b Single–leg hamstring combination								×6–8@	90"
								×6–8@	90"
								×6–8@	

Maximum strength		High Intensity	High Reps	High RI	Medium Intensity	Medium Reps	Medium RI	Low Intensity	Low Reps	Low RI
1a	Squat clean	65%	x5	2'	60%	x6	2'			
		75%	x4	2'	70%	x4	2'			
		75%	x4	2'–3'	80%	x3	2'			
		85%	x3	2'–3'	80%	x3	2'–3'			
		90%	x2		85%	x3	2'–3'			
		92.5%	x2		90%	x2				
1b	Squat clean and press							55%	x6	2'
								65%	x4	2'
								65%	x4	2'
								75%	x3	2'
								75%	x3	2'
2	Bench press (barbell/dumbbells)	70%	x6	2'	70%	x6	2'	65%	x6	2'
		75%	x6	2'	80%	x5	2'	75%	x6	2'
		80%	x4	2'	85%	x4	2'	80%	x4	2'
		85%	x4	2'	85%	x4		85%	x3	
		90%	x3							
3	Resisted slide-board back lunge with overhead press		x5–6@	2'		x6–8@	2'		x6–8@	2'
			x5–6@	2'		x6–8@	2'		x6–8@	2'
			x5–6@	2'		x6–8@	2'		x6–8@	
			x5–6@			x6–8@				
4	Sternum chin-up		x5–6	2'		x6–8	2'		x6–8	2'
			x5–6	2'		x6–8	2'		x6–8	2'
			x5–6			x6–8			x6–8	
5	Single-leg Romanian deadlift and row		x6–8@	90"		x6–8@	90"		x8–10@	90"
			x6–8@	90"		x6–8@	90"		x8–10@	90"
			x6–8@			x6–8@			x8–10@	

TABLE 19.12 (cont.)

Strength-speed		High			Medium			Low		
		Intensity	Reps	RI	Intensity	Reps	RI	Intensity	Reps	RI
1 C O M P L E X	Bulgarian split squat	75%	×5@	2'	70%	×5@	2'	70%	×5@	2'
		75%	×5@	2'	75%	×5@	2'	75%	×5@	2'
		85%	×4@	2'	80%	×4@	2'	80%	×4@	2'
		85%	×4@	2'	85%	×4@	2'	80%	×4@	2'
	Single-leg box jump (SR)		2×4@	2×45"		2×3@	2×45"		2×3@	2×45"
			2×4@	2×45"		2×3@	2×45"		2×3@	2×45"
			2×4@	2×45"		2×3@	2×45"		2×3@	2×45"
			2×4@	45"		2×3@	45"		2×3@	45"
2	Power clean and alternating split jerk	70%	×4	2'	65%	×4	2'	65%	×4	2'
		70%	×4	2'	70%	×4	2'	70%	×4	2'
		80%	×3	2'–3'	75%	×3	2'	75%	×3	2'
		80%	×3		80%	×3		75%	×3	
3	Staggered-stance, one-arm cable press +		×6–8@	/+2'		×6–8@	/+2'		×8–10@	/+2'
			×6–8@	/+2'		×6–8@	/+2'		×8–10@	/+2'
	Staggered-stance, one-arm row		×6–8@			×6–8@			×8–10@	
4	Single-leg Romanian deadlift and row		×6–8@	90"		×6–8@	90"		×8–10@	90"
			×6–8@	90"		×6–8@	90"		×8–10@	90"
			×6–8@			×6–8@			×8–10@	
5	Vertiball slam	2–3 kg MB	3 sets: build up to max speed and stop	90"	2–3 kg MB	3 sets: build up to max speed and stop	90"	2–3 kg MB	3 sets: build up to max speed and stop	90"

Speed-strength

CIRCUIT	High Intensity	High Reps	High RI	Medium Intensity	Medium Reps	Medium RI	Low Intensity	Low Reps	Low RI
Bulgarian split squat	55%	×5@	90"	55%	×5@	90"	55%	×5@	90"
	65%	×5@	90"	62.5%	×5@	90"	60%	×5@	90"
	75%	×4@	90"	70%	×5@	90"	65%	×5@	90"
Battling ropes waves		20"	90"		20"	90"		20"	90"
		20"	90"		20"	90"		20"	90"
		20"	90"		20"	90"		20"	90"
Jump squat	30%	×6	90"	30%	×6	90"	30%	×5	90"
	40%	×5	90"	30%	×6	90"	30%	×5	90"
	50%	×5	90"	30%	×6	90"	30%	×5	90"
Depth jump push-up		×8–10	90"		×6–8	90"		×6–8	90"
		×8–10	90"		×6–8	90"		×6–8	90"
		×8–10	90"		×6–8	90"		×6–8	90"
Resisted sprint	5% BW	30–40 m	2'	10% BW	30–40 m	2'	10% BW	30 m	2'
	5% BW	30–40 m	2'	10% BW	30–40 m	2'	10% BW	30 m	2'
	5% BW	30–40m	2'	10% BW	30–40m	2'	10% BW	30 m	2'
Lateral hurdle jump		2×5	2×45"		2×4	2×45"		2×4	2×45"
		2×5	2×45"		2×4	2×45"		2×4	2×45"
		2×5	2×45"		2×4	2×45"		2×4	2×45"
Single-leg stability ball hamstring combination		×6–8@	2'		×6–8@	2'		×5–6@	2'
		×6–8@	2'		×6–8@	2'		×5–6@	2'
		×6–8@			×6–8@			×5–6@	

TABLE 19.12 (cont.)

Blood flow restriction	High			Medium			Low		
	Intensity	Reps	RI	Intensity	Reps	RI	Intensity	Reps	RI
1 Bulgarian split squat				50%	Until failure	60"	30%	×15@	45"
				50%	Until failure	60"	30%	×12@	45"
				30%	Until failure		30%	×12@	45"
							30%	×12@	
2 Push-up				50%	Until failure	60"	30%	×15	45"
				50%	Until failure	60"	30%	×12	45"
				30%	Until failure		30%	×12	45"
							30%	×12	
3 Back extension				30%	×15	45"	30%	×15	45"
				30%	×15	45"	30%	×12	45"
				30%	×15	45"	30%	×12	45"
				30%	×15		30%	×12	
4 Barbell row				50%	Until failure	60"	30%	×15	45"
				50%	Until failure	60"	30%	×12	45"
				30%	Until failure		30%	×12	45"
							30%	×12	

@ denote for each side.

The in-season is divided into three mesocycles. Over the course of these mesocycles the emphasis progressively shifts from strength endurance in mesocycle one, to the development of strength in mesocycle two, to explosive strength in mesocycle three. Regardless of the mesocycle, the international breaks are used to plan more general work. While specific training results in the greatest short-term effects, general work forms a solid base to achieve optimal performance in the long-term (Bondarchuk 2007). A progressive shift during the in-season from an emphasis on work capacity, hypertrophy, and strength to explosive strength and soccer-specific strength is hence logical. Hypertrophy training sessions are planned during mesocycles one and two, but are not integrated into mesocycle three. The increased cross-sectional area of type II fibers as a result of hypertrophy training will benefit future strength and power output. Towards the end of the in-season the emphasis should be more on short-term training goals and a maximal strength or explosive strength workout is therefore more opportune.

References

Alcaraz PE, Perez-Gomez J, Chavarrias M, Blazevich AJ. Similarity in adaptations to high-resistance circuit vs. traditional strength training in resistance-trained men. *J Strength Cond Res*. 2011 Sep;25(9):2519–27.

Alegre LM, Jiménez F, Gonzalo-Orden JM, Martín-Acero R, Aguado X. Effects of dynamic resistance training on fascicle length and isometric strength. *J Sports Sci*. 2006 May;24(5):501–8.

Alentorn-Geli E, Myer GD, Silvers HJ, Samitier G, Romero D, Lázaro-Haro C, Cugat R. Prevention of non-contact anterior cruciate ligament injuries in soccer players. Part 1: mechanisms of injury and underlying risk factors. *Knee Surg Sports Traumatol Arthrosc*. 2009 Jul;17(7):705–29.

Alfredson H, Pietila T, Jonsson P, Lorentzon R. Heavy-load eccentric calf muscle training for the treatment of chronic Achilles tendinosis. *Am J Sports Med*. 1998 May–Jun;26(3):360–6.

Berger R. Optimum repetitions for the development of strength. *Research Quarterly*. 1962;34:334–8.

Bloomquist K, Langberg H, Karlsen S, Madsgaard S, Boesen M, Raastad T. Effect of range of motion in heavy load squatting on muscle and tendon adaptations. *Eur J Appl Physiol*. 2013 Aug;113(8):2133–42.

Bompa TO, Carrera M. *Periodization training for sports: science-based strength and conditioning plans for 17 sports*. 2nd ed. Champaign, IL: Human Kinetics; 2005. 272 pp.

Bompa TO, Haff G. *Periodization: theory and methodology of training*. 5th ed. Champaign, IL: Human Kinetics; 2009. 480 pp.

Bondarchuk A. *Transfer of training in sports*. Grand Rapids, MI: Ultimate Athlete Concepts; 2007. 218 pp.

Børsheim E, Bahr R. Effect of exercise intensity, duration and mode on post-exercise oxygen consumption. *Sports Med*. 2003;33(14):1037–60.

Brown SP, Miller WC, Eason JM. *Exercise physiology: basis of human movement in health and disease*. Philadelphia, PA: Lippincott Williams & Wilkins; 2006. Chapter 22, Exercise for obesity and weight control; pp. 536–53.

Campos GE, Luecke TJ, Wendeln HK, Toma K, Hagerman FC, Murray TF, Ragg KE, Ratamess NA, Kraemer WJ, Staron RS. Muscular adaptations in response to three different resistance-training regimens: specificity of repetition maximum training zones. *Eur J Appl Physiol*. 2002 Nov;88(1–2):50–60.

Chestnut JL, Docherty D. The effects of 4 and 10 repetition maximum weight-training protocols on neuromuscular adaptations in untrained men. *J Strength Cond Res*. 1999 Nov;13(4):353–9.

Cormie P, McCaulley GO, Triplett NT, McBride JM. Optimal loading for maximal power output during lower-body resistance exercises. *Med Sci Sports Exerc*. 2007 Feb;39(2):340–9.

Cormie P, McGuigan MR, Newton RU. Developing maximal neuromuscular power: part 1 – biological basis of maximal power production. *Sports Med*. 2011 Jan 1;41(1):17–38.

Croisier JL, Forthomme B, Namurois MH, Vanderthommen M, Crielaard JM. Hamstring muscle strain recurrence and strength performance disorders. *Am J Sports Med*. 2002 Mar–Apr;30(2):199–203.

Croisier JL, Ganteaume S, Binet J, Genty M, Ferret JM. Strength imbalances and prevention of hamstring injury in professional soccer players: a prospective study. *Am J Sports Med.* 2008 Aug;36(8):1469–75.

Cronin J, McNair PJ, Marshall RN. Developing explosive power: a comparison of technique and training. *J Sci Med Sport.* 2001 Mar;4(1):59–70.

Da Silva RL, Brentano MA, Kruel LF. Effects of different strength training methods on postexercise energetic expenditure. *J Strength Cond Res.* 2010 Aug;24(8):2255–60.

de Salles BF, Simão R, Miranda F, Novaes Jda S, Lemos A, Willardson JM. Rest interval between sets in strength training. *Sports Med.* 2009;39(9):765–77.

de Salles BF, Simão R, Miranda H, Bottaro M, Fontana F, Willardson JM. Strength increases in upper and lower body are larger with longer inter-set rest intervals in trained men. *J Sci Med Sport.* 2010 Jul;13(4):429–33.

Drinkwater EJ, Lawton TW, Lindsell RP, Pyne DB, Hunt PH, McKenna MJ. Training leading to repetition failure enhances bench press strength gains in elite junior athletes. *J Strength Cond Res.* 2005 May;19(2):382–8.

Dvorak J, Junge A, Derman W, Schwellnus M. Injuries and illnesses of football players during the 2010 FIFA World Cup. *Br J Sports Med.* 2011 Jun;45(8):626–30.

Dvorkin LS. *Tiiazhelaya atletika. Uchebnik dlja vuzov.* Moscow: Sovyetsky Sport Publishers; 2005. 600 pp.

Ebbeling CB, Clarkson PM. Muscle adaptation prior to recovery following eccentric exercise. *Eur J Appl Physiol Occup Physiol.* 1990;60(1):26–31.

Edge J, Hill-Haas S, Goodman C, Bishop D. Effects of resistance training on H+ regulation, buffer capacity, and repeated sprints. *Med Sci Sports Exerc.* 2006 Nov;38(11):2004–11.

Elliot DL, Goldberg L, Kuehl KS. Effect of resistance training on excess post-exercise oxygen consumption. *J Strength Cond Res.* 1992 May;6(2):77–81.

Fleck SJ, Kraemer WJ. *Designing resistance training programs.* 4th ed. Champaign, IL: Human Kinetics; 2014. 520 pp.

Fry AC. The role of resistance exercise intensity on muscle fiber adaptations. *Sports Med.* 2004;34(10):663–79.

Gamble P. *Strength and conditioning for team sports: sport-specific physical preparation for high performance.* 2nd ed. New York: Routledge; 2013. 304 pp.

Gillette CA, Bullough RC, Melby CL. Postexercise energy expenditure in response to acute aerobic or resistive exercise. *Int J Sport Nutr.* 1994 Dec;4(4):347–60.

Goto K, Nagasawa M, Yanagisawa O, Kizuka T, Ishii N, Takamatsu K. Muscular adaptations to combinations of high- and low-intensity resistance exercises. *J Strength Cond Res.* 2004 Nov;18(4):730–7.

Goto K, Ishii N, Kizuka T, Takamatsu K. The impact of metabolic stress on hormonal responses and muscular adaptations. *Med Sci Sports Exerc.* 2005 Jun;37(6):955–63.

Grigg NL, Wearing SC, Smeathers JE. Eccentric calf muscle exercise produces a greater acute reduction in Achilles tendon thickness than concentric exercise. *Br J Sports Med.* 2009 Apr;43(4):280–3.

Haddock BL, Wilkin LD. Resistance training volume and post exercise energy expenditure. *Int J Sports Med.* 2006 Feb;27(2):143–8.

Häkkinen K, Komi PV, Alén M. Effect of explosive type strength training on isometric force- and relaxation-time, electromyographic and muscle fiber characteristics of leg extensor muscles. *Acta Physiol Scand.* 1985 Dec;125(4):587–600.

Harris GR, Stone MH, O'Bryant HS, Proulx CM, Johnson RI. Short-term performance effects of high power, high force, or combined weight-training methods. *J Strength Cond Res.* 2000 Feb;14(1):14–20.

Hoffman JR, Kang J. Strength changes during an in-season resistance-training program for football. *J Strength Cond Res.* 2003 Feb;17(1):109–14.

Johnston RD, Gabbett TJ, Jenkins DG, Hulin BT. Influence of physical qualities on post-match fatigue in rugby league players. *J Sci Med Sport.* 2014 Feb 6. [Epub ahead of print]

Jones K, Bishop P, Hunter G, Fleisig G. The effects of varying resistance-training loads on intermediate- and high-velocity-specific adapatations. *J Strength Cond Res.* 2001 Aug;15(3):349–56.

Kawamori N, Haff GG. The optimal training load for the development of muscular power. *J Strength Cond Res.* 2004 Aug;18(3):675–84.

Kenn J. *The coach's strength training playbook.* Monterey, CA: Coaches Choice; 2003. 160 pp.

Krosshaug T, Nakamae A, Boden BP, Engebretsen L, Smith G, Slauterbeck JR, Hewett TE, Bahr R. Mechanisms of anterior cruciate ligament injury in basketball: video analysis of 39 cases. *Am J Sports Med.* 2007 Mar;35(3):359–67.

LaStayo PC, Woolf JM, Lewek MD, Snyder-Mackler L, Reich T, Lindstedt SL. Eccentric muscle contractions: their contribution to injury, prevention, rehabilitation, and sport. *J Orthop Sports Phys Ther.* 2003 Oct;33(10):557–71.

Liow DK, Hopkins WG. Velocity specificity of weight training for kayak sprint performance. *Med Sci Sports Exerc.* 2003 Jul;35(7):1232–7.

McMahon GE, Morse CI, Burden A, Winwood K, Onambélé GL. Impact of range of motion during ecologically valid resistance training protocols on muscle size, subcutaneous fat, and strength. *J Strength Cond Res.* 2014 Jan;28(1):245–55.

Michaut A, Pousson M, Belleville J, Van Hoecke J. Recovery of muscle contractility after a strength training session: mechanical, neurophysiologic and biochemical approach. *C R Seances Soc Biol Fil.* 1998;192(1):195–208.

Miranda H, Fleck SJ, Simão R, Barreto AC, Dantas EH, Novaes J. Effect of two different rest period lengths on the number of repetitions performed during resistance training. *J Strength Cond Res.* 2007 Nov;21(4):1032–6.

Miranda H, Simão R, Moreira LM, de Souza RA, de Souza JA, de Salles BF, Willardson JM. Effect of rest interval length on the volume completed during upper body resistance exercise. *J Sports Sci Med.* 2009 Sep;8(3):388–92.

Moritani T. Neuromuscular adaptations during the acquisition of muscle strength, power and motor tasks. *J Biomech.* 1993;26 Suppl 1:95–107.

Morrissey MC, Harman EA, Johnson MJ. Resistance training modes: specificity and effectiveness. *Med Sci Sports Exerc.* 1995 May;27(5):648–60.

Murphy E, Schwarzkopf R. Effects of standard set and circuit weight training on excess post-exercise oxygen consumption. *J Strength Cond Res.* 1992 May;6(2):88–91.

Newton RU, Kraemer WJ. Developing explosive muscular power: implications for a mixed methods training strategy. *Strength Cond J.* 1994 Oct;16(5):20–31.

Obst SJ, Barrett RS, Newsham-West R. Immediate effect of exercise on Achilles tendon properties: systematic review. *Med Sci Sports Exerc.* 2013 Aug;45(8):1534–44.

Olbrecht J. *The science of winning: planning, periodizing and optimizing swim training.* 2nd ed. Tienen, Belgium: F&G Partners, Partners in Sports; 2007. 282 pp.

Padulo J, Mignogna P, Mignardi S, Tonni F, D'Ottavio S, Effect of different pushing speeds on bench press. *Int J Sports Med.* 2012 May;33(5):376–80.

Peterson MD, Rhea MR, Alvar BA. Maximizing strength development in athletes: a meta-analysis to determine the dose-response relationship. *J Strength Cond Res.* 2004 May;18(2):377–82.

Pichon C, Hunter GR, Morris M, Bond RL, Metz J. Blood pressure and heart rate response and metabolic cost of circuit versus traditional weight training. *J Strength Cond Res.* 1996 Aug;10(3):153–6.

Pincivero DM, Lephart SM, Karunakara RG. Effects of rest interval on isokinetic strength and functional performance after short-term high intensity training. *Br J Sports Med.* 1997 Sep;31(3):229–34.

Rana SR, Chleboun GS, Gilders RM, Hagerman FC, Herman JR, Hikida RS, Kushnick MR, Staron RS, Toma K. Comparison of early phase adaptations for traditional strength and endurance, and low velocity resistance training programs in college-aged women. *J Strength Cond Res.* 2008 Jan;22(1):119–27.

Rhea MR, Alvar BA, Burkett LN, Ball SD. A meta-analysis to determine the dose response for strength development. *Med Sci Sports Exerc.* 2003 Mar;35(3):456–64.

Robinson JM, Stone MH, Johnson RL, Penland CM, Warren BJ, Lewis RD. Effects of different weight training exercise/rest intervals on strength, power, and high intensity exercise endurance. *J Strength Cond Res.* 1995 Nov;9(4):216–21.

Rooney KJ, Herbert RD, Balnave RJ. Fatigue contributes to the strength training stimulus. *Med Sci Sports Exerc.* 1994 Sep;26(9):1160–4.

Schoenfeld BJ. The mechanisms of muscle hypertrophy and their application to resistance training. *J Strength Cond Res.* 2010 Oct;24(10):2857–72.

Schoenfeld BJ. Postexercise hypertrophic adaptations: a reexamination of the hormone hypothesis and its applicability to resistance training program design. *J Strength Cond Res.* 2013 Jun; 24(6):1720–30.

Schuenke MD, Mikat RP, McBride JM. Effect of an acute period of resistance exercise on excess post-exercise oxygen consumption: implications for body mass management. *Eur J Appl Physiol.* 2002 Mar;86(5):411–17.

Schuenke MD, Herman JR, Gliders RM, Hagerman FC, Hikida RS, Rana SR, Ragg KE, Staron RS. Early-phase muscular adaptations in response to slow-speed versus traditional resistance-training regimens. *Eur J Appl Physiol.* 2012 Oct;112(10):3585–95.

Schuenke MD, Herman J, Staron RS. Preponderance of evidence proves "big" weights optimize hypertrophic and strength adaptations. *Eur J Appl Physiol.* 2013 Jan;113(1):269–71.

Sedlock DA, Fissinger JA, Melby CL. Effect of exercise intensity and duration on postexercise energy expenditure. *Med Sci Sports Exerc.* 1989 Dec;21(6):662–6.

Stanish WD, Rubinovich RM, Curwin S. Eccentric exercise in chronic tendinitis. *Clin Orthop Relat Res.* 1986 Jul;(208):65–8.

Stone MH. Literature review: Explosive exercises and training. *Strength Cond J.* 1993 June;15(3):7–15.

Stoppani J. *Encyclopedia of muscle & strength.* Champaign, IL: Human Kinetics; 2006. 408 pp.

Tanimoto M, Sanada K, Yamamoto K, Kawano H, Gando Y, Tabata I, Ishii N, Miyachi M. Effects of whole-body low-intensity resistance training with slow movement and tonic force generation on muscular size and strength in young men. *J Strength Cond Res.* 2008 Nov;22(6):1926–38.

Thorborg K. Why hamstring eccentrics are hamstring essentials. *Br J Sports Med.* 2012 Jun;46(7):463–5.

Thorborg K, Branci S, Nielsen MP, Tang L, Nielsen MB, Hölmich P. Eccentric and isometric hip adduction strength in male soccer players with and without adductor-related groin pain. An assessor-blinded comparison. *Orthopaedic Journal of Sports Medicine.* 2014 Feb;2(2):1–7.

Thornton MK, Potteiger JA. Effects of resistance exercise bouts of different intensities but equal work on EPOC. *Med Sci Sports Exerc.* 2002 Apr;34(4):715–22.

Tillin NA, Folland JP. Maximal and explosive strength training elicit distinct neuromuscular adaptations, specific to the training stimulus. *Eur J Appl Physiol.* 2014 Feb;114(2):365–74.

Willardson JM, Burkett LN. The effect of rest interval length on the sustainability of squat and bench press repetitions. *J Strength Cond Res.* 2006 May;20(2):400–3.

Woods C, Hawkins RD, Maltby S, Hulse M, Thomas A, Hodson A, Football Association Medical Research Programme. The Football Association Medical Research Programme: an audit of injuries in professional football–analysis of hamstring injuries. *Br J Sports Med.* 2004 Feb;38(1):36–41.

Yamanaka T, Farley RS, Caputo JL. Occlusion training increases muscular strength in division IA football players. *J Strength Cond Res.* 2012 Sep;26(9):2523–9.

Yasuda T, Ogasawara R, Sakamaki M, Ozaki H, Sato Y, Abe T. Combined effects of low-intensity blood flow restriction training and high-intensity resistance training on muscle strength and size. *Eur J Appl Physiol.* 2011 Oct;111(10):2525–33.

Zarins B, Ciullo JV. Acute muscle and tendon injuries in athletes. *Clin Sports Med.* 1983 Mar;2(1):167–82.

Zatsiorsky VM. *Science and practice of strength training.* Champaign, IL: Human Kinetics; 1995. 243 pp.

Zatsiorsky VW, Kraemer WJ. *Science and practice of strength training.* 2nd ed. Champaign, IL: Human Kinetics; 2006. 264 pp.

Zebis MK, Andersen LL, Ellingsgaard H, Aagaard P. Rapid hamstring/quadriceps force capacity in male vs. female elite soccer players. *J Strength Cond Res.* 2011 Jul;25(7):1989–93.

INDEX

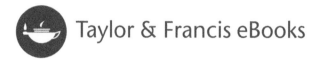